Dangerous Drug
Interactions

Dangerous Drug Interactions

(Previously published as
Deadly Drug Interactions)

How to Protect Yourself from
Harmful Drug/Drug, Drug/Food,
Drug/Vitamin Combinations

Joe Graedon and Teresa Graedon, Ph.D.

St. Martin's Paperbacks

This book was previously published as *Deadly Drug Interactions*.

DANGEROUS DRUG INTERACTIONS

Copyright © 1995, 1999 by Graedon Enterprises, Inc.

Library of Congress Catalog Card Number: 95-34800

ISBN: 0-312-96826-4

Printed in the United States of America

St. Martin's Press edition/1995
St. Martin's Griffin edition/May 1997
St. Martin's Paperbacks revised edition/February 1999

10 9 8 7 6 5 4 3 2 1

9578

ATTENTION: Important Note to Readers

This book is not intended as a substitute for the medical advice of physicians. The reader should regularly consult a physician in matters relating to his or her health and particularly in respect to any symptoms that may require diagnosis or medical attention. Certain drugs with potentially lethal interactions can be successfully used together if appropriate monitoring and other precautions are undertaken. Drug interactions can be highly controversial, and different experts may vary in their interpretations of the degree of danger.

Anyone who discovers an interaction in this book that is of concern must consult a physician before making any changes in drug therapy. **Stopping a medication can be very dangerous. Every reader must consult with his or her physician before starting or stopping any medication.** Any side effects should be reported promptly to a physician.

It is impossible to list all potentially dangerous drug interactions. Information about drug interactions remains incomplete, and new dangers are discovered all the time. In addition, the effects drugs can have vary from person to person. **The reader should not assume that because an interaction is not mentioned in this book, it is therefore safe and cannot be dangerous.**

The authors and the publisher disclaim responsibility for any adverse effects resulting directly or indirectly from the information contained in this book.

CONTENTS

ACKNOWLEDGMENTS

Barbara Anderson, our editor, whose insight and patience made this book possible. Thanks for going to bat for us.

John Barth, who helped us appreciate the power of words.

Charles Branton and Cliff Butler, extraordinary pharmacists.

Maria Carmicino, a fabulous editor who keeps our syndicated newspaper column on track and out of trouble.

Keith Cassell, a wonderfully creative and imaginative designer who made this book far more readable and usable.

Ruth Day, a cognitive psychologist at Duke University whose understanding of how to present data clearly greatly improved the first edition of this book.

Fred Eckel, a pharmacist educator with vision.

Tom Ferguson, the guru of the medical self-care revolution and a soul mate, coauthor, colleague, and friend.

David Flockhart, a clinical pharmacologist with great wisdom about drug interactions and grapefruit.

Heather Jackson, a wise, patient, and thoughtful editor.

David S. McWaters, a pharmacist and lawyer who helped make this book a reality.

Karen Moseley, a great helper and wonderful person.

Charlotte Sheedy, a fabulous agent with boundless energy and enthusiasm who helped move this book through the maze.

Stephanie Shipper, a wonderfully wise woman.

Peter Welling, a superb researcher who helped us understand the importance of food and drug interactions.

Ray Woosley, a clinical pharmacologist who shares our concern about interactions and the lack of adequate safeguards.

Over 1.5 million Americans are hospitalized each year from serious drug reactions. A review of 39 studies over 30 years concluded that prescription medicines are responsible for over 100,000 deaths in hospitals each year (*JAMA* April 15, 1998). These researchers did not include drug-induced deaths outside hospitals or those due to mistakes. It is estimated that at least 125,000 people die annually from medication errors, including the wrong drug, dose, or combination.

If one were to add up these numbers and include fatalities due to side effects and interactions that occur at home, drug reactions would be the third leading cause of death in the United States, after heart disease and cancer. It's hard to imagine that medicines intended to relieve suffering and cure disease could create such an epidemic.

No one knows how many of these deaths are caused by drug interactions. Neither the Food and Drug Administration nor the manufacturers have an organized, systematic way to track such complications. Very little pre-market research is done to predict whether a drug will have any dangerous interactions. Yet it is clear that combining the wrong medicines can lead to disaster.

One blood pressure medication was abruptly removed from pharmacies in June 1998, only a year after its introduction, because of a number of deaths associated with drug interactions. **Posicor** (mibefradil) was incompatible with at least 26 other medicines, including certain antidepressants, cholesterol-lowering drugs (**Mevacor** and **Zocor**), heartburn medication (**Propulsid**) and an antihistamine (**Hismanal**). The gravity of the situation was not fully appreciated until nearly 400,000 people around the world had taken **Posicor**. Even after the drug was recalled, people suffered potentially life-threatening interactions when they were switched too abruptly to other blood pressure pills.

One of the drugs that interacted with **Posicor** was **Viagra** (sildenafil). This impotence pill took off like a rocket ship. Its success was unprecedented, with millions of men lining up to take the pill that promised to improve their love lives. Then reports of deaths and drug interactions began to surface.

Doctors were cautioned that men taking nitrate-type drugs for angina should avoid **Viagra**. The list of medications included nitroglycerin (**Minitran**, **Nitro-Bid**, **Nitro-Dur**, **Nitrogard**, **Nitrolingual**, **Nitrong**, **Nitrostat**, **Transderm-Nitro**), **Imdur**, **ISMO**, **Isordil**, **Monoket** and **Sorbitrate**. But these warnings were inadequate to prevent fatalities from this combination. The number of men who have died while taking **Viagra** has climbed steadily since its introduction.

Drug-interaction experts such as Raymond Woosley, M.D., Ph.D., professor and chairman of the Department of Pharmacology at Georgetown University Medical Center worried that other medications might also interact with **Viagra** in a dangerous way. But even as the death toll mounted, the manufacturer and the FDA continued to reassure the public that **Viagra** was safe.

Unfortunately, the kinds of problems we have observed with **Posicor** and **Viagra** are not unusual. All too often, hazardous combinations are not revealed until people are severely injured or killed. Very few physicians and patients realize that the FDA's drug approval process is flawed in safeguarding against interactions. Even when researchers find incompatibilities, it may take years before pharmaceutical companies or the FDA alert health professionals to the dangers. And after warnings do make it into the official prescribing information, there is no guarantee that doctors will pay attention.

The nonsedating antihistamine **Seldane** was launched in 1985. It took until 1990 before its potential to cause deadly interactions was reported in the medical literature. Once the gravity of the situation was appreciated, letters were sent to physicians and pharmacists warning of the problem. But in January 1997 the FDA conceded that "Although these [educational] efforts have reduced inappropriate prescribing and dispensing of terfenadine [**Seldane**] with other drugs, such events have not been, and almost certainly cannot be, eliminated."

The agency finally threw in the towel on **Seldane** and requested that the drug be withdrawn from the market. Twelve years and countless deaths after its introduction, the manufacturer finally removed **Seldane** from pharmacy shelves. Goodness knows how many **Seldane**-like disasters are still undiscovered.

We wrote *Dangerous Drug Interactions* to help people better protect themselves from the hazards of incompatible drug mixtures. Patients visiting different doctors or shopping at different pharmacies are especially vulnerable, but even those who shop at a single pharmacy can be at risk.

Under managed care, doctors and pharmacies are often pressed for time. With little opportunity to double-check drug references, physicians may be writing more prescriptions for hazardous combinations. And pharmacists, who are expected to save lives by catching such errors, may be too harried to do so. Even in the hospital, patients may not be safe from drug incompatibilities. We know from painful personal experience the tragic consequences that are possible when overworked hospital personnel fail to check for interactions.

When a person—you or someone you love—takes more than one pill, and that includes vitamins, minerals, over-the-counter medications or herbal products, there is a potential for a chemical collision. Don't stand idly by and let such accidents occur.

We have summarized in the Afterword some of the more recent interaction reports uncovered since the hardcover came out. You may wish to scan these pages (431–448) quickly after reading the introduction. To protect yourself and your loved ones, you need information. We hope this book helps.

Joe & Teresa Graedon, October 1998

chapter one

Introduction

Would you want to play Russian roulette? Taking more than one medicine at a time could be very much like loading a gun and spinning the chamber. You may not know if a particular combination will have a lethal outcome.

When the Food and Drug Administration (FDA) set up its standards for approving medications, it did not foresee the possibility that a person might take many different pills together. The FDA, which regulates both prescription and over-the-counter drugs in the United States, does not have its own facilities and funding for drug testing; rather, it issues guidelines and examines the data produced by the companies that make the medicines. It has not required pharmaceutical manufacturers to test new compounds for interaction potential. Consequently, when a new medication is introduced, doctors may not know in advance which other drugs will be incompatible with it.

Each drug is tested under controlled conditions that don't necessarily reflect the real world in which patients take medicine. In fact, for many years most medications were given only on an empty stomach. This may have been convenient for the researchers but it has created trouble for patients. For one thing, some drugs are far better absorbed or less irritating when taken with food. And we are now learning that certain foods and beverages may create hazards when combined with other medications. Although the FDA is now beginning to ask drug companies to look at the effects of food on new drugs, most of the pharmaceuticals on drugstore shelves have few guidelines for how they should be swallowed.

It is common for people to require several different medicines to treat a number of health problems—arthritis, allergies, high blood pressure, depression, and infections, to mention just a few. Because the FDA hasn't known how to deal with the complexity of drug interactions, there is a lack of scientific information about how one drug may affect another.

There are surprisingly few systematic studies of drug interactions in the medical literature. Most of what is published evolves from case reports. An individual physician discovers an unexpected problem in one or a few patients and writes it up. Until someone decides to look further, there is no way to tell if this is truly an interaction hazard or just a coincidence.

Reporting side effects or interactions is not required by any law. Doctors are busy and many are afraid that if they raise a ruckus it may come back to haunt them in the form of a malpractice suit. Former FDA commissioner David Kessler has noted that "only about 1% of serious events are reported to the FDA, according to one study."[1,2] If a physician chooses not to notify the FDA or the drug companies, there's no way other doctors can learn about the situation.

Since the FDA does not have a system for gathering interaction data and drug companies have no incentive to pursue such research, it can take months or years to discover dangerous drug interactions. Hospitalizations and even deaths have occurred before the FDA realized a warning was needed. Undoubtedly, interactions have gone undetected to this day.

Even when the agency finally acknowledges that a particular drug combination poses a risk, there is no good way to bring this information to physicians' attention. It may ultimately show up in the package insert or *Physicians' Desk Reference (PDR)*, but there is no guarantee that the information will be read or appreciated. As a result, doctors must play a dangerous guessing game when they have to prescribe more than one medication.

Types of Drug Interactions

Imagine you are trying to bake a cake with two or three other people and no recipe. Only one of you can be in the kitchen at a time and so none of you knows what the others have put in the batter. Under these circumstances your cake might end up with way too much baking powder or perhaps none at all. If everyone threw in a pinch of salt the cake would taste terrible even if it looked okay. A patient with several doctors may suffer a similar fate.

A person may see three or four different specialists, all prescribing medications for various ailments. The cardiologist could have you on **Lanoxin** (digoxin) and **Vasotec** (enalapril) for your heart, the endocrinologist might have prescribed **Synthroid** (levothyroxine) for thyroid, the rheumatologist may have you on **Indocin** (indomethacin), and on your own you could be taking a multiple vitamin plus aspirin to prevent a heart attack. All these different drugs can interact with one another in a variety of ways to produce toxicity or reduce effectiveness. In the following sections we will describe the three different types of drug interactions that can cause trouble.

Additive Interactions

The drug interaction that most people are familiar with is an additive interaction, which occurs when one drug adds to the effect of another medication. The person who takes **Fiorinal** (aspirin, butalbital, caffeine) for a tension headache and then has a drink to relax could end up spaced out because of the combined effect of the barbiturate (butalbital) and the booze.

A century ago sailors became familiar with additive interactions when they woke up unexpectedly on a ship far from the harbor. They had been slipped a "Mickey Finn." The popular belief is that certain bartenders (in cahoots with sea captains who needed extra hands) put chloral hydrate (a sedative) in with the grog. The combination enhanced the effects of the alcohol, knocked the sailor out, and kept him asleep long enough for the ship to slip anchor.

Antagonistic Interactions

A different kind of interaction occurs when one drug cancels out the benefits of another—the 1+1= 0 effect. For example, birth control pills don't work as well when a woman takes them in conjunction with tuberculosis medicine or antiseizure drugs. She could end up unexpectedly pregnant through no fault of her own because these other drugs change the metabolism of the Pill to reduce its effectiveness. (See pages 164–174 for more details.) A similar interaction involves the popular drug **Prozac**. If it is taken in conjunction with the allergy medicine **Periactin**, **Prozac** may lose its effectiveness as an antidepressant (see page 294). Likewise, the thyroid hormone **Synthroid** may not be absorbed adequately and its effectiveness may be impaired if it is swallowed within two hours of an iron supplement (see page 122).

If a woman becomes pregnant while using birth control pills, doctors often shrug in amazement. Rather than consider a drug interaction as the culprit, they may assume that the woman was at fault for missing a dose. When an antidepressant doesn't seem to relieve depression the assumption is made that the drug isn't working for mysterious and inexplicable reasons. Doctors often chalk up such discouraging results to "biological variability." In other words, some people respond and others don't and no one knows why. Who would ever think to question breakfast as the culprit behind antidepressant failure?

Heart Drug Fails Due to Fiber

Absorption of the heart drug Lanoxin (digoxin) can be reduced when the drug is taken with high-fiber foods.[3] One physician doubled the dose of this drug for a patient who had repeated attacks of atrial fibrillation (a serious heart rhythm disturbance). The doctor should have asked about the patient's diet before changing the dose of Lanoxin. This gentleman was eating a very large bowl of oatmeal with bran every morning at the same time he took his heart pill.

A Canadian researcher has discovered that high-fiber foods can also interfere with the absorption of tricyclic antidepressants such as doxepin (**Adapin,**

Sinequan) and desipramine (**Norpramin**).[4] Dr. Donna Stewart found that patients who had previously improved with these medications did not respond to them after switching to health-conscious diets. High levels of fiber in such foods as wheat bran, rolled oats, sunflower seeds, bran muffins, and wheat germ lowered blood levels of antidepressants. When the diets were modified, the drug levels returned to normal and the depression disappeared. (For more details see page 22.)

If a medication does not produce the anticipated benefit, physicians usually adjust the dose or change drugs. If an antidepressant fails to work, they often write a new prescription. When a blood pressure pill does not adequately control hypertension, out comes another medication, frequently at a higher cost. But sometimes the doctor may not be aware of a therapeutic failure or there may not be enough time to undo the damage of a dangerous drug interaction.

Unpredictable Interactions

Perhaps the scariest type of interaction is what we refer to as the 1+1= 3 reaction. It can take a long time to be discovered. When **Seldane** (terfenadine) was introduced in May 1985 as the first nonsedating antihistamine, it was heralded as "a major advance in the treatment of seasonal allergic rhinitis."[5] Here was a prescription allergy medicine that wouldn't make you drowsy. You could drive, work, think, or make love without feeling like a space cadet. The company bragged that side effects were no more serious with **Seldane** than with an inactive placebo, and no mention was made of any interaction with other drugs.

As a consequence, **Seldane** quickly became the world's number one allergy medicine. In the early 1990s, American doctors wrote more than 16 million prescriptions a year for this drug.[6] But something odd had begun to happen. Reports of dizziness attacks and heart palpitations began trickling in to the Food and Drug Administration (FDA). By June of 1990, enough serious cases of heart rhythm disturbances and cardiac arrest had accumulated for the FDA to call an urgent meeting. Face to face with these data, the experts finally realized that elevated levels of **Seldane**, triggered by overdose, liver disease, or *interactions with certain other drugs*, could lead to a rare but potentially lethal heart condition.

At the FDA's urging, the manufacturer of **Seldane** sent out a letter later that summer warning doctors to be wary of prescribing the antifungal drug **Nizoral** (ketoconazole) together with **Seldane**. The first report in the medical literature appeared in *The Journal of the American Medical Association* on December 5, 1990.[7] Dr. Brian Monahan and his colleagues described a healthy "39-year-old woman who developed lightheadedness and fainting" after only ten days on **Seldane**. She was also taking **Nizoral** for a vaginal yeast infection. When they checked her electrocardiogram (ECG) they discovered a dangerous irregularity called *torsade de pointes* (a French term that describes the way the ECG points seem to twist together).

By April 1, 1992, the FDA had received 25 reports of torsades de pointes. Two of those afflicted had died and the others had to be hospitalized.[8] Of course, no one knows how many cases went unreported. When people drop dead of an apparent heart attack, it may be hard for the doctor to determine whether a medication or combination of medications could have contributed, especially if the drug is as seemingly benign as **Seldane**. Even if a doctor suspects that a patient's symptoms might be related to a combination of medicines, there is no simple way to alert others to this possibility. Getting a written report into the medical literature where other physicians can read it can take years.

Even after an interaction has been reported it may be ignored. Almost three years after the original report on **Seldane**, doctors continued to prescribe this antihistamine in combination with **Nizoral** or the antibiotic erythromycin. Clinical pharmacologists at Georgetown University worried that "in spite of warning letters to physicians and changes in labeling, deaths and cases of torsades de pointes continue to be reported in association with a drug that is often prescribed for what are simply uncomfortable and temporary allergic conditions."[9]

Preventable Tragedy?

"Despite regulatory action, the combination of terfenadine and ketoconazole has continued to be prescribed. The seriousness of the continued occurrence of this drug-drug interaction is illustrated in a recent report to the FDA of a 29-year-old woman who had been taking terfenadine long term for nasal congestion. She was then prescribed ketoconazole for onychomycosis [fingernail and toenail fungus]. One week later, she presented to an emergency department after 'fainting.' Both medications were continued and she suffered a fatal cardiac arrest 3 days later."

Honig, Peter K., et al. "Terfenadine-Ketoconazole Interaction: Pharmacokinetic and Electrocardiographic Consequences." **JAMA** 1993; 269:1513-1518.

The **Seldane** story is just an example of what can go wrong when mixing medicines. It took five years for the FDA and the drug's manufacturer even to realize there was a problem. And the medication stayed on the market for many years afterwards, until it was withdrawn late in 1997. During that time, many people took this antihistamine in combination with erythromycin or ketaconazole, and some of them died as a consequence.[10]

Although **Seldane** is no longer prescribed in the U.S., other potentially lethal interactions may be slipping through the safety net. Pharmacists are supposed to catch dangerous combinations, but many are overworked and too harried to pay close enough attention. In one study, people were sent to 50 pharmacies in the Washington, D.C., area with prescriptions for **Seldane** (terfenadine) and erythromycin. Unfortunately, 16 of the pharmacies filled both prescriptions without any warning whatsoever (*JAMA*, April 10, 1996, p. 1086) because those pharmacists did not catch this potentially lethal interaction. Computer programs that were supposed to alert pharmacists to such interaction problems were in use in 48 of the 50 pharmacies; this, the researchers concluded, "demonstrates that computerized drug-interaction screening programs may not prevent prescribing and filling of potentially dangerous combinations of drugs."

A more extensive survey overseen by Raymond Woosley, M.D., Ph.D., head of the department of pharmacology at Georgetown University Medical Center, confirmed these disturbing findings. In 245 pharmacies in seven cities, "well over half of all the pharmacists failed to warn consumers when presented with prescriptions for drugs that, when taken separately, are safe but when taken together can be at best risky and at worst deadly." (*U.S. News & World Report*, Aug. 26, 1996). This doesn't mean you can't trust your pharmacist, but it strongly suggests that there is no substitute for doing your own homework.

Protecting Yourself from Drug Interaction

- Take charge! It's your body and ultimately you are responsible for swallowing those pills. Make sure *all* your physicians know every drug you take and that they check for interaction potential. There are excellent reference books and computer programs available. Insist that they consult one of these resources.
- Ask your pharmacist for help. This person is a highly trained professional who specializes in drug information and interaction issues. Most pharmacies have computer access to interaction information. Some pharmacists may not want to scare their patients with extra precautions, so be sure to tell them everything you are taking and that you are interested in knowing about potential incompatibility.
- Check this book and report any unusual symptoms immediately. Never start or stop any medication without your doctor's knowledge and supervision. Stopping certain medications suddenly could trigger serious irregular heart rhythms, not to mention convulsions or heart attacks. In addition, discontinuing one drug may have a domino effect, in that it could increase or decrease the effects of other medicines you may be taking.

- Once a drug has been approved for general use, the Food and Drug Administration has no organized system for monitoring drug interactions, and no good way of disseminating interaction information to doctors. The *Physicians' Desk Reference (PDR)* reports some, but not all, dangerous combinations. It may take years for a deadly interaction to make its way into the standard reference books.

- Do not assume that lack of information indicates no interaction. Life-threatening interactions may go undiscovered for months or even years. If you are experiencing a strange or dangerous symptom that cannot easily be explained, ask your physician to contact the drug's manufacturer and to file a report with the FDA.

- We have found the following resources helpful in tracking down drug interactions. We have listed them in the order of their usefulness for us. If you or your physician has a question about anything you find in our book, please check these references. You will discover that there are substantial differences of opinion about the importance of certain interactions:

    Drug Interaction Facts. Tatro, David S., ed. St. Louis: Facts & Comparisons (A Wolters Kluwer Company), 1998.

    Drug Interactions & Updates Quarterly. Hansten, Philip D., John R. Horn, Mary Anne Koda-Kimble, Lloyd Y. Young, eds. Vancouver, Wash.: Applied Therapeutics, 1995.

The Medical Letter Handbook of Adverse Drug Interactions. Rizack, Martin A., with Carol Hillman, D.M., eds. New Rochelle, N.Y.: The Medical Letter, 1997.

Drug Facts and Comparisons. Olin, Bernie R., editor-in-chief. St. Louis: Facts & Comparisons (A Wolters Kluwer Company), 1998.

Evaluations of Drug Interactions. Zucchero, Frederic J., Mark J. Hogan, Amy C. DeWein, eds. St. Louis: Professional Drug Systems, 1994.

Consumer's Guide to Drug Interactions. Schein, Jeffrey R., and Philip Hansten. New York: Collier Books, 1993.

Mosby's GenRx: The Complete Reference for Generic and Brand Drugs. White, Jabin, editor. St. Louis, MO: Mosby, 1998.

Physicians' Desk Reference. Montvale, N.J.: Medical Economics Data Production Company, 1998.

Professional's Guide to Patient Drug Facts. Olin, Bernie R., editor-in-chief. St. Louis: Facts & Comparisons (A Wolters Kluwer Company), 1998.

PDR Guide to Drug Interactions, Side Effects, Indications. Mehta, Mukesh, ed. Montvale, N.J.: Medical Economics Data Production Company, 1998.

The Food and Drug Interaction Guide. Morgan, Brian L.G. New York: Simon & Schuster, 1986.

Drug Interactions Guide Book. Harkness, Richard. Englewood Cliffs, N.J.: Prentice-Hall, 1991.

References

1. Scott, H.D., et al. "Rhode Island Physicians' Recognition and Reporting of Adverse Drug Reactions." *R.I. Med. J.* 1987; 70:311–316.

2. Kessler, David A. "Introducing MEDWatch: A New Approach to Reporting Medication and Device Adverse Effects and Product Problems." *JAMA* 1993; 269:2765–2768.

3. Brown, D.D., et al. "Decreased Bioavailability of Digoxin Due to Hypercholesterolemic Interventions." *Circulation* 1978; 58:164–172.

4. Stewart, Donna E. "High-Fiber Diet and Serum Tricyclic Antidepressant Levels." *J. Clin. Psychopharmacol.* 1992; 12:438–440.

5. "Terfenadine: Separating Sedation from Relief—New Hope for Seasonal Allergic Rhinitis Sufferers." Merrell-Dow, 1985.

6. IMS America Ltd. *1992 National Prescription Audit.* Plymouth Meeting, Pa.: IMS America, 1992.

7. Monahan, Brian P., et al. "Torsades de Pointes Occurring in Association with Terfenadine Use." *JAMA* 1990; 264:2788–2791.

8. Woosley, Raymond L., et al. "Mechanism of the Cardiotoxic Actions of Terfenadine." *JAMA* 1993; 269:1532–1536.

9. Ibid., p. 1535.

10. Honig, Peter K., et al. "Terfenadine-Ketoconazole Interaction: Pharmacokinetic and Electrocardiographic Consequences." *JAMA* 1993; 269:1513–1518.

11. Woosley, op. cit., p. 1536.

12. Ibid.

chapter two

How To Use
This Book

On the following pages you will discover scary stories and horrifying examples of dangerous, potentially lethal drug interactions. But this does not necessarily mean that the combination will be disastrous. Not everyone will experience problems because he or she swallows two theoretically incompatible medications. In many cases, interacting drugs can be used together successfully if the doctor is aware of the potential danger and takes proper precautions. You can help by knowing what to look for; that is why we wrote this book.

One way to avoid interaction problems is to ask your physician if there could be an incompatibility, and, whenever possible, to substitute a drug that is less likely to create difficulties. Remember, however, that each case is special and only your physician has the clinical experience to know if your condition requires these particular drugs. At the risk of being redundant, we emphasize that no one should ever start or stop taking any medicine without first checking with the prescribing doctor. Stopping a pill suddenly can sometimes be far more dangerous than continuing to take a medication.

Don't overreact if you read that you are taking two or three drugs that might interact in a strange, dangerous, or potentially life-threatening way. First check with both your pharmacist and physician to see what you should do. This book will alert you to the possible consequences of combining mismatched medicines. Your doctor's responsibility is to evaluate the situation in light of your special medical history.

How to Read the Guides to Dangerous Drug Interactions

The second part of this book contains detailed descriptions of a number of the most important drug interactions. We used our judgment to select the ones we thought were most common and most serious. If you asked other experts you might get a different selection. It is impossible to list every reported interaction in a book this size.

These descriptions are grouped into categories, such as antidepressants, anticoagulants, and anticonvulsants. For each category, we detail the interactions between the medications. For example, on page 16 you will see a guide to the possible interactions between serotonin-based antidepressants such as **Paxil, Prozac**, and **Zoloft**, and MAO inhibitor antidepressants such as **Nardil** and **Parnate**. Under each drug category you will find brief instructions on how it is best taken (with food or on an empty stomach). At the bottom of the page, the nature of the interaction is described along with some of the symptoms to watch for. Not every interaction has specific side effects, but we try to indicate what precautions should be taken.

Please note that **Prozac** and **Paxil** are sometimes prescribed in combination with other types of antidepressants, even though there are indications that such combinations are occasionally dangerous. For some

Antidepressants	**Antidepressants**
(SEROTONIN-BASED)	(MAO INHIBITORS)

LIFE-THREATENING

BRAND NAME	GENERIC NAME	BRAND NAME	GENERIC NAME
Paxil	paroxetine	**Eldepryl**	selegiline
Prozac	fluoxetine	**Marplan**	isocarboxazid
Zoloft	sertraline	**Nardil**	phenelzine
		Parnate	tranylcypromine

INSTRUCTIONS

Prozac, Paxil, and Zoloft are usually taken once a day, often in the morning. Prozac may be taken without regard to meals. Taking it with food may reduce stomach upset. A few patients experience serious weight loss on these medications. If this occurs, the doctor should be notified.

INSTRUCTIONS

MAO inhibitors can interact in dangerous ways with tyramine-containing foods and beverages. See page 58. Consult your doctor before taking other prescription or over-the-counter drugs. Notify him or her if you notice a skin rash, severe headache, yellow eyes or skin, or dark urine. Do not stop this medicine unless your doctor so advises.

INTERACTION

When a patient does not get adequate relief of depression from one medication, the doctor may add a different antidepressant. The literature accompanying serotonin-based antidepressants warns against this combination. *Fatalities have resulted from this interaction.* Some people who have received this combination experience "serotonin syndrome," a very serious, potentially lethal reaction. Because these drugs last in the body for quite some time, at least two weeks should pass after discontinuing an MAO inhibitor before starting on Prozac, Zoloft, or Paxil. The manufacturer of Prozac recommends waiting five weeks after stopping Prozac before beginning an MAO inhibitor antidepressant. For Zoloft and Paxil, at least two weeks should elapse after stopping the serotonin-based antidepressant before beginning Marplan, Nardil, or Parnate. Eldepryl may also interact with the serotonin-based antidepressants.

Symptoms of Serotonin Syndrome

Severe shivering, agitation, confusion, restlessness, muscle twitches or rigidity, diarrhea, elevated temperature, sweating, changes in blood pressure, and coma. Notify your doctor at once if you experience any of these symptoms.

patients, however, this may represent the best treatment. The potential hazards are worth noting, so that you and your doctor can be alert for any sign of difficulty. Remember, if you become concerned about anything you read here, be sure to *discuss it with your doctor*, so you can understand your treatment and what to do if you detect symptoms of a problem.

How Not to Use This Book

This book contains a summary of many important drug interactions, but it is *not* a bible in which you will find every hazard. You must understand that there is no organized, scientific system for establishing dangerous chemical incompatibilities. Sometimes serious adverse drug reactions are missed or go unreported. Even when an article appears in the medical literature its findings may be ignored or take years to get into reference books or computer data banks.

Once an interaction makes it into the medical manuals there is still uncertainty about the clinical significance of the situation. Physicians and researchers and drug manufacturers often argue for years about the relevance of a particular report. For example, when the cholesterol-lowering drugs **Mevacor** (lovastatin) and **Lopid** (gemfibrozil) are prescribed together, they have on occasion been reported to produce a potentially life-threatening disorder called rhabdomyolysis. In this condition muscle tissue breaks down, resulting in pain, weakness, and possibly even kidney failure. Despite horror stories in the medical literature, admonitions against the combination by experts at the Food and Drug Administration, and strong warnings in the *Physicians' Desk*

Reference (PDR), many cardiologists believe they can combine these drugs safely with careful medical supervision. Who's right? Maybe there is no one right answer. All we can say is that we don't want you to be an unsuspecting guinea pig.

The point is that there are no clear rules when it comes to drug interactions. And there is no good place to turn for guidance. The FDA and the drug companies have left us dangling. Reference books disagree on the facts and their importance.

That makes it virtually impossible for anyone to reassure you that a particular combination is 100 percent safe . . . or warn you that it is definitely hazardous in every case. For example, most interaction guides caution that combining aspirin with the prescription anticoagulant **Coumadin** (warfarin) can be quite dangerous (though some texts are more adamant than others). Information for patients in the *PDR* says unequivocally to avoid salicylates (e.g., aspirin). The fear has been that severe bleeding episodes could occur, leading to fatal hemorrhaging. The risk is real, but some cardiologists may choose to combine these two drugs at low doses with extremely careful monitoring. Far be it from us to second-guess these clinicians.

We hope you understand that we could not include every troublesome, dangerous, or even life-threatening interaction in this book. Our primary references list thousands of potentially problematic drug combinations. One example of a drug interaction we did not discuss, although it is extremely serious and has been associated with deaths, is the combination of **Coumadin** and **Atromid-S** (clofibrate). The reason is that **Atromid-S**, a cholesterol-lowering compound, is prescribed infrequently compared to other such medications. For the same reason, we also left out the interactions of **Coumadin** with **Rythmol** (propafenone), a heart medicine, and with **Antabuse** (disulfiram), a drug that is sometimes given to alcoholics to prevent them from consuming alcohol.

We have generally not covered injectable drugs, which would be administered in the doctor's office or in a hospital. For example, flu vaccine has been reported to interact with **Coumadin** in some patients, and monitoring of prothrombin time is advised. In such a situation, make sure the prescribing physician knows all other medications you are taking.

As you can now tell, evaluating complex combinations is like focusing on a moving target. You never know where it will be next. What was "true" last year may no longer be true this year. Goodness knows what the experts will declare next year. We estimate that more than 20,000 interactions are mentioned in the medical literature. There is no way to include all of them in this work and many are of interest primarily to academic researchers who spend little time with real patients. There are others that have not yet been discovered.

This book is a starting point to alert you to potential dangers, but we don't know your individual situation. No one should ever start or stop any medication without first checking with a physician. Also consult your pharmacist. Chances are good that he or she can look up your medications on a computer to see if there are any flagged interactions. Don't forget to mention any over-the-counter remedies or nutritional supplements you may be taking.

Safety Checklist

Dear Doctor/Pharmacist,

To assist me in taking my medicines properly, and to reduce the risk of dangerous drug interactions, please help me answer these questions:

1) What is the name of my medicine?

      brand: _____

      generic: _____

2) What is the dose? _____

3) What time(s) should I take this medicine?

      _____am   _____ am
      _____ pm   _____ pm   _____ pm

4) Should I take this medicine:

    ☐ with food?
    ☐ at least one hour before or two hours after eating?

5) Are there any special foods I should avoid?

6) Are there any vitamins or supplements I should avoid?

7) Are there any precautions or warnings I should know about?

8) Are there any contraindications that would make this drug inappropriate?

9) Which other medicines should I avoid?

10) Are there any OTC remedies I should avoid?

11) What side effects are common with my medicine?

12) Are there any symptoms that are so serious you would want to know about them immediately?

Photocopy this page and take it to your health care provider.

chapter three

Lethal Drug/
Drug Combinations

What makes a drug interaction dangerous? Lots of combinations create unpleasant consequences. For example, the broad-spectrum antimicrobial drug **Flagyl** (metronidazole) is prescribed for certain digestive tract and vaginal infections and also as part of an exciting new treatment against infectious ulcers. If someone taking **Flagyl** were to drink alcohol, the result might be nausea, flushing, rapid heart beat, and vomiting. This is uncomfortable, but probably not life threatening.

We're more concerned about incompatibilities that have already resulted in one or more reported deaths. We are equally worried about situations that could be so serious someone might die. Since these are often indirect, they may be overlooked and unreported.

The older person who is taking **Valium** (diazepam) or **Xanax** (alprazolam) for nervousness may be a little less steady than his younger counterpart. If he were to receive a prescription for **Tagamet** (cimetidine) for bad heartburn or ulcer pain, the stomach drug could delay elimination of the anti-anxiety agent from the body. That in turn could lead to increased sedation and dizziness as blood levels climbed. If this resulted in a fall and a broken hip, it could be a death sentence for the older person.

Drug interactions can kill in two ways. First, two or more incompatible chemicals can produce an unexpected, disastrous reaction in the body. If you gave a child a chemistry set and turned her loose without an instruction booklet, she might have a great time mixing one chemical with another and watching colors change—until she happened on an explosive combination. Your body won't blow up when you combine chemicals in it, but there have been situations in which blood pressure climbed so high that an artery blew out, resulting in hemorrhage and death.

People also die if one drug blocks another that is crucial to survival. Someone taking an epilepsy drug could have a fatal accident if a competing medicine al-

---

The Case of the Bran Muffins

We were intrigued to read about the 42-year-old woman who, like her father, had suffered from severe depression. Over nine years she had four bad bouts of the blues that required antidepressant therapy. Her psychiatrist had prescribed 75 mg of desipramine (Norpramin) with excellent results.

The physician was puzzled when her patient didn't improve on this drug a fifth time. The dose was the same but after three weeks the patient wasn't getting any better. Blood tests revealed that less than half the usual amount of desipramine was circulating in her body; this was too little to be effective.

Upon questioning, the patient said her family doctor had recommended bran to overcome constipation. She was eating only a bran muffin at breakfast and another at lunch. The fiber dramatically interfered with the absorption of her medicine. Thanks to an alert psychiatrist, the patient gave up the muffins, her blood levels returned to normal, and the depression soon lifted.

Stewart, Donna E. "High-Fiber Diet and Serum Tricyclic Antidepressant Levels." *J. Clin. Psychopharmacol.* 1992; 12:438–440.

ters the anticonvulsant's effectiveness. An infection that progresses because an antibiotic is inactivated could be lethal. An anticoagulant prescribed to prevent blood clots may not thin the blood adequately as a result of an interaction. The resulting stroke might be a killer.

Therapeutic failures are hard to track. For example, people who are depressed sometimes commit suicide. If someone takes his life while on an antidepressant, the automatic assumption is made that the medicine wasn't strong enough to overcome feelings of hopelessness. Family and friends are left wondering what went wrong and what more they might have done. Few would think to look for an interaction as a contributing factor in such a suicide.

Antidepressant (MAO Inhibitor) Hazards

When a depressed patient doesn't seem to be getting better on a particular antidepressant, the physician may add another type of drug to the program. There are several different kinds of medicines to choose from. They work through distinct pathways in the brain and affect separate neurochemicals, such as serotonin, dopamine, and norepinephrine. Combining the wrong classes of antidepressants can lead to disaster.

In one case a physically healthy 34-year-old engineer was being treated with **Parnate** (tranylcypromine) for serious depression. Although this drug had worked in the past, this time the engineer was still feeling extremely depressed, even suicidal. His doctor added **Anafranil** (clomipramine), hoping that the two drugs together would be helpful. Instead, the engineer felt awful. After two doses he felt nauseated and began sweating profusely. When he called his doctor to com-

plain about these symptoms, he was reassured and
told to keep taking both medications.

The combination of **Anafranil** and **Parnate** led to
further problems. The engineer became confused and
anxious; other symptoms included rapid heart beat,
shivering, fever, and breathing difficulty. Two days
later he was admitted to the hospital and put in intensive care where he lost consciousness. His condition
deteriorated rapidly and he died 30 hours later.[1]
Apparently these two drugs triggered hemorrhaging
throughout his body.

This isn't the first time an antidepressant has killed
someone because of a bad interaction. The class of
medications called MAO (monoamine oxidase) inhibitors includes **Nardil** (phenelzine), **Marplan** (isocarboxazid), and **Parnate** (tranylcypromine). These
drugs are prescribed for a range of problems including
depression, agoraphobia (fear of crowds), panic, and
bulimia (an eating disorder that involves bingeing).

Deaths have been reported when other types of antidepressants are prescribed with MAO inhibitors. For
example, tricyclic antidepressants such as those in the
box can be extremely dangerous in combination with MAO inhibitors. Symptoms
of the interaction in-
clude confusion, fe-
ver, rapid heart rate,
fast breathing, sweat-
ing, agitation, sei-
zures, flushing, head-
ache, and coma. It is
safest to allow at

Tricylic Antidepressants

Asendin	(amoxapine)
Aventyl	(nortriptyline)
Elavil	(amitriptyline)
Norpramin	(desipramine)
Pamelor	(nortriptyline)
Sinequan	(doxeprin)
Surmontil	(trimipramine)
Tofranil	(imipramine)
Vivactil	(protriptyline)

least two weeks after stopping an MAO inhibitor before starting one of these other antidepressants.

Even some of the newer medications for depression such as **Prozac** (fluoxetine) and **Zoloft** (sertraline) may provoke a severe interaction when taken with MAO inhibitors.[2, 3, 4] People may develop restlessness, nausea, shivering, double vision, confusion, and uncontrollable muscle contractions. Deaths have been reported.[5] Because **Prozac** lasts a long time in the body, its manufacturer recommends allowing at least five weeks to pass between stopping **Prozac** and starting any MAO inhibitor.

Prozac Interactions

Other drugs that may interact with Prozac include other antidepressants like **Desyrel** (trazodone), **Tofranil** (imipramine), **Norpramin** (desipramine), and **Pamelor** (nortriptyline); pain relievers like **Talwin** (pentazocine); anti-anxiety agents like **Valium** (diazepam) and **Xanax** (alprazolam); major tranquilizers such as **Haldol** (haloperidol); and the antiseizure drug **Tegretol** (carbamazepine).[6] (See page 284 for specifics.)

A number of other prescription drugs can interact in a dangerous or life-threatening way with MAO inhibitors. Perhaps the most famous case is that of Libby Zion. This 18-year-old woman was admitted to New York Hospital on the evening of March 4, 1984, with a fever and an earache. Although she told physicians that she had been taking **Nardil** for depression, they administered a pain reliever called **Demerol** (meperidine) to calm her down. Instead, it made her more agitated. Because she was thrashing around, hospital personnel tried to control her with a restraining jacket and tied her hands and feet to the bed. Her condition continued to deteriorate and by 6:30 A.M. her temperature had reached 108°F. Libby Zion died around 7:45 A.M.

The physician on duty did not realize that **Nardil** and **Demerol** do not mix. This combination can cause agitation, seizures, and fever, and lead to coma or death. The cause of Libby Zion's tragic death remains controversial, but it is clear that she never should have been given **Demerol**. On February 6, 1995, a jury technically awarded Libby Zion's parents $750,000 for their daughter's pain and suffering.

We too have experienced a terrible drug interaction with **Demerol**. Joe's mother required angioplasty to open a single clogged coronary artery. She was at one of the top-ranked hospitals in the United States. Hospital personnel were informed that she should never receive morphine or similar drugs because she could not tolerate narcotics; nevertheless, she was given **Demerol** after the procedure. This narcotic interacted with the **Eldepryl** she had been taking before admission, and as a result, she suffered involuntary muscle twitching, hyperexcitability, and agitation. In an attempt to restrain her, the nurse tied her feet to the bed.

Cardiologists know that it is crucial for patients to be kept calm after angioplasty to prevent internal bleeding. Helen Graedon died the following day. According to the death certificate, her heart stopped due to loss of blood pressure because of retroperitoneal hemorrhage (internal bleeding).

Such lethal interactions are not limited to medications. Foods can also trigger deadly reactions in combination with certain drugs.

Someone taking **Nardil** or **Parnate** could die if they ate cheddar cheese, pepperoni, pickled herring, guacamole, or even soy sauce. Such foods contain a substance called tyramine that, in combination with these drugs, can raise blood pressure so high it could cause a stroke. For a more complete discussion of this interaction, turn to Chapter 4.

Over-the-counter remedies can also be hazardous in combination with MAO inhibitors. Nonprescription diet pills and cold remedies contain the decongestant phenylpropanolamine (PPA). It is found in everything from **Acutrim**, **Dexatrim**, and **Stay Trim** to **Alka-Seltzer Plus Night-Time Cold Medicine**, **Contac 12 Hour Capsules**, **Dimetapp Cold and Flu Caplets**, and **Tylenol Cold Effervescent Tablets**. One patient on **Nardil** developed a severe heart rhythm disturbance and another died when they added cold remedies containing PPA.[7] Pseudoephedrine (an ingredient in **Actifed**, **Advil Cold and Sinus**, **Dristan Sinus Caplets**, **NyQuil**, **Sudafed**, etc.) has been implicated in stroke and death when taken with an MAO inhibitor such as **Nardil**.

Cough medicine could also be dangerous in conjunction with MAO inhibitors. One 26-year-old woman on **Nardil** died after swallowing two ounces of cough syrup containing dextromethorphan.[8] Another person experienced an adverse reaction after taking two teaspoons of a cough medicine together with **Marplan**.[9] The culprit appears to be dextromethorphan, an ingredient found in most over-the-counter cough remedies. Nausea, dizziness, muscle spasms, and loss of consciousness are symptoms of this interaction.

Digitalis Dangers

Lanoxin (digoxin) is one of the most commonly prescribed, herb-based medicines in the world. It is derived from digitalis, the foxglove plant, which has a long history of medicinal use. Digitalis was used by the ancient Egyptian and Roman physicians as a heart tonic. Today digoxin is employed primarily to treat congestive heart failure and certain heart rhythm disturbances such as atrial fibrillation and flutter. Although digoxin started to fall into disfavor in the 1980s, new research suggests that this time-honored agent still plays a significant role in heart treatment.

Getting the dose of digoxin correct is tricky, however, and can be a little like walking a tightrope. Too much digoxin can be extremely hazardous. Symptoms can include loss of appetite, nausea, vomiting, diarrhea, headache, confusion, depression, weakness, drowsiness, disturbed vision, and disorientation. Hallucinations, seizures, and ultimately life-threatening disruptions of heart rhythm can be consequences of digoxin toxicity. Death can be the ultimate result of overdose.

Because digoxin levels can be altered by other drugs, including antidepressants such as **Prozac** and antibiotics like **Biaxin**, a physician might not realize that an older person is getting too much of this medicine. Symptoms may be attributed to aging or to the underlying heart problem. Let's face it, confusion, weakness, and disorientation might be mistaken for the onset of Alzheimer's disease. If someone dies suddenly of an apparent heart attack, most people would assume this unfortunate event occurred despite his many medicines, rather than because of them.

Because people taking **Lanoxin** often have other heart problems, they may also be using other heart medications. Quinidine (**Cardioquin**, **Quinalan**,

Quinaglute, **Quinidex**, **Quinora**) is frequently pre-scribed for a variety of arrhythmias. But quinidine and digoxin is a dangerous mix unless the cardiologist is extremely careful. Quinidine can increase blood levels of digoxin into the danger zone.[10] It took more than 60 years for physicians to discover this dangerous inter-action. Doctors who believe they can anticipate trouble just by doing blood tests may be kidding themselves and putting their patients at risk. New research suggests that even when serum digoxin levels are in the so-called normal therapeutic range, electrocardiograms may show evidence of toxicity.[11]

Another heart drug that may cause life-threatening problems in conjunction with **Lanoxin** is **Cordarone** (amiodarone). **Cordarone** may cause digoxin levels to soar into the toxic range. In addition, when some patients took this combination their hearts stopped beating (asystole).[13] Their lives were saved, but the sight of an electrocardiogram strip showing only a flat line can be very scary.

Diuretic Dangers

Physicians consider water pills (diuretics) so safe and effective that they are among the most widely used drugs in the world. Such medications are frequently the first step in treating high blood pressure and may be used to combat fluid buildup due to many different causes, including congestive heart failure.

It is quite common for people with serious heart trouble to be taking both **Lanoxin** and a diuretic such as **Lasix** (furosemide). The trouble is that many water pills deplete the body of minerals, including sodium, potassium, and magnesium. We can probably do without the sodium, but both potassium and magnesium

Drugs That May Increase Digoxin Levels[12]

(Never stop Lanoxin [digoxin] or any other medicine without careful medical supervision. Have your doctor and pharmacist evaluate the interaction potential of digoxin with the following medications.)

Achromycin V (tetracycline)
Adalat (nifedipine)*
Calan (verapamil)
Cardizem (diltiazem)*
Cordarone (amiodarone)
Declomycin (demeclocycline)
E.E.S. (erythromycin)
E-Mycin (erythromycin)
ERYC (erythromycin)
EryPed (erythromycin)
Ery-Tab (erythromycin)
Erythrocin (erythromycin)
Ilosone (erythromycin)
Isoptin (verapamil)
Minocin (minocycline)

Orinase (tolbutamide)
PCE (erythromycin)
Plaquenil (hydroxychloroquine)
Procardia (nifedipine)*
Quinamm (quinine)
Rythmol (propafenone)
Sandimmune (cyclosporine)
Sporanox (itraconazole)
Tambocor (flecainide)
Terramycin (oxytetracycline)
Valium (diazepam)
Vascor (bepridil)*
Verelan (verapamil)
Vibramycin (doxycycline)
Xanax (alprazolam)*

*These interactions are controversial and confusing. Please ask your doctor to monitor your progress carefully for any signs of toxicity.

are crucial for normal heart function. Cortisone (**Cortone**) and similar drugs such as betamethasone (**Celestone**), dexamethasone (**Decadron**), hydrocortisone (**Cortef**, **Hydrocortone**), prednisone, prednisolone (**Delta-Cortef**), and methylprednisolone (**Medrol**) may also deplete potassium, so close monitoring is essential if this combination is necessary.

Physicians are aware that low potassium levels can make digitalis-type drugs extremely hazardous, even lethal. The heart can suddenly stop beating. That's why doctors are usually very careful to monitor blood levels of this mineral when someone is on

Lanoxin. If potassium drops too low they may pre-scribe a potassium supplement (**K-Lor**, **K-Lyte**, **K-Tab**, **Micro-K**, **Slow-K**, etc.) or switch the patient to a potassium-preserving diuretic such as **Dyazide**, **Moduretic,** or **Maxzide**.

If all this sounds complicated, hang on to your seat. It gets worse. The problem is that too *much* potassium may be just as hazardous as too little and can also cause cardiac arrest. Think about Goldilocks and the porridge. Getting it just right is not easy. Combining diuretics such as **Aldactone**, **Aldactazide**, **Dyazide**, **Maxzide,** or **Moduretic** (which keep potassium levels up) with heart and blood pressure pills such as **Accupril** (quinapril), **Altace** (ramipril), **Capoten** (captopril), **Lotensin** (benazepril), **Monopril** (fosinopril), **Prinivil** (lisinopril), **Vasotec** (enalapril), and **Zestril** (lisinopril) can be very tricky. It is not uncommon for people taking digoxin to be taking such medications as well, but this combination can lead to a buildup of excess potassium that may trigger life-threatening changes in heart rhythms. People who use potassium-containing salt substitutes could also end up in trouble.

Too Much Potassium (hyperkalemia)

- Serum potassium above 5mEq/L
- Palpitations, heart rhythm changes
- Tingling or numbness in lips, feet, or hands
- Breathing difficulty
- Weakness
- Slow pulse
- Confusion

Too Little Potassium (hypokalemia)

- Serum potassium below 3.5 mEq/L
- Irregular pulse
- Muscle cramps
- Breathing difficulty
- Weakness

When people are on diuretics, magnesium levels may also drop. This mineral is often overlooked, but it can be as important as potassium for people on **Lanoxin**. Make sure your physician is checking your blood magnesium as well as potassium if you are on digoxin and a diuretic. That way he or she may be able to spot a problem before it becomes life-threatening. For additional information see the diuretic section in the Guides to Dangerous Drug Interactions at the end of this book (pages 345 and 353).

Arthritis Drug Interactions

Millions of people rely on their daily dose of pain medicine to make it through the day. These drugs are used for everything from tennis elbow and bursitis to headaches and arthritis. They are called nonsteroidal anti-inflammatory drugs, or NSAIDs for short. While they can relieve discomfort, they can also do nas-

NSAIDS	
NAME	GENERIC
Advil	ibuprofen
Aleve	naproxen
Anaprox	naproxen
Ansaid	flurbiprofen
Butazolidin	phenylbutazone
Clinoril	sulindac
Dolobid	diflunisal
Feldene	piroxicam
Indocin	indomethacin
Indocin SR	
Lodine	etodolac
Meclomen	meclofenamate
Motrin	ibuprofen
Motrin IB	
Nalfon	fenoprofen
Naprosyn	naproxen
Nuprin	ibuprofen
Orudis	ketoprofen
Relafen	nabumetone
Rufen	ibuprofen
Tolectin	tolmetin
Voltaren	diclofenac

ty things to the stomach, kidneys, and liver.

It is estimated that every year at least 70,000 people are hospitalized because of digestive diseases brought on by NSAIDs. Experts report that these medications are responsible for anywhere between 7,600 and 20,000 deaths annually.[14, 15]

Anticoagulants

Blood thinners such as **Coumadin** (warfarin) save lives. They prevent blood clots that can lead to strokes and heart attacks. But thinning the blood too much can lead to life-threatening hemorrhage. Up to a third of those on long-term anticoagulant therapy experience bouts of serious bleeding. [16]

That's cause for concern by itself, but add an arthritis drug to the mix and you are playing with fire. Anti-inflammatory drugs often cause stomach irritation and ulceration. When someone taking one of these pain relievers also takes an anticoagulant such

Anticoagulants and NSAIDS

"Our data show that compared with nonusers of either drug, concurrent users of NSAIDs and oral anticoagulants had nearly a 13-fold increase in the risk of developing hemorrhagic peptic ulcer disease and that approximately 10% of the hospitalizations for hemorrhagic ulcer disease in users of anticoagulants were attributable to NSAID exposure. These findings provide clear evidence that NSAIDs increase the risk of hemorrhagic complications in elderly users of anticoagulants, and they should be used with extreme caution in patients receiving anticoagulants."

Shorr, Ronald I., et al. "Concurrent Use of Nonsteroidal Anti-Inflammatory Drugs and Oral Anticoagulants Places Elderly Persons at High Risk for Hemorrhagic Peptic Ulcer Disease." *Arch. Intern. Med.* 1993; 153:1665-1670.

as **Coumadin,** the risk of a bleeding ulcer becomes much greater. This could be a deadly complication, especially in older people.

Methotrexate

NSAIDs create extra problems when they are mixed with certain other medications. Some of these interactions may be fatal. One in particular concerns us. It is the combination of anti-inflammatory drugs and methotrexate (**Abitrexate**, **Folex**, **Rheumatrex**), a powerful chemotherapeutic agent for cancer treatment. In recent years it has gained much wider use against psoriasis and rheumatoid arthritis. The problem is that cases of serious toxicity are cropping up. There have even been deaths reported.

A few people who took both methotrexate and a drug such as **Ansaid**, **Butazolidin**, **Indocin**, **Naprosyn**, **Orudis**, or even aspirin have experienced complications such as diarrhea, fever, severe ulceration of the mouth and gastrointestinal tract, nausea, vomiting, kidney failure, blood abnormalities due to bone marrow damage, and death.[17] Apparently NSAIDs can boost blood levels of methotrexate, sometimes to dangerous levels.

If you suffer from severe arthritis or psoriasis, you should be alert to the dangers of this interaction because these medications might be prescribed together for someone with your condition. No one seems to know how often this interaction proves fatal, and it may be quite rare. Nevertheless, it is serious enough to warrant careful attention. Unless a physician is monitoring methotrexate closely it could be a recipe for disaster when combined with NSAIDs.

Lithium

People who suffer from bipolar mood disorder (previously called manic-depression) are usually treated with lithium (**Cibalith-S**, **Eskalith**, **Lithobid**, **Lithonate**, **Lithotabs**). This medication is supposed to smooth out the wild mood swings typical of this problem, blunting the highs and interrupting the lows.

Under the best of conditions, lithium can be a difficult drug. Adverse reactions may include thirst, hand tremor, nausea, irregular heart rhythms, muscle twitches, dizziness, slurred speech, confusion, forgetfulness, hair loss, fatigue, and impotence. Fortunately, such complications are rare when blood levels are carefully controlled. But many arthritis medicines may interfere with normal elimination of lithium and lead to toxicity.[18, 19, 20]

Signs of Lithium Poisoning

diarrhea	blurred vision
drowsiness	incoordination
weakness	seizures
slurred speech	fatigue
blackouts	kidney failure
vomiting	coma
confusion	death

Thiazide diuretics such as hydrochlorothiazide may also raise lithium levels and lead to symptoms of overdose. Careful monitoring is essential!

Be Vigilant

There are far too many possible interactions for your doctor to know them all by heart. Anytime you add another medication to what you are already taking, ask her to look it up to see if it is compatible. Then make sure you ask the pharmacist as well. Don't overlook vitamins, minerals, or nonprescription drugs. Remember, even something as seemingly innocuous as a cold or allergy remedy could be lethal in combination with an antidepressant such as **Nardil** (an MAO inhibitor). (See page 129 for more details.)

Hospitalization is another potential risk. You would think that a place with so many health professionals would be good protection against the kind of problems we are talking about in this book, but bureaucracies can create confusion. In hospitals it is quite possible for the left hand not to know what the right hand is doing. People often get more medicines in a hospital than they do at home. Some experts have estimated that the average hospital patient receives nine different drugs simultaneously. And surgery poses special risks. A "simple" antibiotic such as tetracycline could interact with the general anesthetic **Penthrane** (methoxyflurane) to cause kidney damage. Three deaths have been reported as a result of this combination.[21]

The following table lists drugs that have been reported to interact in especially hazardous ways. Some of these combinations have resulted in fatal outcomes. There is not enough space to discuss every serious interaction in this book, but we make this information available to you so that you can check with your pharmacist and physician about your particular situation. Remember, NEVER start or stop any medication without medical supervision. If you want further details on the nature of some of the most common and serious interactions, check the individual drug listings in Guides to Dangerous Drug Interactions at the back of this book.

Hazardous Drug Interactions*

*Each person may react differently, and your doctor may have an excellent reason to prescribe certain drugs together. Be sure to discuss your individual situation with your physician.

THIS DRUG	CAN INTERACT WITH
Advil (ibuprofen)	**Coumadin** (warfarin)
Advil (ibuprofen)	lithium
Advil (ibuprofen)	methotrexate
Aldactone (spironolactone)	potassium supplements/salt substitutes
Aleve (naproxen)	**Coumadin** (warfarin)
Aleve (naproxen)	lithium
Aleve (naproxen)	methotrexate
Anafranil (clomipramine)	**Hismanal** (astemizole)
Anafranil (clomipramine)	**Nardil** (phenelzine)
Anafranil (clomipramine)	**Parnate** (tranylcypromine)
Anafranil (clomipramine)	**Prozac** (fluoxetine)
Anafranil (clomipramine)	**Seldane** (terfenadine)
Anaprox (naproxen)	**Coumadin** (warfarin)
Anaprox (naproxen)	lithium
Anaprox (naproxen)	methotrexate
Ansaid (flurbiprofen)	**Coumadin** (warfarin)
Ansaid (flurbiprofen)	methotrexate
Antabuse (disulfiram)	**Coumadin** (warfarin)
Anturane (sulfinpyrazone)	**Coumadin** (warfarin)
Asendin (amoxapine)	**Nardil** (phenelzine)
Asendin (amoxapine)	**Parnate** (tranylcypromine)
aspirin	**Coumadin** (warfarin)
Bactrim (co-trimoxazole)	**Coumadin** (warfarin)
barbiturates	**Coumadin** (warfarin)

THIS DRUG	CAN INTERACT WITH
Bronkaid tablets (theophylline, etc.)	**Cipro** (ciprofloxacin)
Bronkaid tablets (theophylline, etc.)	**Noroxin** (norfloxacin)
Bronkaid tablets (theophylline, etc.)	**Tagamet** (cimetidine)
Butazolidin (phenylbutazone)	**Coumadin** (warfarin)
Butazolidin (phenylbutazone)	methotrexate
Calan (verapamil)	**Lanoxin** (digoxin)
Cardioquin (quinidine)	**Cordarone** (amiodarone)
Cardioquin (quinidine)	**Lanoxin** (digoxin)
Cardizem (diltiazem)	**Cordarone** (amiodarone)
Catapres (clonidine)	**Norpramin** (desipramine)
Catapres (clonidine)	**Pertofrane** (desipramine)
Catapres (clonidine)	**Tofranil** (imipramine)
Choloxin (dextrothyroxine)	**Coumadin** (warfarin)
Cipro (ciprofloxacin)	theophylline
Cordarone (amiodarone)	**Cardizem** (diltiazem)
Cordarone (amiodarone)	**Coumadin** (warfarin)
Cordarone (amiodarone)	**Lanoxin** (digoxin)
Cordarone (amiodarone)	quinidine
Cordarone (amiodarone)	**Sandimmune** (cyclosporine)
Coumadin (warfarin)	androgens (male hormones)
Coumadin (warfarin)	**Antabuse** (disulfiram)
Coumadin (warfarin)	**Anturane** (sulfinpyrazone)
Coumadin (warfarin)	aspirin and other NSAIDs
Coumadin (warfarin)	**Bactrim** (co-trimoxazole)
Coumadin (warfarin)	barbiturates
Coumadin (warfarin)	**Butazolidin** (phenylbutazone)
Coumadin (warfarin)	**Choloxin** (dextrothyroxine)
Coumadin (warfarin)	**Cordarone** (amiodarone)
Coumadin (warfarin)	**Danazol** (danocrine)

THIS DRUG	CAN INTERACT WITH
Coumadin (warfarin)	**Diflucan** (fluconazole)
Coumadin (warfarin)	**Flagyl** (metronidazole)
Coumadin (warfarin)	**Monistat** (miconazole)
Coumadin (warfarin)	**Nolvadex** (tamoxifen)
Coumadin (warfarin)	**Septra** (co-trimoxazole)
Coumadin (warfarin)	**Tagamet** (cimetidine)
Cytovene (ganciclovir)	**Retrovir** (zidovudine)
Danocrine (danazol)	**Coumadin** (warfarin)
Darvocet-N (propoxyphene/APAP)	**Tegretol** (carbamazepine)
Darvon (propoxyphene)	**Tegretol** (carbamazepine)
Demerol (meperidine)	**Nardil** (phenelzine)
Demerol (meperidine)	**Parnate** (tranylcypromine)
Desyrel (trazodone)	**Prozac** (fluoxetine)
dextromethorphan	**Nardil** (phenelzine)
dextromethorphan	**Parnate** (tranylcypromine)
Diflucan (fluconazole)	**Coumadin** (warfarin)
Diflucan (fluconazole)	**Hismanal** (astemizole)
Diflucan (fluconazole)	**Seldane** (terfenadine)
Dilantin (phenytoin)	isoniazid
Duraquin (quinidine)	**Cordarone** (amiodarone)
Dyazide (triamterene+HCTZ)	potassium supplements/salt substitutes
E.E.S. (erythromycin)	**Hismanal** (astemizole)
E.E.S. (erythromycin)	**Mevacor** (lovastatin)
E.E.S (erythromycin)	**Norpace** (disopyramide)
E.E.S. (erythromycin)	**Pravachol** (pravastatin)
E.E.S. (erythromycin)	**Seldane** (terfenadine)
E.E.S (erythromycin)	**Tegretol** (carbamazepine)

THIS DRUG	CAN INTERACT WITH
E.E.S (erythromycin)	**Zocor** (simvastatin)
Effexor (venlafaxine)	**Parnate** (tranylcypromine)
Elavil (amitriptyline)	**Eldepryl** (selegiline)
Elavil (amitriptyline)	**Isuprel** (isoproterenol)
Elavil (amitriptyline)	**Nardil** (phenelzine)
Elavil (amitriptyline)	**Parnate** (tranylcypromine)
Eldepryl (selegiline)	**Elavil** (amitriptyline)
Eldepryl (selegiline)	**Luvox** (fluvoxamine)
Eldepryl (selegiline)	**Paxil** (paroxetine)
Eldepryl (selegiline)	**Prozac** (fluoxetine)
Eldepryl (selegiline)	**Vivactil** (protriptyline)
Eldepryl (selegiline)	**Zoloft** (sertraline)
E-Mycin (erythromycin)	**Hismanal** (astemizole)
E-Mycin (erythromycin)	**Mevacor** (lovastatin)
E-Mycin (erythromycin)	**Norpace** (disopyramide)
E-Mycin (erythromycin)	**Pravachol** (pravastatin)
E-Mycin (erythromycin)	**Seldane** (terfenadine)
E-Mycin (erythromycin)	**Tegretol** (carbamazepine)
E-Mycin (erythromycin)	**Zocor** (simvastatin)
ERYC (erythromycin)	**Hismanal** (astemizole)
ERYC (erythromycin)	**Mevacor** (lovastatin)
ERYC (erythromycin)	**Norpace** (disopyramide)
ERYC (erythromycin)	**Pravachol** (pravastatin)
ERYC (erythromycin)	**Seldane** (terfenadine)
ERYC (erythromycin)	**Tegretol** (carbamazepine)
ERYC (erythromycin)	**Zocor** (simvastatin)
EryPed (erythromycin)	**Hismanal** (astemizole)
EryPed (erythromycin)	**Mevacor** (lovastatin)
EryPed (erythromycin)	**Norpace** (disopyramide)

THIS DRUG	CAN INTERACT WITH
EryPed (erythromycin)	**Pravachol** (pravastatin)
EryPed (erythromycin)	**Seldane** (terfenadine)
EryPed (erythromycin)	**Tegretol** (carbamazepine)
EryPed (erythromycin)	**Zocor** (simvastatin)
Ery-Tab (erythromycin)	**Hismanal** (astemizole)
Ery-Tab (erythromycin)	**Mevacor** (lovastatin)
Ery-Tab (erythromycin)	**Norpace** (disopyramide)
Ery-Tab (erythromycin)	**Pravachol** (pravastatin)
Ery-Tab (erythromycin)	**Seldane** (terfenadine)
Ery-Tab (erythromycin)	**Tegretol** (carbamazepine)
Ery-Tab (erythromycin)	**Zocor** (simvastatin)
Eskalith (lithium)	NSAIDs
Flagyl (metronidazole)	**Coumadin** (warfarin)
Folex (methotrexate)	NSAIDs
Haldol (haloperidol)	**Prozac** (fluoxetine)
Hismanal (astemizole)	**Diflucan** (fluconazole)
Hismanal (astemizole)	erythromycin
Hismanal (astemizole)	**Luvox** (fluvoxamine)
Hismanal (astemizole)	**Nizoral** (ketoconazole)
Hismanal (astemizole)	**Prozac** (fluoxetine)
Hismanal (astemizole)	**Sporanox** (itraconazole)
Imuran (azathioprine)	**Zyloprim** (allopurinol)
Indocin (indomethacin)	**Coumadin** (warfarin)
Indocin (indomethacin)	lithium
Indocin (indomethacin)	methotrexate
isoniazid	**Dilantin** (phenytoin)
Isoptin (verapamil)	**Lanoxin** (digoxin)
Isuprel (isoproterenol)	**Elavil** (amitriptyline)
K-Dur (potassium)	potassium-sparing diuretics

THIS DRUG	CAN INTERACT WITH
K-Tab (potassium)	potassium-sparing diuretics
Klor-Con (potassium)	potassium-sparing diuretics
Lanoxin (digoxin)	**Cardioquin** (quinidine)
Lanoxin (digoxin)	**Cordarone** (amiodarone)
Lanoxin (digoxin)	**Quinaglute** (quinidine)
Lanoxin (digoxin)	**Quinalan** (quinidine)
Lanoxin (digoxin)	**Quinidex** (quinidine)
Lanoxin (digoxin)	quinidine
Lanoxin (digoxin)	**Quinora** (quinidine)
Lanoxin (digoxin)	**Rythmol** (propafenone)
Lanoxin (digoxin)	**Sandimmune** (cyclosporine)
Lanoxin (digoxin)	**Vascor** (bepridil)
Lanoxin (digoxin)	**Verelan** (verapamil)
Larodopa (levodopa)	**Nardil** (phenelzine)
Larodopa (levodopa)	**Parnate** (tranylcypromine)
lithium	**Indocin** and other NSAIDs
Lithobid (lithium)	NSAIDs
Lithonate (lithium)	NSAIDs
Lithotabs (lithium)	NSAIDs
Lopid (gemfibrozil)	**Mevacor** (lovastatin)
Luvox (fluvoxamine)	**Eldepryl** (selegiline)
Luvox (fluvoxamine)	**Hismanal** (astemizole)
Luvox (fluvoxamine)	**Nardil** (phenelzine)
Luvox (fluvoxamine)	**Parnate** (tranylcypromine)
Luvox (fluvoxamine)	**Seldane** (terfenadine)
Maxzide (triamterene + HCTZ)	potassium supplements/salt substitutes
methotrexate	**Indocin** and other NSAIDs
Mevacor (lovastatin)	**Biaxin** (clarithromycin)

THIS DRUG	CAN INTERACT WITH
Mevacor (lovastatin)	erythromycin
Mevacor (lovastatin)	**Lopid** (gemfibrozil)
Mevacor (lovastatin)	niacin
Mevacor (lovastatin)	**Sandimmune** (cyclosporine)
Micro-K (potassium)	potassium-sparing diuretics
Midamor (amiloride)	potassium supplements/salt substitutes
Moduretic (amiloride + HCTZ)	potassium supplements/salt substitutes
Monistat (miconazole)	**Coumadin** (warfarin)
Motrin (ibuprofen)	**Coumadin** (warfarin)
Motrin (ibuprofen)	lithium
Motrin (ibuprofen)	methotrexate
Naprosyn (naproxen)	**Coumadin** (warfarin)
Naprosyn (naproxen)	lithium
Naprosyn (naproxen)	methotrexate
Nardil (phenelzine)	**Anafranil** (clomipramine)
Nardil (phenelzine)	**Asendin** (amoxapine)
Nardil (phenelzine)	**Demerol** (meperidine)
Nardil (phenelzine)	dextromethorphan
Nardil (phenelzine)	diet pills/decongestants
Nardil (phenelzine)	**Elavil** (amitriptyline)
Nardil (phenelzine)	**Larodopa** (levodopa)
Nardil (phenelzine)	**Norpramin** (desipramine)
Nardil (phenelzine)	phenylpropanolamine
Nardil (phenelzine)	**Prozac** (fluoxetine)
Nardil (phenelzine)	pseudoephedrine
Nardil (phenelzine)	**Tofranil** (imipramine)
Nizoral (ketoconazole)	**Hismanal** (astemizole)

THIS DRUG	CAN INTERACT WITH
Nizoral (ketoconazole)	**Seldane** (terfenadine)
Nolvadex (tamoxifen)	**Coumadin** (warfarin)
Noroxin (norfloxacin)	theophylline
Norpace (disopyramide)	erythromycin
Norpramin (desipramine)	**Catapres** (clonidine)
Norpramin (desipramine)	**Nardil** (phenelzine)
Norpramin (desipramine)	**Parnate** (tranylcypromine)
Norpramin (desipramine)	**Prozac** (fluoxetine)
Nuprin (ibuprofen)	**Coumadin** (warfarin)
Nuprin (ibuprofen)	lithium
Nuprin (ibuprofen)	methotrexate
Orudis (ketoprofen)	**Coumadin** (warfarin)
Orudis (ketoprofen)	methotrexate
Pamelor (nortriptyline)	**Prozac** (fluoxetine)
Parnate (tranylcypromine)	**Anafranil** (clomipramine)
Parnate (tranylcypromine)	**Asendin** (amoxapine)
Parnate (tranylcypromine)	**Demerol** (meperidine)
Parnate (tranylcypromine)	dextromethorphan
Parnate (tranylcypromine)	diet pills/decongestants
Parnate (tranylcypromine)	**Effexor** (venlafaxine)
Parnate (tranylcypromine)	**Elavil** (amitriptyline)
Parnate (tranylcypromine)	**Larodopa** (levodopa)
Parnate (tranylcypromine)	**Luvox** (fluvoxamine)
Parnate (tranylcypromine)	**Norpramin** (desipramine)
Parnate (tranylcypromine)	**Paxil** (paroxetine)
Parnate (tranylcypromine)	phenylpropanolamine
Parnate (tranylcypromine)	**Prozac** (fluoxetine)
Parnate (tranylcypromine)	pseudoephedrine
Parnate (tranylcypromine)	**Tofranil** (imipramine)

THIS DRUG	CAN INTERACT WITH
Parnate (tranylcypromine)	**Zoloft** (sertraline)
Paxil (paroxetine)	**Eldepryl** (selegiline)
Paxil (paroxetine)	**Nardil** (phenelzine)
Paxil (paroxetine)	**Parnate** (tranylcypromine)
PCE (erythromycin)	**Hismanal** (astemizole)
PCE (erythromycin)	**Mevacor** (lovastatin)
PCE (erythromycin)	**Norpace** (disopyramide)
PCE (erythromycin)	**Pravachol** (pravastatin)
PCE (erythromycin)	**Seldane** (terfenadine)
PCE (erythromycin)	**Tegretol** (carbamazepine)
PCE (erythromycin)	**Zocor** (simvastatin)
Pertofrane (desipramine)	**Catapres** (clonidine)
phenylpropanolamine	**Nardil** (phenelzine)
phenylpropanolamine	**Parnate** (tranylcypromine)
potassium-sparing diuretics	**Micro-K** (potassium)
potassium-sparing diuretics	**Slow-K** (potassium)
potassium supplements/ salt substitutes	**Dyazide** (triamterene + HCTZ)
potassium supplements/ salt substitutes	**Maxzide** (triamterene + HCTZ)
potassium supplements/ salt substitutes	**Midamor** (amiloride)
potassium supplements/ salt substitutes	**Moduretic** (amiloride + HCTZ)
potassium-wasting diuretics	**Lanoxin** (digoxin)
Primatene Tablets (theophylline, etc.)	**Cipro** (ciprofloxacin)
Primatene Tablets (theophylline, etc.)	**Noroxin** (norfloxacin)

THIS DRUG	CAN INTERACT WITH
Primatene Tablets (theophylline, etc.)	**Tagamet** (cimetidine)
Prozac (fluoxetine)	**Anafranil** (clomipramin)
Prozac (fluoxetine)	**Desyrel** (trazodone)
Prozac (fluoxetine)	**Eldepryl** (selegiline)
Prozac (fluoxetine)	**Haldol** (haloperidol)
Prozac (fluoxetine)	**Nardil** (phenelzine)
Prozac (fluoxetine)	**Norpramin** (desipramine)
Prozac (fluoxetine)	**Pamelor** (nortriptyline)
Prozac (fluoxetine)	**Parnate** (tranylcypromine)
Prozac (fluoxetine)	**Tegretol** (carbamazepine)
Prozac (fluoxetine)	**Tofranil** (imipramine)
Prozac (fluoxetine)	**Valium** (diazepam)
Prozac (fluoxetine)	**Xanax** (alprazolam)
pseudoephedrine	**Nardil** (phenelzine)
pseudoephedrine	**Parnate** (tranylcypromine)
Purinethol (mercaptopurine)	**Zyloprim** (allopurinol)
Quinaglute (quinidine)	**Cordarone** (amiodarone)
Quinaglute (quinidine)	**Lanoxin** (digoxin)
Quinalan (quinidine)	**Cordarone** (amiodarone)
Quinalan (quinidine)	**Lanoxin** (digoxin)
Quinidex (quinidine)	**Cordarone** (amiodarone)
Quinidex (quinidine)	**Lanoxin** (digoxin)
quinidine	**Cordarone** (amiodarone)
quinidine	**Lanoxin** (digoxin)
Quinora (quinidine)	**Cordarone** (amiodarone)
Quinora (quinidine)	**Lanoxin** (digoxin)
Retrovir (zidovudine)	**Cytovene** (ganciclovir)

THIS DRUG	CAN INTERACT WITH
Rheumatrex (methotrexate)	NSAIDs
Sandimmune (cyclosporine)	**Cordarone** (amiodarone)
Sandimmune (cyclosporine)	**Lanoxin** (digoxin)
Seldane (terfenadine)	**Diflucan** (fluconazole)
Seldane (terfenadine)	erythromycin
Seldane (terfenadine)	**Luvox** (fluvoxamine)
Seldane (terfenadine)	**Nizoral** (ketoconazole)
Seldane (terfenadine)	**Prozac** (fluoxetine)
Seldane (terfenadine)	**Sporanox** (itraconazole)
Septra (co-trimoxazole)	**Coumadin** (warfarin)
Slo-bid (theophylline)	**Tagamet** (cimetidine)
Slow-K (potassium)	potassium-sparing diuretics
Slo-bid (theophylline)	**Cipro** (ciprofloxacin)
Slo-bid (theophylline)	**Noroxin** (norfloxacin)
Sporanox (itraconazole)	**Hismanal** (astemizole)
Sporanox (itraconazole)	**Seldane** (terfenadine)
Tagamet (cimetidine)	**BiCNU** (carmustine)
Tagamet (cimetidine)	**Coumadin** (warfarin)
Tagamet (cimetidine)	theophylline
Tedral (theophylline, etc.)	**Cipro** (ciprofloxacin)
Tedral (theophylline, etc.)	**Noroxin** (norfloxacin)
Tedral (theophylline, etc.)	**Tagamet** (cimetidine)
Tegretol (carbamazepine)	**Biaxin** (clarithromycin)
Tegretol (carbamazepine)	**Darvocet-N** (propoxyphene/APAP)
Tegretol (carbamazepine)	**Darvon** (propoxyphene)
Tegretol (carbamazepine)	erythromycin
Tegretol (carbamazepine)	**Tagamet** (cimetidine)

THIS DRUG	CAN INTERACT WITH
Theo-Dur (theophylline)	**Cipro** (ciprofloxacin)
Theo-Dur (theophylline)	**Noroxin** (norfloxacin)
Theo-Dur (theophylline)	**Tagamet** (cimetidine)
theophylline	**Tagamet** (cimetidine)
Tofranil (imipramine)	**Catapres** (clonidine)
Tofranil (imipramine)	**Marplan** (isocarboxazid)
Tofranil (imipramine)	**Nardil** (phenelzine)
Tofranil (imipramine)	**Parnate** (tranylcypromine)
Tofranil (imipramine)	**Prozac** (fluoxetine)
Tolectin (tolmetin)	**Coumadin** (warfarin)
Tolectin (tolmetin)	methotrexate
Valium (diazepam)	**Prozac** (fluoxetine)
Vivactil (protriptyline)	**Eldepryl** (selegiline)
Voltaren (diclofenac)	**Coumadin** (warfarin)
Voltaren (diclofenac)	lithium
Voltaren (diclofenac)	methotrexate
Xanax (alprazolam)	**Prozac** (fluoxetine)
Zoloft (sertraline)	**Eldepryl** (selegiline)
Zoloft (sertraline)	**Nardil** (phenelzine)
Zoloft (sertraline)	**Parnate** (tranylcypromine)
Zyloprim (allopurinol)	**Imuran** (azathioprine)
Zyloprim (allopurinol)	**Purinethol** (mercaptopurine)

References

1. Tackley, R.N., and B. Tregaskis. "Fatal Disseminated Intravascular Coagulation Following a Monoamine Oxidase Inhibitor/Tricyclic Interaction." *Anaesth.* 1987; 42:760–763.

2. Westermeyer, Joseph. "Fluoxetine-Induced Tricyclic Toxicity: Extent and Duration." *J. Clin. Pharmacol.* 1991; 31:388–392.

3. Otton, S. Victoria, et al. "Inhibition by Fluoxetine of Cytochrome P450 2D6 Activity." *Clin. Pharmacol. Ther.* 1993; 53:401–409.

4. Reidenberg, Marcus M. "Clinical Pharmacology." *JAMA* 1993; 270:192–194.

5. Hansten, Philip D., and John R. Horn. *Drug Interactions & Updates.* Malvern, Pa.: Lea & Febiger, 1993, pp. 491–492.

6. Otton, op. cit.

7. Ibid.

8. Rivers, N., et al. "Possible Lethal Reaction Between Nardil and Dextromethorphan." *Can. Med. Assoc. J.* 1970; 103:85.

9. Sovner, R., et al. "Interaction Between Dextromethorphan and Monoamine Oxidase Inhibitor Therapy with Isocarboxazid." *N. Engl. J. Med.* 1988; 319:1671.

10. Reiffel, J.A., et al. "A Previously Unrecognized Drug Interaction Between Quinidine and Digoxin." *Clin. Cardiol.* 1979; 2:40–42.

11. Mordel, Amnon, et al. "Quinidine Enhances Digitalis Toxicity at Therapeutic Serum Digoxin Levels." *Clin. Pharmacol. Ther.* 1993; 53:457–462.

12. Tatro, David S., et al. *Drug Interaction Facts.* St. Louis, Mo.: Facts and Comparisons, 1993.

13. Klein, H.O., et al. "Asystole Produced by the Combination of Amiodarone and Digoxin." *Am. Heart J.* 1987; 113: 399–400.

14. Fries, James F. "NSAID Gastropathy: Epidemiology." *J. Musculoskeletal Med.* 1991: 8(2):21–28.

15. Paulus, H.E. "FDA Arthritis Advisory Committee Meeting: Post-Marketing Surveillance of Non-Steroidal Anti-Inflammatory Drugs." *Arthritis Rheum.* 1985; 28:1168–1169.

16. Levine, M.N., et al. "Hemorrhagic Complications of Long-Term Anticoagulant Therapy." *Chest* 1989; 95:26S–36S.

17. Hansten, Philip D., et al., eds. *Drug Interactions and Updates Quarterly.* Vancouver, Wa.: Applied Therapeutics, 1993, pp. 415–418.

18. Herschberg, S.N., and F.S. Sierles. "Indomethacin-Induced Lithium Toxicity." *Am. Fam. Phys.* 1983; 28(2):155–157.

19. Reiman, N.I.W., and J.C. Frolich. "Effects of Diclofenac on Lithium Kinetics." *Clin. Pharmacol. Ther.* 1981; 30:348–352.

20. Simard, M., et al. "Lithium Carbonate Intoxication." *Arch. Int. Med.* 1989; 144:36–46.

21. Kuzucu, E.Y. "Methoxyflurane, Tetracycline, and Renal Failure." *JAMA* 1970; 211:1162.

chapter four

Eat, Drink, and Be Wary! Food/Drug Interactions

Who would ever guess that taking your blood pressure medicine with grapefruit juice instead of orange juice could make you sick? Or that licorice could be lethal when eaten with **Lanoxin** or **Lasix**? How could cheddar cheese, pepperoni pizza, or pickled herring combined with an antidepressant create a hypertensive crisis? Yet all of these interactions are real and could lead to disaster.

Hidden Hazards of Grapefruit Juice

Most people don't think twice about how they swallow their pills. But the beverage used to wash them down or the food that is eaten at the same time may produce unexpected, even fatal, results. Grapefruit juice contains ingredients called flavonoids and bergamottin, a furanocoumarin. Grapefruit has an impact on the metabolism of certain drugs through its effect on a crucial intestinal enzyme.[1]

Calcium channel blockers such as felodipine (**Plendil**) and nifedipine (**Adalat, Procardia**) have become extremely popular for treating high blood pressure and angina. But grapefruit juice can dramatically increase the concentration of such medications.[2] One study examined blood levels of **Plendil** taken with Old South grapefruit juice, with water, and with

Minute Maid orange juice. While neither water nor orange juice had a measurable impact on blood levels of the drug, grapefruit juice tripled the amount of drug in the circulation.[3] Increased blood levels of the drug were associated with headaches, flushing, and light-headedness. Nifedipine bioavailability was boosted by 134 percent.

People who take drugs such as nifedipine and verapamil (**Calan**, **Isoptin**, and **Verelan**) are rarely told what beverages to avoid. Because grapefruit juice can affect the rate at which the drugs are metabolized, boosting their levels in the bloodstream, the possibility of side effects is increased. Be prudent: choose another liquid for swallowing those pills.

As far as we know, the complications associated with **Plendil** and **Procardia** are not life threatening. But before **Seldane** (terfenadine) was removed from the market, concern was raised that it might interact with grapefruit juice.[4] Because ingredients in grapefruit juice can interfere with the enzymes that process the antihistamine terfenadine, some individuals might end up with unusually high levels of **Seldane** circulating in the body. In susceptible people, this could provoke a dangerous change in heart rhythm called "torsade de pointes."[5]

Until a few years ago, doctors didn't know that they should even ask their patients if they drank grapefruit juice, and it's certainly not something that would show up on a patient's medical record. As difficult as it may be to get information about drug/drug interactions, it is even more difficult to try to track down drug/food interactions. Researchers are actively investigating the grapefruit juice connection.[6, 7, 8] Dr. David

Flockhart at Georgetown University Medical Center is an authority on this interaction. His research suggests that grapefruit juice can indeed have an important impact on both **Seldane** and **Hismanal**.[9] We urge you not to contribute to medical science by getting written up in a case report. Choose something else with which to swallow your **Hismanal**. See the afterword (page 431) for the latest on grapefruit/drug interactions.

Sandimmune (cyclosporine) is a powerful immune-suppressing drug that is frequently prescribed for patients who have received organ transplants. It has also been tried experimentally for a range of serious health problems including Crohn's disease, lupus, multiple sclerosis, rheumatoid arthritis, and severe psoriasis. The dose of **Sandimmune** has to be adjusted carefully and frequent tests of kidney and liver function are crucial. Adverse reactions such as kidney problems, high blood pressure, diarrhea, tremor, numbness, and convulsions may occur.

Since the solution has to be diluted in a beverage, people are frequently advised to disguise the flavor with milk or juice. If they select grapefruit juice, however, it could have a profound impact on the blood levels of the medicine. Researchers at the University of California, San Francisco, have found that an ingredient in grapefruit juice slows the body's ability to metabolize cyclosporine. A study with transplant patients shows that an eight-ounce glass of grapefruit juice together with the cyclosporine can boost blood levels of the drug by about one third, on average.[10] Such an increase could lead to toxicity if blood levels are not monitored very carefully. On the other hand, some scientists have suggested that this interaction could be used to the patient's advantage. Because **Sandimmune** is very expensive, a patient whose dose is lowered through coadministration with grapefruit juice might be able to achieve the desired effect with less medicine. One individual told us that over a period of several months, his doctors reduced his dose of cyclosporine gradually to about half of his initial dose. This is not a do-it-yourself project, and requires extremely careful monitoring and close coordination with the transplant follow-up team.

Although orange juice does not appear to interact with **Plendil**, **Procardia**, **Seldane**, or **Sandimmune**, it may affect aluminum absorption from some common antacids. For decades, researchers assumed that the aluminum in antacids was not absorbed into the body. Doctors became alarmed, however, when they discovered that an aluminum overload was responsible for dementia in kidney dialysis patients when they were given aluminum antacids or when the water was not purified to remove aluminum. While no research demonstrates a causal connection, this mineral is also found in higher concentrations in the brains of Alzheimer's disease victims.

Aluminum remains very controversial, but it appears prudent to minimize the amount of aluminum absorbed into the body. Taking an aluminum-containing antacid with orange juice increases aluminum absorption substantially. British scientists at the Institute of Food Research found that "there was an approximately 10-fold increase in 24 hour urinary aluminium excretion following the **Aludrox** plus orange juice." They concluded, "**Aludrox** and other aluminium-containing medicines should not be taken together with citric acid because of the increase in aluminium absorption. Patients should therefore be advised not to consume food or drinks containing citric acid (such as citrus fruits and juices) at the same time as their antacid preparation but to leave an interval of at least 2–3 hours between them."[11]

Another fruit juice interaction involves antibiotics. Penicillin and erythromycin should not be taken with citrus juice or soft drinks, because these acidic beverages could interfere with proper absorption and effectiveness of the drug.

Liabilities of Licorice

Licorice lovers of the world, beware! Your favorite candy could be a killer. The ingredient in natural licorice that gives people problems is glycyrrhizin. It has been used as a drug for centuries. Folk wisdom has it that licorice can be helpful against indigestion and ulcers.[12] Russian researchers suggest that it lowers cholesterol in rabbits.[13] Chinese scientists find that it controls coughs. Japanese investigators are looking into the immune-stimulating properties of this herbal remedy.[14]

So far, so good. Licorice sounds terrific, and, as connoisseurs ourselves, we were delighted to learn about these benefits. But too much licorice can cause serious medical complications. Regular indulgence in more than an ounce of natural black licorice daily can lead to muscle pain, fluid retention, weakness, hormonal imbalance, fatigue, hypertension, sexual complications, paralysis, and, worst of all, potassium depletion. There is a case of one woman who experienced cardiac arrest because her licorice binges produced excessive potassium loss from her system.[15]

People can really get themselves into serious trouble if they are on diuretics that deplete potassium and if they also indulge in licorice treats. This combination has been reported to produce dangerously low potassium levels, leading to such adverse reactions as weakness, muscle pain, and paralysis.[16, 17]

If a regular licorice eater were also taking **Lanoxin** (digoxin), it could easily become a prescription for disaster. Irregular heart rhythms and cardiac arrest are a distinct possibility. One reader of our syndicated newspaper column wrote to tell us that she had an extreme reaction to such a combination: "The doctors in the emergency room had no idea what was wrong, but a friend of my granddaughter's asked about licorice. Not one doctor ever heard of such a thing. Since then I have heard of several people who have had this problem."

Don't assume that licorice is found only in candy. We heard from another reader who wondered about smokeless tobacco: "My husband chews tobacco. Since he started, his blood pressure has really gone up. Is there any licorice in this product?" The answer is yes. Licorice is frequently used to flavor tobacco and it can be absorbed into the body. Licorice also appears in other unlikely places. As one woman told us, "For years I sucked on licorice 'chips' from England to relieve chronic throat irritation. They worked fine for my throat, but I ended up with hypertension and went into a coma. Beware of licorice!"

Where to Look for Licorice
Candy
Smokeless tobacco products
Cough drops
Chinese medicine
Sweetening additive in foods and drinks

Treacherous Tyramine: The Cheese Effect

There are a few drugs that absolutely demand that you pay strict attention to what you eat because of the potential for a fatal drug/food interaction. The MAO (monoamine oxidase) inhibitors are unquestionably the most notorious, because they can interact with a substance called tyramine, which is found in certain foods. This interaction can cause extreme elevations in blood pressure and has led to fatalities.

By the time physicians realized that these medications could interact with common foods such as cheddar cheese, avocado, pepperoni, salami, and soy sauce, scores of people had experienced strokes and at least 15 had died.[18] And those were the reported cases. No one knows how many strokes and deaths went unreported.

What makes this reaction so bizarre is that the tyramine content of a food can vary dramatically. For example, liver is safe if it is very fresh. But a liver pâté that has sat around for a few days may contain a hazardous level of tyramine for someone taking an MAO inhibitor. A firm avocado may be okay, while a ripe one might be high enough in tyramine to induce a hypertensive crisis.[19]

When MAO inhibitors first became popular for treating depression, physicians had no idea of the dangers. Anecdotes started accumulating in the medical literature. In 1964 Welsh physicians reported the following case:

On September 3, 1963, a 40-year-old man was put on Parnate (tranylcypromine) for serious depression. A month later he complained of a slight headache but ate supper with his family. He consumed beef casserole, cheese, and crackers. The cheese was cheddar, Caerphilly (a Welsh cheese similar to cheddar), and some Danish blue. During the night he felt much worse. He was dizzy, nauseated, and his headache was unbearable. By morning he felt well enough to eat breakfast with his family and consumed two or three large slices of cheese. Shortly thereafter he became distressed and incoherent. He started bleeding from his nose and was agitated, aggressive, and confused. By the time he got to the hospital he was incoherent, his temperature was 104.5°F, and his pulse and blood pressure were elevated. He died at 8:30 P.M. On autopsy his brain was found to be swollen with intense vascular congestion. The physicians concluded that it was the combination of the cheese and his medicine that killed him.

Cuthill, J.M., et al. "Death Associated with Tranylcypromine and Cheese." *Lancet* 1964; i:1076–1077.

Physicians began to realize that certain foods, especially cheese, could get patients into trouble when eaten in conjunction with an MAO inhibitor. In 1965 a fascinating episode took place at a psychiatric hospital in Hartford, Connecticut. On the afternoon of October 21, a patient complained of severe headache, nausea, dizziness, and heart palpitations shortly after eating lunch. His blood pressure was also elevated. Within an hour, five other patients "experienced similar severe symptoms." Some blood pressures reached stratospheric levels with systolic numbers soaring over 200 (normal is around 120).

The similarity of the reactions led physicians to question what these patients had in common. All six had eaten chicken livers for lunch and they were all on **Parnate**. The leftover chicken livers were analyzed, and they turned out to be quite high in tyramine. This incident raised medical awareness that chicken livers (especially if not perfectly fresh) in combination with an MAO inhibitor could trigger a dangerous hypertensive crisis.[20]

Because this reaction is so serious, there are at least four types of foods that must be strictly avoided while taking an MAO inhibitor. They include **broad bean pods** (also known as fava beans or Italian green beans—not ordinary green beans or lima beans); **yeast concentrates** such as Marmite, as well as brewer's yeast and yeast supplements; salted, smoked, or pickled fish, especially **pickled herring**; and **aged cheeses**, including blue types such as Stilton and Roquefort, soft varieties such as Camembert or Brie, and other popular kinds including cheddar, Swiss, brick, and Parmesan. Cottage cheese, farmer's cheese,

Foods That May Interact with MAO Inhibitors

Avocados	Fish (pickled, salted, or smoked)
Bananas (overripe)	
Beef liver (stored)	Gruyère cheese
Blue cheese	Meat concentrate (in gravy or soup)
Bologna	
Brick cheese	Miso soup
Brie	Mozzarella cheese
Brewer's yeast	Parmesan cheese
Broad beans	Pepperoni
Caffeine (large quantities)	Protein dietary supplements
Camembert	Provolone cheese
Caviar	Romano cheese
Chartreuse liqueur	Roquefort cheese
Cheddar	Salami
Chianti	Soy sauce
Chicken liver (stored)	Stilton cheese
Chocolate (large quantities)	Summer sausage
Drambuie liqueur	Vermouth
Emmenthaler cheese	Yeast extract (Marmite, etc.)
Figs (canned or overripe)	Yeast supplements

and cream cheese, or Neufchâtel, aren't aged and therefore pose little if any threat.[21]

Other tyramine-containing foods warrant caution. The action of bacteria on protein produces tyramine, so any meat, including fish or chicken, should be avoided if you are not convinced of its freshness. This warning usually extends to liver pâtés and chopped chicken liver if they have

Signs of Hypertensive Crisis	
Severe headache	Chills
Stiff neck	Pale appearance
Palpitations	Chest pain
Anxiety	Sweating
High blood pressure	Collapse
Nausea	Coma

been stored any length of time, and to aged sausages such as salami, pepperoni, and bologna. One young man on **Nardil** had a hypertensive reaction to the spicy chicken nuggets he ate in a restaurant, presumably due to the MSG in the seasoning mix.[22] Fermented soybean products, such as miso, and oriental fish or shrimp pastes may pose hazards.

Chianti wine is high in tyramine, and one person died from an MAO inhibitor/vermouth interaction, so it is smart to avoid Chianti and vermouth. Experts counsel moderation when it comes to other drinks: not more than one or two bottles of beer or eight ounces of wine. Nonalcoholic brands may contain relatively high levels of tyramine and are not a good substitute. Some imported beers are also high in tyramine and ought to be avoided. Since not all brands have been tested, it is wise to eschew them all.

As a result of these kinds of reactions, MAO inhibitors such as **Nardil** (phenelzine) and **Parnate** (tranylcypromine) lost their luster in the 1970s and 1980s. The tricyclic class of antidepressants became far more popular because they seemed safer. But in recent years there has been a resurgence of interest in the MAO inhibitors. For one thing, not everyone responds to one class of medicine. Some people may actually get better faster on a drug like **Nardil** or **Parnate** than with **Elavil** (amitriptyline) or even **Prozac** (fluoxetine). Another reason is that physicians have found that MAO inhibitors may help some patients who suffer from eating disorders such as bulimia (in which people may binge and then throw up the food they have eaten). They may also be beneficial in treating panic attacks, agoraphobia, obsessive-compulsive disorder, posttraumatic stress syndrome, and narcolepsy.

Antidepressants aren't the only medications that possess the ability to block the enzyme monoamine oxidase—and therefore require users to follow a diet low in tyramine. Another such drug is isoniazid, a tuberculosis medication being used with increasing frequency as TB makes a comeback. Brand names include **Laniazid**, **Nydrazid**, **Rifamate**, and **Rimactane/INH**. Others include the antibiotic **Furoxone** (furazolidone); **Matulane** (procarbazine), a chemotherapeutic agent used against cancer; and the blood pressure pill **Eutonyl** (pargyline). All of these drugs can interact with tyramine-containing foods to cause stimulation and raised blood pressure. Any person taking a drug that blocks the enzyme monoamine oxidase should avoid or restrict the foods in the table on page 59.

Hazards of Healthy Foods

We often seem to fall into the habit of thinking about certain foods as especially good for us. When something fits into our mental category of "health," we encourage people to clean their plate, and eat that food often. The idea that anyone could overdose on broccoli, spinach, or brussels sprouts is almost unthinkable. But in combination with particular medications, a wonderful Dr. Jekyll food could turn into a dangerous Mr. Hyde.

Salt Substitutes

One example of a "healthy" food that can potentially cause harm is the salt substitute. By now, most people are aware that too much sodium in the diet can be dangerous, especially when there's a tendency to fluid retention or high blood pressure. As a result, those worried about their blood pressure may turn to using one of the salt alternatives found in the grocery store.

One man was admitted to the Veterans Administration Hospital in Madison, Wisconsin, "complaining of sudden onset of shortness of breath, severe weakness, and dizziness." He had been taking Lasix (furosemide), Aldactone (spironolactone), and digoxin. On admission the physicians noted the patient "appeared lethargic, and weak, with labored respirations." His blood pressure was dangerously low and his pulse was only 12 to 15 beats per minute. The electrocardiogram revealed a person on the verge of cardiac arrest. His serum potassium level was perilously high—7.8.

Intensive treatment saved his life but the physicians were puzzled as to how he could have ended up in such a state. Then, they reported "the patient's wife told us that her husband was liberally using a commercially available salt substitute for several days prior to admission."

Yap, Vicente, et al. "Hyperkalemia with Cardiac Arrhythmia: Induction by Salt Substitutes, Spironolactone, and Azotemia." *JAMA* 1976; 236:2775–2776.

A good idea? Yes, but only if they are not also taking medicine that leads to potassium buildup in the body. Most of the salt substitutes rely on potassium to provide the missing "salty" flavor.

What happened to this Wisconsin patient was a drug/food interaction between his salt substitute and the potassium-sparing diuretic **Aldactone**. Other drugs that can also cause a dangerous elevation of potassium in combination with either a salt substitute or potassium supplement include **Accupril, Altace, Mavik, Aldactazide, Capoten, Dyazide, Lotensin, Maxzide, Moduretic, Monopril, Prinivil, Vasotec,** and **Zestril**. If you are taking any of these drugs, make sure to check with your physician about any salt substitutes and have your blood level of potassium monitored frequently.

Overdosing on Oatmeal

After years of hearing that eating oatmeal is "the right thing to do," it is difficult to imagine that anything so wholesome could cause trouble. But one reader must have had an inkling when he wrote: "I take **Lanoxin** to control atrial fibrillation [an irregular heart rhythm that can lead to blood clots that cause strokes]. I have had nine attacks within the last four years. Three of those attacks were within just one month. Since then, my doctor increased the **Lanoxin** from 0.25 to 0.50 mg. Are there any liquids, foods, fruits, vegetables, or vitamins that may interfere with the **Lanoxin** being effective in controlling the heartbeat? (I eat a very large dish of Mother's oats and bran every morning.)"

Bran, oatmeal, and other high-fiber foods may interfere with absorption of the crucial heart medicine **Lanoxin** (digoxin). Because it can be tricky to get the dose of **Lanoxin** adjusted properly, anything that affects its absorption may reduce this drug's effectiveness. According to clinical pharmacologist Brian F. Johnson, M.D., and his colleagues, ". . . concurrent administration of digoxin tablets with a meal high in fiber content has been demonstrated to decrease the extent of absorption. This may be a frequent problem in view of the current campaigns of medical organizations and manufacturers to promote greater consumption of fiber-rich foods."[23] These researchers found that **Lanoxicaps** were not as strongly affected by fiber as **Lanoxin** tablets. Don't stop your cereal suddenly, however. If you do, blood levels of digoxin could soar and lead to toxicity. Consult with your doctor to develop a plan for adjusting your diet and dosage.

Large amounts of fiber can interfere with other drugs as well, including certain antidepressants. When antidepressants are affected, mood disorders may not respond.[24] Because of the potential for suicide, this drug/food interaction must be taken seriously.

Broccoli, Brussels Sprouts and Blood Clots

It doesn't seem fair that eating healthy food like oatmeal could get people into trouble with their medicine. How about those old standbys liver and spinach, together with today's vegetable superstars—broccoli, cabbage, and brussels sprouts? These healthy foods are all quite rich in vitamin K, and while they are indeed nutritious, they could have a dangerous impact on a person taking a blood-thinning drug such as **Coumadin** (warfarin).

Coumadin works partly by counteracting the vitamin K essential to the blood's clotting action. But when it is overwhelmed by too much vitamin K from a huge helping of kale or kohlrabi, the usual dose might be inadequate. The consequence could be a life-threatening blood clot in the brain, lung, or heart. All of the vegetables in the entire cabbage family, as well as asparagus, lettuce, and the already-mentioned liver, are high in vitamin K; these foods should be eaten only in modest quantities by anyone on **Coumadin**. Periodic blood tests (prothrombin times) are also a good idea.

Although it is not usually thought of as rich in vitamin K, large quantities of avocado can also reduce the effectiveness of **Coumadin**.[25] As with vitamin-K–rich foods, overindulging could be a mistake with serious consequences. It would, at least in theory, be possible for someone taking **Coumadin** to experience a dangerous blood clot as a result of pigging out on too much guacamole.

When Milk Does A Body Harm

Health-conscious dieters know that milk and other dairy products have many nutritional benefits, especially for women trying to maintain adequate calcium intake. But dairy products can interact with certain antibiotics to render them virtually useless. Milk can reduce blood levels of tetracyclinelike drugs such as **Achromycin V**, as well as **Cipro** (ciprofloxacin) and **Noroxin** (norfloxacin) by 50 percent or more. That's enough to sabotage their impact.

A woman taking tetracycline for a *Chlamydia* infection (a very common sexually transmitted disease that can cause infertility) might not realize her medicine was ineffective when taken within an hour of her breakfast yogurt. Someone with the life-threatening tick-borne disease Rocky Mountain spotted fever could continue to get sicker or even die if he took his tetracycline in the morning and then had milk in his coffee or pancakes made with powdered milk.

Another medicine that may not do its job effectively when taken with milk or dairy products is **Didronel** (etidronate). This drug is being prescribed for osteoporosis prevention. But if calcium is consumed within two hours of taking **Didronel**, the medicine cannot be absorbed adequately.

Milk can also interfere with the planned action of laxatives containing bisacodyl, such as **Carter's Little Pills**, **Dulcolax,** or **Fleet**. Normally, these pills are coated to keep them from dissolving in the acid environment of the stomach, so that they go to work in the lower intestine. Drinking milk at the same time as you take the drug may lower stomach acidity enough that the coating dissolves there. This could result in stomach irritation and a big bellyache.

Coffee Complaints

Most of us have learned how much coffee we can handle before getting into trouble with jitters, insomnia, or heart palpitations. But some drugs may interact with caffeine to give you more of a java jolt than expected. **Cipro** (ciprofloxacin), **Penetrex** (enoxacin), and **Noroxin** (norfloxacin) may all slow elimination of caffeine from the body and produce unexpected stimulation. Even oral contraceptives and the popular stomach medicine **Tagamet** (cimetidine) could give someone more clout from their cup. That may be okay during a morning coffee break but could be an unwelcome effect at bedtime.

Anyone taking the asthma drug theophylline (**Bronkaid** tablets, **Bronkodyl**, **Primatene** tablets,

Slo-bid, Theo-Dur) should limit caffeine from all sources. Since theophylline and caffeine are chemical cousins and produce similar effects in the body (caffeine can even help open airways), taking them together would be like getting an overdose.

Caffeine can crop up in some of the most unexpected places. You might not even realize that you are taking a hefty dose of caffeine when you swallow two **Bayer Select Headache Pain Relief** pills. But at 130 mg of caffeine per dose, you would be getting the equivalent of a strong cup of coffee. Be suspicious of herbal products that claim to boost energy. They may contain naturally occurring caffeine-like ingredients that could interact with other medications.

Sources of Caffeine

Anacin (32mg/pill)
Bayer Select Headache (65mg/pill)
BC Powder (32mg/powder)
Coffee 8 oz (100 to 150 mg/cup)
Cola beverages 12 oz (38-46 mg)
Excedrin (65mg/pill)
Midol Max-Strength (60mg/pill)
NoDoz (100mg/tab)
Tea 6 oz brewed 3 minutes (36 mg)
Vanquish (33mg/pill)
Vivarin (200mg/pill)

Coffee and tea can get some people into trouble in an entirely different way. Both beverages (but especially tea) may interact with supplements taken to combat iron deficiency anemia. The tannins in the tea grab on to the iron in the supplement and keep it from being absorbed. Whether the iron is in a pill all by itself, such as **Feosol** or **Femiron**, or combined with other nutrients as a vitamin supplement with iron, it will be wasted if it is taken at breakfast with coffee or tea.

Iced tea lovers will also have to be wary. Someone who has a healthy spinach salad or an egg salad sandwich will not absorb the iron if they drink iced tea with their lunch. In fact, tea is so effective at blocking iron absorption it is sometimes prescribed for people with excess iron buildup in the blood.

Food and Asthma Medications

One of the strangest drug/food interactions we have ever heard of is the alteration of asthma medicine by meat cooked over coals. Theophylline (**Bronkaid** tablets, **Bronkodyl**, **Primatene** tablets, **Slo-bid**, **Theobid**, **Theo-Dur**, **Theolair**, **Theo-24**, **Uniphyl**, etc.) is eliminated from the body up to 42 percent more rapidly when a person has been eating a diet high in char-broiled foods.[26] Apparently the compounds formed when food is "blackened" by grilling make the liver work harder and faster. This means that some medicines, particularly theophylline, may not work as well as they should. That could lead to worsening of symptoms or an asthma attack.

Another potential interaction that is undeniably peculiar involves red peppers. Experiments with rabbits indicate that a hot pepper suspension (perhaps along the lines of **Tabasco** sauce?) increases the blood levels of theophylline for quite some time after the two substances are taken together.[27] We have no idea whether this could spell trouble for jalapeño junkies, but be forewarned.

Food can also make certain asthma preparations far more hazardous. Drug companies have developed slow-release theophylline for the sake of convenience. Products such as **Theo-24**, **Theochron**, **Theo-X**, and **Uniphyl** are designed to linger in the body so that only one or two doses will be needed in a day. In some cases, food can change the rate of release and raise the risk of side effects. When **Theo-24**, for example, is taken with a high-fat breakfast (or within an hour of such a meal) absorption and blood levels of the drug are boosted substantially. Symptoms such as nausea, vomiting, loss of appetite, anxiety, irritability, headache, palpitations, and muscle contractions could occur after a meal containing fried eggs, bacon, buttered toast, or whole milk. Taking a different theophylline product, however, may have the opposite effect. If someone swallows **Theolair** with a high-fat breakfast, it may reduce the amount of theophylline available to fight asthma symptoms.

There is some evidence that **Uniphyl** absorption increases when the drug is swallowed at mealtime, but the effect is not nearly so impressive as that seen with **Theo-24.** Maintaining consistency (same time of day, same type of food) seems logical. The situation is so complicated that you should check and double-check with both your physician and your pharmacist as to exactly how your brand of theophylline should be taken. Then follow the instructions consistently. Always taking this medicine the same way, whether it is with food or without, will help the doctor establish the proper dose, and should lower the likelihood of unpleasant surprises.

Pudding and Dilantin

Patients who don't swallow pills well may sometimes be given their medicine crushed and mixed with food to mask the taste. A research team in San Antonio discovered that it made a big difference whether that food was applesauce or vanilla pudding. Some ingredient in the pudding interfered with the absorption of **Dilantin Infatabs** (phenytoin) so that the appropriate dose did not get into the bloodstream. The resulting blood levels were only half as high as those achieved when the **Dilantin Infatabs** were mixed in applesauce.[28]

The researchers found that a similar interaction occurred when phenytoin was administered with a special solution used for tube feeding. The common ingredients include caseinates, corn oil starch, coconut oil, and carrageenan. Many foods may contain one or more of these ingredients, but we do not know if they would also interact with **Dilantin Infatabs**.

Which Medicines to Take with Food— or Without Food

The next time you get a prescription from your physician that says "take three times a day," it's time to arrange a conference with your doctor and pharmacist. Such instructions are woefully inadequate. Find out if you should be taking your medicine with meals or on an empty stomach, and if there are any specific foods or beverages that might interfere with its proper action. You have learned that such simple pleasures as licorice, grapefruit juice, chicken nuggets, and vanilla pudding can have unexpected and undesirable consequences when taken with certain drugs.

You would think that physicians have ready access to basic dosing instructions. After all, how you take your pills can have a profound effect on how well they get into your bloodstream and work in your body. Despite the importance of this essential information, it's not readily available. Only a few entries in the *Physicians' Desk Reference* specify how a pill should be swallowed in relation to meals.

The problem goes back to when the Food and Drug Administration set up its guidelines for drug testing. To keep things simple, the scientists wanted the drugs given at the same time and in the same way to everyone in a laboratory setting. That usually meant on an empty stomach. While this might have made sense once, it has nothing to do with real life. Who has time to get up early so you can take your pill an hour before breakfast? Fitting it in two hours after a meal in the midst of a hectic afternoon is just as improbable.

Because the FDA was slow to recognize the importance of the food/drug connection, and even slower to require research on the issue, the available data is sketchy at best. There is no one place doctors can check, and if they search the literature as we did, they will discover confusion and contradiction. This is also a constantly changing arena. Acetaminophen, for example, is one of the most common drugs in the world. It is not only available as **Anacin-3**, **Tylenol**, and **Panadol**, but also can be found in hundreds of OTC combination products. Although acetaminophen has been used for decades, it wasn't until 1994 that researchers discovered that fasting greatly enhanced its potential to cause liver damage.[29] This may not be an esoteric concern. When people are sick with the flu or are suffering from chronic pain, they may not feel like eating for days. The acetaminophen/food question demonstrates how important this whole issue is and how badly it has been neglected.

We contacted most major pharmaceutical manufacturers to ask them how their most popular drugs should be taken. In a shocking number of cases we learned there were inadequate or no data available. Frequently the companies had no recommendations as to how and with what their medicines should be swallowed.

We have gathered the information we were able to find into the following table. If your doctor gives you other instructions, check with her and your pharmacist to find out if they know something we don't. There may be special circumstances that apply in your case. Make sure you ask them to fill out the form on page 20, which specifies instructions on taking your medication.

Medicines that are to be taken without food should be swallowed at least one hour before eating or two hours afterward ("on an empty stomach"). If a medication upsets your stomach, you may experience less discomfort if you take it with food. Consult your physician and pharmacist as to whether that is appropriate. Other medications may be absorbed best with food, and the kind of food you take it with (high fat versus low fat) might make a difference.

In the table that begins on page 73, drugs that are absorbed better with food are marked with a single asterisk. This is somewhat unusual, because food often delays or interferes with drug absorption. Better absorption generally increases the levels of a medication in the bloodstream and enhances the effectiveness of the drug. It may also increase the risk of side effects. Drugs that are marked with a double asterisk are absorbed better without food, but may cause stomach upset. If you experience stomach distress, please check with your doctor to see if you should take your medicine with food to reduce this side effect. Drug companies that make certain diabetes medications often advise that these be taken 15 to 30 minutes before a meal. Such drugs are marked with a triple asterisk in the table.

Food and Drug Compatibility

DRUG	TAKE WITH FOOD	TAKE WITHOUT FOOD	TAKE WITHOUT REGARD TO FOOD
Accutane	■		
acetaminophen			■
acetaminophen + codeine	■		
acetazolamide	■		
Achromycin V		■	
Actifed	■		
Adalat		■	
Adapin	■		
Advil	■		
Agoral		■	
Alazine	■*		
Aldactazide	■*		
Aldactone	■*		
Aldoclor	■*		
Aldoril	■		
Allerest	■		
allopurinol	■		
Alupent	■		
Amcill		■	
aminophylline	■		
amitriptyline	■		
amoxicillin		■	
Amoxil			■
ampicillin		■	

* Absorbed better with food.

** Absorbed better without food; may be taken with food to reduce stomach upset.

*** To be taken 15 to 30 minutes before a meal.

DRUG	TAKE WITH FOOD	TAKE WITHOUT FOOD	TAKE WITHOUT REGARD TO FOOD
Anacin-3			■
Anafranil	■		
Anaprox	■		
Antivert	■		
Anturane	■		
APAP			■
Apresazide	■*		
Apresoline	■*		
Aralen	■		
Aristocort	■		
Artane	■		
A.S.A. Enseals			■
Ascriptin w/Codeine	■		
Asendin	■		
aspirin	■		
aspirin (coated)		■	
Atabrine	■		
atenolol			■
Ativan	■		
Atromid-S	■		
Augmentin			■
Aventyl	■		
Azo Gantanol		■	
Azo Gantrisin		■	
Azolid	■		
Azulfidine	■		

* Absorbed better with food.

** Absorbed better without food; may be taken with food to reduce stomach upset.

*** To be taken 15 to 30 minutes before a meal.

DRUG	TAKE WITH FOOD	TAKE WITHOUT FOOD	TAKE WITHOUT REGARD TO FOOD
Bactocill		■	
Bactrim		■**	
Beepen-VK		■**	
Benadryl	■		
Benemid	■		
Bentyl	■		
Benylin	■		
benztropine	■		
betamethasone	■		
Betapen-VK		■**	
bethanechol		■	
Bicillin		■	
Bonine	■		
Brethine	■		
Bricanyl	■		
brompheniramine	■		
Bronkodyl	■		
Butazolidin	■		
Calan SR	■		
calcium carbonate	■		
Capoten		■	
Carafate		■	
Cardioquin	■		
Cardizem		■	
Cardizem SR			■
Ceclor		■**	

* Absorbed better with food.

** Absorbed better without food; may be taken with food to reduce stomach upset.

*** To be taken 15 to 30 minutes before a meal.

DRUG	TAKE WITH FOOD	TAKE WITHOUT FOOD	TAKE WITHOUT REGARD TO FOOD
Ceftin	■*		
Celestone	■		
cephalexin			■**
chlorothiazide	■*		
chlorpheniramine	■		
chlorpromazine	■		
Chlor-Trimeton	■		
chlorzoxazone	■		
Cipro		■**	
Claritin		■	
Cleocin			■
Clinoril	■		
clofibrate	■		
cloxacillin		■	
Cloxapen		■	
codeine	■		
Cogentin	■		
Cognex		■**	
Colace	■		
ColBenemid	■		
Colestid			■
Compazine	■		
Corgard			■
Cortef	■		
cortisone	■		
Corzide	■*		

* Absorbed better with food.

** Absorbed better without food; may be taken with food to reduce stomach upset.

*** To be taken 15 to 30 minutes before a meal.

DRUG	TAKE WITH FOOD	TAKE WITHOUT FOOD	TAKE WITHOUT REGARD TO FOOD
Coumadin			■
Cuprimine		■	
Darvocet-N 100	■*		
Darvon	■*		
Darvon Compound	■*		
Decadron	■		
Declomycin		■	
Delta-Cortef	■		
Deltapen-VK		■**	
Deltasone	■		
Demulen			■
Depakene	■		
Depen		■	
desipramine	■		
Desyrel	■		
dexamethasone	■		
DiaBeta	■***		
Diabinese	■		
Dialose	■		
Diamox	■		
dicloxacillin	■		
dicumarol	■*		
dicyclomine	■		
Didrex		■	
Didronel		■	
diethylpropion		■	

* Absorbed better with food.

** Absorbed better without food; may be taken with food to reduce stomach upset.

*** To be taken 15 to 30 minutes before a meal.

DRUG	TAKE WITH FOOD	TAKE WITHOUT FOOD	TAKE WITHOUT REGARD TO FOOD
digoxin	■		
Dilantin	■*		
dimenhydrinate	■		
Dimetane	■		
Dimetapp	■		
diphenhydramine	■		
dipyridamole		■	
Diupres	■*		
Diuril	■*		
docusate	■		
Dolene	■*		
Dolobid	■		
Dopar		■**	
doxepin	■		
doxycycline	■		
Dramamine	■		
Drixoral	■		
Dulcolax		■	
Duricef			■
Duvoid		■	
Dyazide	■*		
Dycill		■	
Dymelor	■		
Dynapen		■	
Dyrenium	■*		
Ecotrin		■	

* Absorbed better with food.

** Absorbed better without food; may be taken with food to reduce stomach upset.

*** To be taken 15 to 30 minutes before a meal.

DRUG	TAKE WITH FOOD	TAKE WITHOUT FOOD	TAKE WITHOUT REGARD TO FOOD
Edecrin	■		
E.E.S.	■		
Elavil	■		
Elixophyllin	■		
Empirin w/Codeine	■		
E-Mycin			■
Endep	■		
Entex LA	■		
Equanil	■		
Eramycin		■	
ERYC		■	
Erypar		■	
EryPed	■*		
Erythrocin		■	
erythromycin		■	
erythromycin estolate	■		
erythromycin ethylsuccinate	■		
erythromycin stearate		■	
Esimil	■		
Eskalith	■*		
Evac-Q-Kwik		■	
Fastin		■	
Feldene	■		
Femiron	■		
Feosol	■		

* Absorbed better with food.

** Absorbed better without food; may be taken with food to reduce stomach upset.

*** To be taken 15 to 30 minutes before a meal.

DRUG	TAKE WITH FOOD	TAKE WITHOUT FOOD	TAKE WITHOUT REGARD TO FOOD
Fergon	■		
Fer-in-Sol	■		
Fiorinal w/Codeine	■		
Flagyl	■		
Flexeril	■		
Fulvicin	■*		
Furadantin	■*		
Furalan	■*		
furosemide		■**	
Gantanol		■	
Gantrisin		■	
Gastrocrom	1/2 hour before meals and at bedtime		
Geocillin		■	
Glucotrol	■***		
Grifulvin	■*		
Grisactin	■*		
Gris-PEG	■*		
griseofulvin	■*		
Halcion			■
Haldol	■		
haloperidol	■		
Hexadrol	■		
Hismanal		■	
hydralazine	■*		
hydrochlorothiazide	■		
hydrocodone	■		

* Absorbed better with food.
** Absorbed better without food; may be taken with food to reduce stomach upset.
*** To be taken 15 to 30 minutes before a meal.

DRUG	TAKE WITH FOOD	TAKE WITHOUT FOOD	TAKE WITHOUT REGARD TO FOOD
hydrocortisone	■		
Hygroton	■		
Ibuprin	■		
ibuprofen	■		
Ilosone	■*		
imipramine	■		
Imuran	■		
Inderal	■*		
Inderide	■*		
Indocin	■		
indomethacin	■		
INH		■	
iron	■		
Ismelin	■		
isoniazid		■	
Isoptin		■	
Isordil		■	
Kaochlor	■		
Kaon	■		
Kato	■		
Kay Ciel	■		
Keflex			■**
Kenacort	■		
K-Lor	■		
Klorvess	■		
Klotrix	■		

* Absorbed better with food.

** Absorbed better without food; may be taken with food to reduce stomach upset.

*** To be taken 15 to 30 minutes before a meal.

DRUG	TAKE WITH FOOD	TAKE WITHOUT FOOD	TAKE WITHOUT REGARD TO FOOD
K-Lyte	■		
labetalol	■*		
Laniazid		■	
Lanoxicaps			■
Lanoxin	■		
Larodopa		■**	
Larotid		■	
Lasix		■**	
Ledercillin VK		■**	
levodopa		■**	
Levothroid		■	
Levsin		■	
Levsinex		■	
Libritabs	■		
Librium	■		
Lincocin		■	
lithium	■*		
Lithobid	■*		
Lithonate	■*		
Lithotabs	■*		
Lodine	■		
Lo/Ovral	■		
Lopid	■***		
Lopressor	■*		
Lorabid		■	
Lorelco	■*		

* Absorbed better with food.

** Absorbed better without food; may be taken with food to reduce stomach upset.

*** To be taken 15 to 30 minutes before a meal.

DRUG	TAKE WITH FOOD	TAKE WITHOUT FOOD	TAKE WITHOUT REGARD TO FOOD
Lozol	■		
Ludiomil	■		
Macrodantin	■*		
Mandelamine	■		
maprotiline	■		
Marax	■		
Maxzide			■
meclizine	■		
Meclomen	■		
Medrol	■		
Mellaril	■		
meprobamate	■		
methenamine	■		
methylprednisolone	■		
Meticorten	■		
metoprolol	■		
metronidazole	■		
Mevacor	■*		
Mexitil	■		
Micro-K	■		
Micronase	■***		
Midamor	■*		
milk of magnesia		■	
Miltown	■		
Moduretic	■*		
Motrin	■		

* Absorbed better with food.

** Absorbed better without food; may be taken with food to reduce stomach upset.

*** To be taken 15 to 30 minutes before a meal.

DRUG	TAKE WITH FOOD	TAKE WITHOUT FOOD	TAKE WITHOUT REGARD TO FOOD
Motrin IB	■		
Mysoline	■		
Nafcil		■	
nafcillin		■	
Nalfon	■		
Naprosyn	■		
Nardil	■		
Naturetin			■
Navane	■		
NegGram		■	
niacin	■		
Nicobid	■		
Nicolar	■		
nitrofurantoin	■*		
Nitrostat		■	
Nizoral	■*		
Noctec	■		
Normodyne	■*		
Norpramin	■		
nortriptyline	■		
Nuprin	■		
Nydrazid		■	
Omnipen		■	
Orinase		■**	
Ornade	■		
Ortho-Novum			■

* Absorbed better with food.

** Absorbed better without food; may be taken with food to reduce stomach upset.

*** To be taken 15 to 30 minutes before a meal.

DRUG	TAKE WITH FOOD	TAKE WITHOUT FOOD	TAKE WITHOUT REGARD TO FOOD
oxacillin		■	
Oxalid	■		
Oxsoralen	■*		
Oxycodan	■		
oxycodone	■		
oxyphenbutazone	■		
oxytetracycline		■	
Pamelor	■		
Panmycin		■	
papaverine	■		
Paraflex	■		
paraminosalicylic acid	■		
Parnate	■		
P.A.S.	■		
Pavabid	■		
Paxipam	■		
PBZ	■		
PCE		■	
Pediazole	■*		
penicillamine		■	
penicillin G		■	
penicillin V		■	
penicillin V K		■**	
pentaerythritol tetranitrate		■	
Pentids		■	
Pen-V		■**	

* Absorbed better with food.
** Absorbed better without food; may be taken with food to reduce stomach upset.
*** To be taken 15 to 30 minutes before a meal.

DRUG	TAKE WITH FOOD	TAKE WITHOUT FOOD	TAKE WITHOUT REGARD TO FOOD
Pen-Vee K		■**	
Pepcid			■
Percocet	■		
Percodan	■		
Periactin	■		
Peritrate		■	
Permitil	■		
Persantine		■	
Pertofrane	■		
phentermine		■	
phenylbutazone	■		
phenytoin	■*		
Placidyl	■		
Plaquenil	■		
Polycillin		■	
Polymox		■	
Pondimin		■	
Ponstel	■		
potassium	■		
prednisolone	■		
prednisone	■		
Preludin		■	
Premarin	■		
primidone	■		
Principen		■	
Prinivil			■

* Absorbed better with food.

** Absorbed better without food; may be taken with food to reduce stomach upset.

*** To be taken 15 to 30 minutes before a meal.

DRUG	TAKE WITH FOOD	TAKE WITHOUT FOOD	TAKE WITHOUT REGARD TO FOOD
Priscoline	■		
Pro-Banthine		■	
probenecid	■		
procainamide		■**	
Procan SR		■**	
Procardia		■	
Prolixin	■		
Proloprim			■
Pronestyl		■**	
propantheline		■	
propoxyphene w/acetaminophen	■		
propranolol	■*		
Propulsid	■***		
Prostaphlin		■	
Protostat	■		
Provera	■		
Prozac			■**
Quadrinal	■		
Quibron-T	■		
Quinaglute	■		
Quinidex	■		
quinidine	■		
quinine	■		
Quinora	■		
Reglan	30 min before meals		

* Absorbed better with food.

** Absorbed better without food; may be taken with food to reduce stomach upset.

*** To be taken 15 to 30 minutes before a meal.

DRUG	TAKE WITH FOOD	TAKE WITHOUT FOOD	TAKE WITHOUT REGARD TO FOOD
reserpine	■		
Rifadin		■	
Rifamate		■	
rifampin		■	
Rimactane		■	
Ritalin	Children: At mealtime		
	Adults: 30 to 45 min before meals		
Rondomycin		■	
Rufen	■		
Rythmol	■		
Salutensin	■		
Sandimmune	■		
Seldane			■
Seldane-D	■		
Septra		■**	
Ser-Ap-Es	■*		
Serax	■		
Serpasil	■		
Sinequan	■		
Slo-bid			■
Slow-K	■		
Somophyllin	■		
Sorbitrate		■	
Spectrobid		■	
spironolactone	■*		
Sporanox	■*		

* Absorbed better with food.

** Absorbed better without food; may be taken with food to reduce stomach upset.

*** To be taken 15 to 30 minutes before a meal.

DRUG	TAKE WITH FOOD	TAKE WITHOUT FOOD	TAKE WITHOUT REGARD TO FOOD
Stelazine	■		
sulfamethoxazole		■	
sulfasalazine	■		
sulfinpyrazone	■		
sulfisoxazole		■	
Sumycin		■	
Surmontil	■		
Synalgos	■		
Synthroid		■	
Tagamet	■		
Talwin Compound	■		
TAO		■	
Tavist-D	■		
Tedral	■		
Tegison	■		
Tegopen		■	
Tegretol	■*		
Tenoretic			■
Tenormin			■
Tenuate		■	
Tepanil		■	
Terramycin		■	
tetracycline		■	
Tetralan		■	
Theo-24		■	
Theo-Dur	■		

* Absorbed better with food.

** Absorbed better without food; may be taken with food to reduce stomach upset.

*** To be taken 15 to 30 minutes before a meal.

DRUG	TAKE WITH FOOD	TAKE WITHOUT FOOD	TAKE WITHOUT REGARD TO FOOD
Theo-Dur Sprinkle		▣	
Theobid	▣		
Theolair	▣		
theophylline	▣		
thioridazine	▣		
Thorazine	▣		
Thyrolar		▣	
Ticlid	▣*		
Tofranil	▣		
Tolectin		▣**	
Tolinase	▣		
Trandate	▣*		
Tranxene	▣		
Trental	▣		
triamcinolone	▣		
triamterene	▣		
Triavil	▣		
trifluoperazine	▣		
trihexyphenidyl	▣		
Trilafon	▣		
Trimox			▣
Tuss-Ornade	▣		
Tylenol			▣
Tylenol w/codeine	▣		
Tylox	▣		
Unipen		▣	

* Absorbed better with food.
** Absorbed better without food; may be taken with food to reduce stomach upset.
*** To be taken 15 to 30 minutes before a meal.

DRUG	TAKE WITH FOOD	TAKE WITHOUT FOOD	TAKE WITHOUT REGARD TO FOOD
Uniphyl	■*		
Unipres	■*		
Urecholine		■	
Uri-Tet		■	
Urobiotic-250		■	
Valium	■		
valproic acid	■		
Vasotec			■
V-Cillin K		■**	
Veetids		■**	
Velosef			■
Vibramycin	■		
Vicodin	■		
Videx		■	
Visken			■
Vivactil	■		
Voltaren	■		
Wyamycin S		■	
Wygesic	■		
Xanax	■		
Zantac	■		
Zestril			■
Zoloft	■*		
Zovirax			■
Zyloprim	■		

* Absorbed better with food.

** Absorbed better without food; may be taken with food to reduce stomach upset.

*** To be taken 15 to 30 minutes before a meal.

References

1. Guengerich, F.P., and D.H. Kim. "In Vitro Inhibition of Dihydropyridine Oxidation and Aflatoxin B1 Activation in Human Liver Microsomes by Naringenin and Other Flavonoids." *Carcinogen* 1992; 11:2275–2279.

2. Edgar, B., et al. "Acute Effects of Drinking Grapefruit Juice on the Pharmacokinetics and Dynamics of Felodipine—and its Potential Clinical Relevance." *Eur. J. Clin. Pharmacol.* 1992; 42:313–317.

3. Bailey, David G., et al. "Interaction of Citrus Juices with Felodipine and Nifedipine." *Lancet*. 1991; 337:268–270.

4. Woosley, Raymond L., et al. "Mechanism of the Cardiotoxic Actions of Terfenadine." *JAMA* 1993; 269:1532–1536.

5. Ibid., pp. 1535–1536.

6. Soons, P.A., et al. "Grapefruit Juice and Cimetidine Inhibit Stereoselective Metabolism of Nitrendipine in Humans." *Clin. Pharmacol. Ther.* 1991; 50:394–403.

7. Miniscalco, A., et al. "Inhibition of Dihydropyridine Metabolism in Rat and Human Liver Microsomes by Flavonoids Found in Grapefruit Juice." *J. Pharmacol. Exp. Ther.* 1992; 261:1195–1199.

8. Fuhr, Uwe, et al. "Inhibitory Effect of Grapefruit Juice and Its Bitter Principal, Naringenin, on CYP1A2 Dependent Metabolism of Caffeine in Man." *Br. J. Clin. Pharmacol.* 1993; 35:431–436.

9. Flockhart, David. Personal communication, November 16, 1993.

10. Ducharme, M.P., et al. "Trough Concentrations of Cyclosporine in Blood Following Administration with Grapefruit Juice." *Br. J. Clin. Pharmacol.* 1993; 36:457–459.

11. Fairweather-Tait, S., et al. "Orange Juice Enhances Aluminum Absorption from Antacid Preparation." *European J. Clin. Nutr.* 1994; 46:71–73.

12. Tarnawski, Andrzej, et al. "Cytoprotective Drugs: Focus on Essential Fatty Acids and Sucralfate." *Scand. J. Gastroenterol.* 1987; 22(Suppl. 127):39–43.

13. Mezenova, T.D. "Hypolipidemic Activity of Licorice Root Extract." *Pharm. Chem. J.*(USSR) 1984; 17:275–277.

14. Shinada, Masahiro, et al. "Enhancement of Interferon-α Production in Glycyrrhizin-Treated Human Peripheral Lymphocytes in Response to Concanavalin A and to Surface Antigen of Hepatitis B Virus (42241)." *Proc. Soc. Exp. Biol. Med.* 1986; 181:205–210.

15. Bannister, B., et al. "Cardiac Arrest Due to Licorice Induced Hypokalemia." *Br. Med. J.* 1977; 2:738–739.

16. Shintani, Shuzo, et al. "Glycyrrhizin (Licorice)-Induced Hypokalemic Myopathy." *Eur. Neurol.* 1992; 32:44–51.

17. Farese, Robert V., et al. "Licorice-Induced Hypermineralocorticoidism." *N. Engl. J. Med.* 1991; 325:1223–1227.

18. Baldessarini, Ross J. "Drugs and the Treatment of Psychiatric Disorders," in *Goodman and Gilman's The Pharmacological Basis of Therapeutics*, 8th ed. Gilman, Alfred, et al., eds. New York: Pergamon, 1990, pp. 417.

19. Generali, J.A., et al. "Hypertensive Crisis Resulting from Avocados and a MAO Inhibitor." *Drug Intell. Clin. Pharm.* 1981; 15:904–906.

20. Hedberg, David L., et al. "Six Cases of Hypertensive Crisis in Patients on Tranylcypromine after Eating Chicken Livers." *Am. J. Psychiatry.* 1966; 122:933–937.

21. Brown, Candace, et al. "The Monoamine Oxidase

Inhibitor-Tyramine Interaction." *J. Clin. Pharmacol.* 1989; 29:529–532.

22. Pohl, R., et al. "Reaction to Chicken Nuggets in a Patient Taking an MAOI." *Am. J. Psychiatry* 1988; 145:651.

23. Johnson, Brian F., et al. "The Effect of Dietary Fiber on the Bioavailability of Digoxin in Capsules." *J. Clin. Pharmacol.* 1987; 27:487–490.

24. Stewart, Donna E. "High-Fiber Diet and Serum Tricyclic Antidepressant Levels." *J. Clin. Psychopharmacol.* 1992; 12:438–440.

25. Wells, Philip S., et al. "Interactions of Warfarin with Drugs and Food." *Ann. Int. Med.* 1994; 121:676–683.

26. Kappus, A., et al. "Effect of Charcoal-Broiled Beef on Antipyrine and Theophylline Metabolism." *Clin. Pharmacol. Ther.* 1978; 23:445–449.

27. Bouraoui, A., et al. "Effects of Capsicum Fruit on Theophylline Absorption and Bioavailability in Rabbits." *Drug-Nutrient Interactions* 1988; 5:345–350.

28. Jann, M. W., et al. "Interaction of Dietary Pudding with Phenytoin." *Pediatrics* 1986; 78:952–953.

29. Whitcomb, David C., et al. "Association of Acetaminophen Hepatoxicity with Fasting and Ethanol Use." *JAMA* 1994; 272:1845–1850.

chapter five

Drug/Vitamin and Drug/Mineral Interactions

People often take their vitamins for granted. They don't think of them as medicines and may not mention them when the doctor asks what else they are taking. In fact, some people are afraid to discuss vitamin supplements with their physician because they worry that he or she will be scornful or dismissive. Sometimes this concern is justified. Many medical schools do not give nutrition an important place in the curriculum; some do not teach it at all. As a consequence, the doctor may not know much more than the patient about vitamins, minerals, and their potential impact on health.

Treating nutritional supplements casually or keeping them a secret from the physician could be a mistake, however. Some medications are known to interact with minerals or vitamins in a negative manner, but the doctor or pharmacist probably won't think to give you advice on avoiding these dangers unless he or she knows you take vitamins. The popularity of vitamin and mineral supplements has increased dramatically over the past decade or so, as women try to prevent osteoporosis with extra calcium and vitamin D, as middle-aged baby boomers learn that beta carotene pills may reduce the risk of heart attack or cancer, and as other people take high doses of vitamin C to prevent and treat the common cold. With more and more people popping vitamin pills, the potential for interactions with popular drugs also increases.

How Drugs Affect Nutrition

Unfortunately, researchers have not devoted enormous amounts of time and energy to the study of how nutrients interact with drugs, partly because the practical benefits are not immediately apparent. The Food and Drug Administration has not required drug companies to spend the time or resources required to uncover such interactions. Federal bureaucrats generally have been skeptical about the need for supplements or the existence of nutritional problems. Unless people start developing classic deficiency diseases such as scurvy, pellagra, or beriberi, no one is likely to worry.

Such clear-cut and dramatic cases of deficiency disease are almost unknown in the United States today. We have heard that there were cases of pellagra on hospital wards in the American South until the early 1960s, but none has been seen for decades. In some impoverished pockets of the country there still may be children suffering from the weak bones of rickets, or people with gums and old scars bleeding from scurvy. But there may be millions more people with deficiencies far more subtle.

One careful study showed that the potent ulcer and heartburn medicine **Prilosec** (omeprazole) can reduce absorption of vitamin B_{12} dramatically.[1] **Zantac** (ranitidine) and **Tagamet** (cimetidine) may also affect vitamin B_{12} absorption. Over a long period of time, it is certainly possible that the chronic depletion of vitamin B_{12} could have a negative effect on a person's health, even resulting in pernicious anemia.

Neurological problems may also result. Symptoms to be alert for include burning tongue or feet, numbness or tingling, depression, and irritability.

Some deficiencies may be so common that they are hardly noticed. Several studies over the past few years have demonstrated a strong link between high blood levels of homocysteine and low levels of the B vitamins folic acid, B_6 and B_{12}.[2, 3]

You may be wondering what homocysteine is and why anyone would get excited about it. This toxic amino acid has gotten relatively little public attention, but it may be almost as important as cholesterol in determining who is at risk of heart attack, stroke, or other vascular diseases:

"Why should we care about homocysteine? Early studies showed that individuals with very high levels of homocysteine (due to genetic metabolic defects) often died of severe vascular disease in their teens or twenties. More recent work has shown that even moderately elevated levels are associated with increased risk of cardiovascular disease . . . an elevated homocysteine concentration may contribute to a substantial fraction of myocardial infarctions [heart attacks] (and perhaps other cardiovascular outcomes) in the United States."

Stampfer, Meir J., and Willett, Walter C. "Homocysteine and Marginal Vitamin Deficiency: The Importance of Adequate Vitamin Intake." (Editorial) *JAMA* 1993; 270:2726–2727.

The suggestion of a connection between vitamin intake, homocysteine levels, and the risk of heart attack is not brand new. It was presented to the public over a decade ago in the fascinating book, *Beyond Cholesterol: Vitamin B_6, Arteriosclerosis, and Your Heart*, by Edward R. Gruberg and Stephen A. Raymond, but despite this, the hypothesis has not captured people's attention as cholesterol has. Not only does this recent research, part of the far-reaching Framingham study, confirm the connection between low B-vitamin levels and high levels of homocysteine, but it also indicates that inadequate B-vitamin status may be far more common than expected, at least among the elderly.

Biochemists have known for years that certain medications can alter nutritional balance, creating a relative deficiency of one vitamin or another. A number of drugs reduce the levels of vitamin B_6 and folic acid circulating in the bloodstream. Anticonvulsants, especially **Dilantin**, are the best-known culprits, but oral contraceptives; estrogen replacement drugs such as **Premarin**, **Estrace**, and **Estraderm**; aspirin; and blood pressure drugs such as **Apresoline**, **Dyazide**, and **Maxzide** may also lower the amounts of one or another of these crucial B vitamins in the body. Cholesterol medicines such as **Questran**, corticosteroids, the potent rheumatoid arthritis medicine methotrexate, and even alcohol can also have this effect.

Eminent epidemiologists Meir J. Stampfer and Walter C. Willett point out that we can't even be sure that low B-vitamin levels are responsible for high homocysteine, but "several investigators have demonstrated that elevated levels of homocysteine can often be normalized with nutritional supplements, particularly with folate; thus, the associations observed by Selhub et al. are very likely to be causal."[4]

So far as we know, researchers have not yet examined the possibility that many of these medications might be indirectly connected to high homocysteine levels and an elevated risk of heart attack. This appears theoretically possible, though. What a shame it would be if people were taking medicines such as

Dyazide or even **Premarin** to protect their hearts, and these drugs ended up lowering folate levels, raising homocysteine, and thus increasing the risk of a heart attack. If you want to err on the side of caution, you might check whether the medication you take could affect your nutritional status. The table at the end of this chapter is a good place to start. Another precaution might be vitamin supplements. Drs. Gruberg and Raymond recommended an intake of 10 to 25 mg of vitamin B_6 supplement daily, because the average American diet rarely supplies more than 2 mg of this vitamin. Various experts suggest that supplementation of folic acid, for whatever reason, usually should be 400 to 800 micrograms (0.4 to 0.8 mg) daily.

How Supplements Affect Drugs

Doctors and pharmacists are unquestionably interested in one type of interaction between nutrients and drugs. When nutritional supplements interfere with a medication and make it less effective, they tend to sit up and take notice. You should, too, because taking a medicine with supplements that counteract it is a waste of money and potentially damaging to your health. One of the clearest examples of such an interaction is tetracycline and calcium.

Mineral Supplements and Tetracycline

Tetracycline is one of the most commonly prescribed antibiotics in the world. It is cheap and quite effective for treating all kinds of maladies from acne to sexually transmitted diseases. It is the drug of choice against a *Chlamydia* infection, which can cause scarring of the fallopian tubes and infertility. Tetracycline is also the primary treatment for Rocky Mountain spotted fever, a potentially deadly disease transmitted by wood ticks.

When tetracycline (**Achromycin V**, **Sumycin**, etc.) or one of its common relatives (**Declomycin [demeclocycline]**, **Terramycin [oxytetracycline]**, etc.) is dispensed by a pharmacist, it usually comes with a warning on the label to avoid milk and dairy products. Calcium can inactivate tetracycline and prevent its absorption into the bloodstream.

The patient may not realize that antacids, laxatives, and, most important, nutritional supplements should also be shunned. Few physicians and pharmacists realize how many women now swallow calcium pills to prevent osteoporosis. In addition, they may be taking vitamin and mineral supplements with iron, magnesium, and zinc. These minerals can all bind to tetracycline, forming an insoluble precipitate and preventing the drug's absorption if they are taken with it. How many people take their supplements and antibiotic together? Most of us find it much easier just to swallow the whole handful of pills at once and forget about it until it's time for the afternoon dose of tetracycline. But once you learn about minerals, you won't want to take them at the same time as this antibiotic.

A woman being treated for *Chlamydia* infection might not know it was not clearing up. Her doctor might not realize it, either. Weeks and months could go by before he discovered the problem, and by then serious complications that can lead to infertility might be in progress.

An even more dangerous situation could occur if a person had Rocky Mountain spotted fever. This disease can kill if it is not treated quickly and appropriately, preferably with tetracycline. Inactivating the antibiotic by taking a vitamin and mineral supplement with it could lead to tragedy, although we don't know of any actual fatalities due to this potential oversight.

Another class of antibiotics also interacts poorly with mineral supplements. The quinolones, including **Cipro**, **Floxin**, **Maxaquin**, **Noroxin**, and **Penetrex**, are not absorbed efficiently if the minerals calcium, zinc, or iron are taken at the same time. Certain vitamin and mineral formulations now feature zinc because of its reputation for speeding healing and protecting against macular degeneration (an eye disorder). A number of antacids also contain minerals and should be avoided when a person is taking one of these strong new antibiotics. See page 134–137 for a more complete discussion.

B Vitamin Supplements and Anticonvulsants

As we mentioned, the epilepsy medicine **Dilantin** (phenytoin) can lower folic acid and vitamin B_6 levels in the body. If it were severe enough, this interaction could lead to blood abnormalities; it is possible that it might contribute to high homocysteine levels as well. Correcting the vitamin deficit requires medical supervision, however, because high levels of either folic acid or vitamin B_6 might interfere with the efficacy of the medication and result in seizures. This is why communicating with the doctor is so crucial. Although he may be well aware that 80 mg of vitamin B_6 can halve the effectiveness of the anticonvulsant, he may not know that the patient is taking this vitamin on her own to treat premenstrual symptoms. Supplementation with folic acid or vitamin B_6 can also diminish the effectiveness of barbiturates, especially phenobarbital.

Since the risk of a seizure is so serious, no one on these anticonvulsants should take supplements containing the B vitamins for any reason unless the doctor is supervising.

Vitamins E and K and Coumadin

Vitamins also interact in a dangerous manner with the anticoagulant **Coumadin** (warfarin). Vitamin E has been praised for its antioxidant properties and is getting attention for its possible role in preventing heart disease. Investigators have documented that vitamin E supplements seem to lower the risk of heart disease by about one third and boost the cardioprotective action of beta carotene.[5] Vitamin E, like aspirin, also helps blood flow freely by promoting factors that prevent clots. Vitamin E could create havoc when taken with **Coumadin**, because this vitamin apparently adds to the effect of the blood thinner. Clearly, if you take an anticoagulant, don't undertake self-treatment with vitamin E. Your doctor should be monitoring any such supplementation very closely.

Vitamin K has the opposite effect on **Coumadin**, but fortunately it is not widely available as a supplement. If you are on this anticoagulant, though, keep in mind that excessive amounts of foods rich in vitamin K (mostly vegetables, but also some other foods such as liver) can block the activity of **Coumadin** and allow clots to form. Rather than avoid these healthy foods altogether, it makes most sense to try to keep your intake fairly constant from one day and one week to the next. If you plan to alter your diet, ask your doctor to monitor your prothrombin time a little more closely. See pages 64 and 224 for summaries of these **Coumadin** interactions.

Another nutritional supplement that interacts with **Coumadin** (warfarin) is something called coenzyme Q_{10} (ubiquinone). This is a natural substance found in the body. It has become a very hot item in health food stores and mail-order vitamin catalogs. Research suggests that this antioxidant may be beneficial in helping to treat congestive heart failure, cardiovascular conditions, gum disease, and a number of other disorders. How effective it is remains to be determined, but judging from sales figures, this is a very successful product taken by lots of folks.

Researchers in Sweden have observed that when patients on a stable regimen of **Coumadin** to prevent blood clots started taking coenzyme Q_{10}, their bleeding time changed significantly. Their blood became more prone to clotting, and the **Coumadin** appeared less effective.[6] This interaction could be extremely dangerous, because a person might have a life-threatening clot as a consequence. Anyone taking coenzyme Q_{10} together with **Coumadin** should consult a physician before stopping the supplement. Sudden discontinuation of coenzyme Q_{10} might trigger an unexpected alteration in clotting time.

Foods Rich in Vitamin K (more than 50 mcg/100g)	
Bran	Liver
Broccoli	Mung Beans
Cabbage	Oats
Cauliflower	Seaweed
Chick-peas	Soybean Oil
Corn Oil	Soybeans
Eggs	Spinach
Lentils	Turnip Greens
Lettuce	Watercress

Source: Adapted from Pennington, Jean A. T., ed. *Bowes & Church's Food Values of Portions Commonly Used,* 15th ed. New York: Harper & Row, 1989.

Potentially Dangerous Nutrient/Nutrient Interactions

Potassium and Vitamin B₁₂

Relatively few doctors or patients are aware that prescription potassium supplements such as **K-Dur, K-Tab, Micro-K,** and **Slow-K** can interfere with the absorption of vitamin B_{12}. This vitamin is stored in the body and does not become depleted quickly, so a short course of potassium therapy poses little cause for concern. But long-term use—by people taking diuretic blood pressure pills who are simultaneously prescribed potassium supplements, for example—could eventually result in depletion of body stores of this crucial vitamin. Ask your doctor to evaluate your situation, as injections are usually the most effective means of supplementing vitamin B_{12}.

Beta Carotene, Vitamin E, and Alcohol

Little red capsules of beta carotene are popular items on the vitamin shelf these days. Some researchers hypothesize that this precursor to vitamin A may help protect the body against a number of different cancers, and that it may help reduce the risk of heart attack. As a result, there may be millions of people taking it in the hope of warding off heart disease or cancer.

This probably makes good sense. Beta carotene is an excellent antioxidant, and the toxicity of this vitamin building block is very low. It is, for example, far safer than preformed vitamin A, which is stored in the body and can build up to dangerous levels. Beta carotene has one important and little-known interaction, however. Long-term supplementation (15 mg daily up to 60 mg) lowers blood levels of vitamin E significantly. These two antioxidants seem to work together, for beta carotene protects from heart attack most strongly when people also have high vitamin E levels.[7] Therefore, it would be prudent, if you plan to take beta carotene as a preventive measure, to take vitamin E as well. This should keep your levels of both antioxidants in the normal range or above.

Beta carotene is also reported to interact negatively with alcohol. The combination may increase liver damage well over that found with alcohol alone. The research was done in baboons who were given a substantial dose of alcohol as a proportion of their daily calories over an extended period of time.[8] As a consequence, we don't have good information on how much alcohol might trigger this response in humans. It is chilling, however, to think of someone maintaining a moderate drinking habit (between one and three drinks a day) because of research showing this may reduce the risk of heart disease, and adding a beta carotene supplement for the same reason. Liver disease is devastating, so if you drink regularly, it might be prudent not to make beta carotene a habit.

Drug/Nutrient Interactions

The table of Drug/Nutrient Interactions on the following pages summarizes information on how drugs affect nutrient status and which nutritional supplements may interfere with optimal drug benefits. This field is still evolving and we expect more information to become available over the next several years. (The table does not include discussion of most cancer drugs, however, as these are administered primarily in the hospital under close supervision. Many of them have significant effects on nutritional status, but in some cases that contributes to their effectiveness.) Please remember to keep your physician informed of your concerns and of any supplements you plan to take in conjunction with prescribed medications.

Drug/Nutrient Interactions

DRUG	INTERACTION	NUTRIENT
Acne Medicine Accutane	Because **Accutane** is related to vitamin A, taking these two compounds together could increase toxicity. Avoid this combination.	Vitamin A
Alcohol	Research in baboons indicates that beta carotene can increase the liver damage caused by chronic alcohol intake.	Beta Carotene
	Alcohol has numerous effects on the body. Some of these, such as changes in liver and intestinal function, may impact several nutrients. One consequence of long-term alcohol abuse is brain damage—Wernicke-Korsakoff syndrome. Lack of the B vitamin thiamine plays an important role in the development of this problem.	Folic Acid Thiamine
	Absorption or utilization of vitamins B_6, B_{12}, and C is affected by regular alcohol intake. In addition, drinkers may	Vitamin B_6 Vitamin B_{12} Vitamin C Iron Zinc

DRUG	INTERACTION	NUTRIENT
	absorb too much iron and too little zinc, putting additional stress on the system. These nutritional problems occur when a person drinks alcohol too much or too often.	
Aluminum-Based Antacids **Di-Gel** **Gelusil** **Maalox** **Mylanta** **Riopan,** and others	The aluminum and magnesium in antacids can form a complex with phosphate and deplete the body of calcium. Weakened bones may result. Anyone at risk of osteoporosis should be cautious about this interaction. Aluminum-based antacids may inactivate thiamine. Don't take them at mealtime.	**Calcium** **Phosphate** **Thiamine**
Antibiotics **Bactrim** **Mandol** **Moxam** Neomycin **Septra** and others	Broad-spectrum antibiotics can mess up the good intestinal bacteria that make vitamin K. In some people this could lead to unusual bleeding. Check with your physician and pharmacist to see whether vitamin K supplementation is a good idea.	**Vitamin K**

DRUG	INTERACTION	NUTRIENT
Quinolones **Cipro** **Floxin** **Maxaquin** **Noroxin** **Penetrex**	These high-powered antibiotics may not work as well as expected if they are taken at the same time as certain minerals. This includes antacids as well as nutritional supplements. Check with your doctor and pharmacist, because this interaction could be serious.	**Calcium** **Iron** **Zinc**
Tetracyclines **Achromycin** **Aureomycin** **Minocin** **Panmycin** **Terramycin** and others	Calcium and other minerals can combine with tetracyclines so that the antibiotics are not absorbed into the body. Make sure you don't take any mineral supplements or mineral-containing antacids within two hours of a tetracycline pill. Long-term use of tetracycline may deplete these nutrients and require supplementation. Expert Daphne Roe, M.D., suggests 5 mg of riboflavin, 100 to 200 mg vitamin C, and 800 to 1,500 mg calcium daily, to be taken at least two hours before or after the tetracycline.	**Calcium** **Iron** **Magnesium** **Riboflavin** **Vitamin C** **Zinc**

DRUG	INTERACTION	NUTRIENT
Arthritis Medicines Aspirin **Anacin** **Ascriptin** **Bayer** **Bufferin** **Excedrin** and others	Studies suggest aspirin may block vitamin C from getting into cells. Questions remain about the importance of this interaction. Until more is known, it seems logical to increase daily consumption of vitamin-C–containing foods or consider a supplement (50 to 100 mg) while taking aspirin regularly. It is not clear whether extra vitamin C will correct this imbalance.	**Vitamin C**
	Folic acid levels are lower when people rely on large doses of aspirin. Regular users may need a folic acid supplement. Check with your physician for the right amount. Dr. Roe suggests 0.4 to 1.0 mg.	**Folic Acid**
	Small amounts of blood are regularly lost from the stomach when aspirin is taken. This can add up over time and deplete the body of iron. This actually may be beneficial for people at risk of heart disease since some research suggests that excess iron increas-	**Iron**

DRUG	INTERACTION	NUTRIENT
	es the risk of heart attack. If anemia results, however, iron supplementation (20 to 50 mg) may be necessary. A blood test is needed for this diagnosis.	
Indomethacin **Indocin**	Indomethacin irritates the stomach lining even more than aspirin. Over time, continued low-level blood loss could lead to iron deficiency. If anemia occurs, a supplement of 20 to 50 mg of iron daily may be needed.	**Iron**
Methotrexate **Folex Methotrate Mexate Rheumatrex**	Methotrexate affects the intestinal wall so that these nutrients are not absorbed efficiently. Nutritional imbalances may result. Since methotrexate is being used more aggressively against arthritis, psoriasis, and cancer, patients must discuss this issue with their physicians.	**Folic Acid Vitamin B$_{12}$ Beta Carotene**

DRUG	INTERACTION	NUTRIENT
Penicillamine **Cuprimine Depen**	Penicillamine may not be as well absorbed if it is taken at the same time as iron or magnesium. Supplements often contain these minerals, so it may make sense to wait several hours before you take your multivitamin preparation. This medicine may also deplete the body of copper or zinc, causing a loss of the sense of taste. Ask about supplements, including 24- to 100-mg tablets of vitamin B$_6$.	**Iron Magnesium Copper Zinc Vitamin B$_6$**
Beta Carotene	As people learn more about the potential benefits of antioxidant vitamins, many are taking beta carotene at levels much higher than those normally found in the vegetables in their diets. Regular doses of beta carotene (from 15 to 60 mg daily) can lead, over a period of months, to lowered levels of vitamin E in the blood. Because vitamin E is itself an important antioxidant, it might be wise to add a supple-	**Vitamin E**

DRUG	INTERACTION	NUTRIENT
Beta Carotene (continued)	ment of 100 to 400 IU if you are taking beta carotene.	
Birth Control Pills Demulen Norlestrin Ortho-Novum Ovcon Ovral Tri-Norinyl and others	Women using combination oral contraceptives may need more of these vitamins. Both folic acid and B$_6$ levels may be low, and too little vitamin B$_6$ could be responsible for depression. Ask your doctor about a supplement. Vitamin C (1 gram or more) may increase blood levels of estrogen. Side effects may become more noticeable. This interaction is controversial and may not be significant.	**Vitamin B$_6$** **Folic Acid** **Vitamin E** **Vitamin C**
Blood Pressure Medicines ACE Inhibitors **Accupril** **Altace** **Capoten** **Lotensin** **Monopril** **Prinivil** **Vasotec**	These popular blood pressure medications tend to maximize potassium levels. This is fine unless a person is getting extra potassium through a potassium supplement or a potassium-based salt substitute. Too much of this important mineral is just as bad as not enough. If you are taking	**Potassium**

DRUG	INTERACTION	NUTRIENT
Zestril	one of these medicines, you should probably avoid extra potassium unless your doctor is supervising closely. Your physician should periodically test your blood levels of potassium.	
Hydralazine-containing **Apresazide** **Apresoline** Hydralazine **Ser-Ap-Es** and others	This medicine can deplete the body of vitamin B_6 through its effect on an essential enzyme. Reduced vitamin B_6 may result in depression or nerve damage (leading to numbness or tingling of hands or feet). Supplementation may be advisable. Dr. Daphne Roe suggests 25 to 100 mg daily.	**Vitamin B_6**
Loop Diuretics **Bumex** **Edecrin** **Lasix**	These strong diuretics (water pills) may cause the loss of important minerals from the body. Periodic blood tests are essential to see whether supplements are needed.	**Calcium** **Magnesium** **Potassium**

DRUG	INTERACTION	NUTRIENT
Thiazide Diuretics **Aldoril** **Diuril** Hydrochloro- thiazide **Hydro- DIURIL** **Ser-Ap-Es** and others	These diuretics promote urination. Minerals are often lost in the process. This could actually prove counterproductive, since both potassium and mag- nesium appear to help regulate blood pressure. Periodic blood checks to keep track of mineral lev- els are a good idea.	**Magnesium** **Potassium** **Zinc**
Triamterene- containing **Dyazide** **Dyrenium** **Maxzide**	Folic acid deficiency could become a problem unless a supplement (0.4 to 1.0 mg) is taken. These drugs conserve potassium. Taking a po- tassium supplement at the same time could result in an overload of this mineral.	**Folic Acid** **Potassium**
Blood Thinners **Coumadin** **Panwarfin** Warfarin	Very large amounts (5 grams or more) of vita- min C could interfere with the effectiveness of this medicine. This inter- action is uncertain.	**Vitamin C**
Blood Thinners **Coumadin**	Vitamin E itself acts as an anticoagulant, and the combination may thin	**Vitamin E**

DRUG	INTERACTION	NUTRIENT
Panwarfin Warfarin	the blood too much and lead to bruises or excessive bleeding. Less than 400 IU daily does not appear to be a problem. Vitamin K counteracts these medications and makes them less effective. Don't go overboard on foods high in this vitamin (see list on page 103). For any of these interactions, your doctor can check bleeding time with a test.	**Vitamin K**
Cholesterol Medicines **Cholybar Colestid Questran**	"Bile acid sequestrants" such as **Questran** can interfere with the absorption of fats and fat-soluble vitamins. Some animal studies suggest that vitamin E and even iron absorption may also be adversely affected. Because of their impact on vitamin K, these drugs could cause complications in combination with blood thinners. Blood tests are advised. Supplements of 2,000 to 5,000 IU vitamin A, 200 to 800 IU vitamin D, and 0.4 to 1.0 mg folic acid	*Fat-Soluble Vitamins* **Vitamin A Vitamin D Vitamin E Vitamin K** *Water-Soluble Vitamins* **Vitamin B$_{12}$ Folic Acid**

DRUG	INTERACTION	NUTRIENT
	should be taken at a different time from the cholesterol medicine.	
Colchicine ColBenemid	Absorption of these nutrients may be impaired. Check with your physician about supplementation.	**Vitamin B$_{12}$** **Beta Carotene** **Magnesium** **Potassium**
Corticosteroids **Aristocort** **Cortef** **Decadron** **Delta-** **Cortef** **Deltasone** **Kenacort** **Medrol** Prednisone and others	Cortisonelike drugs can deplete the body of vitamin D$_3$ and interfere with calcium absorption and metabolism. Long-term use may result in bone loss. Such medications may also lead to depletion of potassium and vitamins B$_6$, B$_{12}$, or folic acid. Check with your doctor about a supplement.	**Calcium** **Vitamin D$_3$** **Potassium** **Vitamin B$_6$** **Vitamin B$_{12}$** **Folic Acid**
Epilepsy *Drugs* Barbiturates Phenobarbital	Either folic acid or vitamin B$_6$ supplements can reduce blood levels of this anticonvulsant, potentially leading to seizures. If supplementation is needed, it should be carefully monitored.	**Folic Acid** **Vitamin B$_6$**

DRUG	INTERACTION	NUTRIENT
Epilepsy Drugs Barbiturates Phenobarbital	Barbiturates such as phenobarbital interfere with the normal metabolism of vitamin D, and as a consequence calcium may be lost from bones. Rickets or osteomalacia are a hazard. Check with your doctor about vitamin D supplements.	**Vitamin D Calcium**
Dilantin	Patients on Dilantin (phenytoin) may become deficient in folic acid or vitamin B_6. Supplementation is very tricky, however, and must be directed by a knowledgeable physician. Too much folic acid (more than 2 mg/day) or vitamin B_6 can interfere with effectiveness so that the drug would fail to prevent seizures. At doses of 80 mg daily of vitamin B_6, Dilantin is only 50 percent as effective as it is without the vitamin B_6. Periodic blood tests for anemia are needed.	**Folic Acid Vitamin B_6**
	Dilantin interferes with vitamin D, and thus with calcium. The consequence could be rickets	**Vitamin D Calcium**

DRUG	INTERACTION	NUTRIENT
Dilantin (continued)	in children or osteomalacia (weak bones) in adults. A supplement of 400 to 800 IU of vitamin D daily is appropriate.	
	Blood levels of vitamin K may be reduced. A supplement of 1 to 5 mg daily may be advisable. Ask your doctor.	**Vitamin K**
Mysoline	Levels of vitamin K may be lower. The doctor might prescribe a supplement of 1 to 5 mg daily to overcome this.	**Vitamin K**
	Like other barbiturates, Mysoline (primidone) alters the metabolism of vitamin D and can lead to the loss of calcium from bones. A vitamin D supplement (400 to 800 IU daily) may be necessary.	**Calcium Vitamin D**
***Etidronate* Didronel**	Minerals such as calcium, magnesium, and iron react with this medicine to prevent its absorption if they are taken within 2 hours of taking the drug. However, the drug changes vitamin D me-	**Calcium Iron Magnesium Vitamin D**

DRUG	INTERACTION	NUTRIENT
	tabolism, so adequate calcium and vitamin D intake must be maintained.	
Hormone Replacement Therapy **Estrace** **Estratab** **Menest** **Premarin** and others	Women using estrogen replacement therapy may need more of these vitamins. Both folic acid and B_6 levels may be low, and too little vitamin B_6 could be responsible for depression. Ask your doctor about a supplement such as 1.5 to 5 mg vitamin B_6 and 0.4 to 1.0 mg folic acid.	**Vitamin B_6** **Folic Acid** **Vitamin E**
Iron **Femiron** **Feosol** **Fer-in-Sol** **Mol-Iron** and others	Taking a calcium supplement at the same meal with an iron supplement or a multivitamin containing iron can reduce the amount of iron absorbed. To minimize interference, take these pills at different times.	**Calcium**
Laxatives Mineral Oil **Agoral** **Mikinol** **Neo-Cultol**	Regular use of a mineral oil laxative interferes with proper absorption of the fat-soluble vitamins. A lack of vitamin D	*Fat-Soluble Vitamins* **Vitamin A** **Vitamin D** **Vitamin E**

DRUG	INTERACTION	NUTRIENT
and others	can affect calcium and phosphate balance, and bone loss may occur.	**Vitamin K**
Levodopa **Dopar** **Larodopa**	Vitamin B_6 can reduce the effectiveness of this anti-Parkinson's disease drug. Supplementation should be avoided.	**Vitamin B_6**
Major *Tranquilizers* Chlorproma-zine **Thorazine** Fluphenazine **Permitil** **Prolixin** and others	The B vitamins riboflavin and B_{12} (cyanocobal-amin) may become depleted. A supplement may be required to prevent deficiency. A high dose of vitamin C reduced the serum level of Prolixin in one case, however, so caution is suggested. Dr. Daphne Roe suggests 2 to 5 mg of riboflavin daily.	**Riboflavin** **Vitamin B_{12}** **Vitamin C**
Potassium **Kaon-Cl** **Klotrix** **K-Tab** **Micro-K** **Slow-K** and others	Potassium supplements can interfere with the absorption of vitamin B_{12}. Because these medications are often taken for many weeks or months, a deficiency of this crucial vitamin could develop. Research has	**Vitamin B_{12}**

DRUG	INTERACTION	NUTRIENT
	shown that some older people show cognitive or neurological effects of inadequate vitamin B_{12} even before their blood tests show a deficiency.	
Sleeping Pills **Doriden**	Long-term use of this sleeping pill can interfere with vitamin D metabolism, which in turn affects calcium balance. The result could be osteomalacia, or weakened bones. A vitamin D supplement might be appropriate.	**Vitamin D Calcium**
Sulfasalazine **Azulfidine**	This medicine for inflammatory bowel disease interferes with the proper absorption of folic acid. Talk to your doctor about a supplement in the range of 0.4 to 1 mg daily.	**Folic Acid**

DRUG	INTERACTION	NUTRIENT
Thyroid Hormone Levothyroxine **Levo-T** **Levothroid** **Levoxine** **Synthroid**	Iron supplements taken at the same time as thyroid replacement hormone can reduce the hormone's effectiveness, as judged by blood tests and clinical symptoms. Take these pills at different times.	**Iron**
	Case reports suggest that calcium may also interfere with levothyroxine absorption. Take these pills at least four hours apart.	**Calcium**
Tuberculosis Drugs Isoniazid **INH** **Laniazid** **Nydrazid** **Rifamate**	Deficiencies of niacin and vitamin B_6 are possible, and may require supplementation. Do *not* take supplements without supervision, as too much vitamin B_6 might diminish the effectiveness of the drug. (Recommended daily doses range from 6 to 50 mg of B_6, and from 15 to 25 mg of niacin.)	**Niacin** **Vitamin B_6**
	Drug-induced changes in vitamin D metabolism may also affect calcium and phosphate balance. Check with your doctor about a vitamin D supplement of 400 or 800 IU daily.	**Vitamin D** **Calcium** **Phosphate**

DRUG	INTERACTION	NUTRIENT
Paraamino-salicylate **P.A.S.**	A vitamin B_{12} deficiency is possible. Folic acid may also become depleted. Ask your doctor if supplements are advisable.	**Vitamin B_{12}** **Folic Acid**
Ulcer Medicines **Prevacid Prilosec Tagamet Zantac**	These acid-suppressing drugs, and possibly others including Axid and Pepcid, can reduce the absorption of vitamin B_{12} that is chemically bound to protein. The effect may depend upon dose and seems to disappear after the drug is discontinued. Ask your doctor about supplementation.	**Vitamin B_{12}**
Tagamet Zantac	A controversial theory suggests that reducing acid as effectively as these medications do could allow bacteria to survive in the stomach. These "bugs" may produce carcinogenic chemicals called nitrosamines, which might increase the risk of stomach cancer. We suggest vitamin insurance: the antioxidants vitamin C (500 mg 3 or 4	**Vitamin C** **Vitamin E**

DRUG	INTERACTION	NUTRIENT
	times daily) and vitamin E (400 IU daily) may help protect the stomach.	
Urinary Anti-Infectives **Furadantin Furalan Macrodantin** and others	Nitrofurantoin medications for urinary tract infections interfere with folic acid metabolism. Folic acid deficiencies are unusual, perhaps because the drugs are usually prescribed for less than two weeks. If you need the drug long-term, ask your doctor about supplementation.	**Folic Acid**

References

1. Marcuard, S. P., et al. "Omeprazole Therapy Causes Malabsorption of Cyanocobalamin (vitamin B_{12})." *Ann. Intern. Med.* 1994; 120:211–215.

2. Selhub, Jacob, Paul F. Jacques, et al. "Vitamin Status and Intake as Primary Determinants of Homocysteinemia in an Elderly Population." *JAMA* 1993; 270:2693–2698.

3. Selhub, Jacob, et al. "Association Between Plasma Homocysteine Concentrations and Extracranial Carotid-Artery Stenosis." *N. Engl. J. Med.* 1995; 332:286–291.

4. Stampfer, Meir J., and Walter C. Willett. "Homocysteine and Marginal Vitamin Deficiency: The Importance of Adequate Vitamin Intake." (Editorial) *JAMA* 1993; 270:2726–2727.

5. Kardinaal, A. F. M., F. J. Kok, et al. "Antioxidants in adipose tissue and risk of myocardial infarction: The EURAMIC study." *Lancet* 1993; 342:1379–1384.

6. Spigset, Olav. "Reduced Effect of Warfarin Caused by Ubidecarenone." (Letter) *Lancet* 1994; 344:1372–1373.

7. Kardinaal, op.cit. p. 1382.

8. Leo, M. A., et al. "Interaction of Ethanol with b-Carotene: Delayed Blood Clearance and Enhanced Hepatotoxicity." *Hepatology* 1992; 15:883–891.

References for the Drug/Nutrient Interactions Chart

Campbell, Norman R.C., et al. "Ferrous Sulfate Reduces Thyroxine Efficacy in Patients with Hypothyroidism." *Ann. Intern. Med.* 1992; 117:1010–1013.

Cook, J.D., S.A. Dassenko, and P. Whittaker. "Calcium Supplementation: Effect on Iron Absorption." *Am. J. Clin. Nutr.* 1991 (Jan.); 53:106–111.

Garrison, Robert H., Jr., and Elizabeth Somer. *The Nutrition Desk Reference,* 2nd ed. New Canaan, Conn.: Keats Publishing, 1990, pp. 273–283.

Hansten, Philip D., and John R. Horn, eds. *Drug Interactions & Updates.* Vancouver, Wash.: Applied Therapeutics, 1990.

Olin, Bernie R., ed. *Drug Facts and Comparisons.* St. Louis: Facts & Comparisons, 1991.

Roe, Daphne A. "Diet, Nutrition and Drug Reactions," in *Modern Nutrition in Health and Disease,* 7th ed. Shils, Maurice E., and Vernon R. Young, eds. Philadelphia: Lea & Febiger, 1988, pp. 630–645.

Tatro, David S., ed. *Drug Interaction Facts.* St. Louis: Facts & Comparisons, 1992.

chapter six

Prescription Drug/ Over-the-Counter Drug Interactions

Most people perceive nonprescription remedies as wimpy drugs. After all, if the Food and Drug Administration allows everyone access to such products in pharmacies, supermarkets, and convenience stores, surely they must be safe. We hate to burst another bubble, but nothing could be further from the truth.

Over-the-counter (OTC) medications, like all drugs, can cause side effects. Sometimes the complications are merely a minor annoyance, such as drowsiness from an antihistamine. Other times an adverse reaction could land you in the emergency room, as in the case of the man who swallowed a decongestant cold remedy and subsequently couldn't urinate. The label (which he read carefully) did not warn him that if he had an enlarged prostate gland he should avoid this medicine. When his bladder felt like it would burst, he rushed to the hospital (and broke an arm in the process when, in his haste, he slipped on some ice). A catheter had to be inserted to provide him some relief.

The medication this gentleman used was **Sudafed** (pseudoephedrine), an oral decongestant that works by constricting blood vessels. Once upon a time it was available only by prescription. Physicians presumably warned people about complications and interactions to prevent this kind of adverse event from occurring.

When we notified **Sudafed's** manufacturer that its label was inadequate for OTC use, and unreadable at that, there was some initial defensiveness. Fortunately, changes were eventually made and the **Sudafed** label now reads: "Do not take this preparation if you have high blood pressure, heart disease, diabetes, thyroid disease, or difficulty in urination due to enlargement of the prostate gland, except under the advice and supervision of a physician."

Lethal Prescription Drug/ OTC Drug Interactions

Unfortunately, many people don't take time to read the cautions and warnings on OTC medications. First, they assume there is no possibility for problems, and second, the print is usually so small you need a magnifying glass to read it, and even when you *can* read it, the precautions are often totally inadequate or nonsensical. Read a little further on the **Sudafed** box and you will find the words "Drug Interaction Precaution: Do not use this product if you are now taking a prescription monoamine oxidase inhibitor (MAOI) (certain drugs for depression, psychiatric or emotional conditions, or Parkinson's disease)."

Most people wouldn't know if they were taking a pill containing a monoamine oxidase inhibitor. Medical mumbo jumbo may be okay in the *Physicians' Desk Reference*, or *PDR*, but it doesn't belong on OTC labels. In the case of **Sudafed** (and lots of other cold and cough remedies) the monoamine oxidase (MAO) inhibitor warning is serious indeed. If someone were to take pseudoephedrine, ephedrine, phenylephrine, or phenylpropanolamine (PPA) while they were on an antidepressant such as **Nardil** or **Parnate**, blood pressure could soar. Such a hypertensive crisis could lead to a stroke. One person taking **Nardil** experienced a terrible headache, heart palpitations, and an extremely dangerous elevation in blood pressure to 240/120 (normal is 120/80) after downing only 2 teaspoons of an OTC product containing the decongestant phenylephrine.[1] Phenylpropanolamine (a decongestant and appetite suppressant) has also been linked to lethal hypertensive crisis.

Even something as seemingly simple as a cough remedy may produce an extremely hazardous reaction with MAO inhibitor drugs. The combination could bring on symptoms such as nausea, fever, agitation, dizziness, changes in blood pressure, seizures, and coma. A death has been linked with the combination of **Nardil** and two ounces of a dextromethorphan-containing cough remedy.[2] The box below lists the OTC drugs that don't mix with MAO inhibitors.

OTC Drugs That Don't Mix With MAO Inhibitors

(The following is a partial list of OTC drugs containing dextromethorphan, ephedrine, phenylephrine, PPA, or pseudoephedrine.)

Acutrim Late Day Strength Appetite Suppressant	Alka-Seltzer Plus Cough & Cold Medicine
Acutrim II Maximum Strength Appetite Suppressant	Alka-Seltzer Plus Night-Time Cold Medicine
Acutrim 16 Hour Steady Control Appetite Suppressant	Alka-Seltzer Plus Sinus Allergy Medicine
Actifed Plus	Allerest Headache Strength
Actifed Sinus Daytime/Nighttime	Allerest Maximum Strength
Actifed Syrup	Allerest No Drowsiness
Advil Cold and Sinus	Allerest Sinus Pain Formula
Afrin Tablets	Allerest 12 Hour
Alka-Seltzer Plus Cold Medicine	

OTC Drugs That Don't Mix With MAO Inhibitors, Con't

A.R.M. Allergy Relief Medicine

Bayer Select Sinus Pain Relief Formula

BC Cold Powder Multi-Symptom Formula

BC Cold Powder Non-Drowsy Formula

Benadryl Allergy Sinus Headache Formula

Benadryl Cold Nighttime Formula

Benadryl Cold Tablets

Benadryl Decongestant

Benylin Decongestant

Benylin Expectorant

Bronkaid Tablets

Bronkotabs

Cheracol-D Cough Formula

Cheracol Plus Head Cold/Cough Formula

Chlor-Trimeton Allergy Decongestant

Chlor-Trimeton Allergy-Sinus Headache

Comtrex Multi-Symptom Cold Reliever

Contac Continuous Action Decongestant/Antihistamine

Contac Day & Night Cold & Flu

Contac Maximum Strength Continuous Action Decongestant/Antihistamine

Contac Severe Cold and Flu Formula

Coricidin 'D' Decongestant

Cough Formula Comtrex

Delsym Cough Formula

Dexatrim Maximum Strength Caffeine-Free

Dexatrim Maximum Strength Extended Duration Time

Dexatrim Maximum Strength Plus Vitamin C/Caffeine-free

Dimetapp Cold & Allergy

Dimetapp Cold & Flu

Dimetapp DM Elixir

Dimetapp Elixir

Dimetapp Extentabs

Dimetapp Liquid-Gels

Dimetapp Sinus

Dristan Cold

Dristan Cold, Maximum Strength Multi-Symptom Formula

Dristan Juice Mix-In

Dristan Sinus

Drixoral Cold and Allergy

Drixoral Sinus

4-Way Cold Tablets

Hold DM Cough Suppressant Lozenge

Maximum Strength Dristan Cold Multi-Symptom Formula

Maximum Strength Dristan Cold No Drowsiness Formula

Medi-Flu

Primatene Tablets

Robitussin Cough Calmers

Robitussin Maximum Strength Cough & Cold

OTC Drugs That Don't Mix With MAO Inhibitors, Con't

Robitussin Maximum Strength
Cough Suppressant
Robitussin-CF
Robitussin-DM
Robitussin-PE
Sinarest
Sine-Off Maximum Strength
Sine-Off Sinus Medicine Tablets
Sinus Excedrin Analgesic,
Decongestant
Sinutab Sinus Allergy
Sudafed Plus
Sudafed Severe Cold Formula
Sudafed Sinus
Tavist-D
TheraFlu Flu and Cold Medicine
Triaminic Allergy Medicine
Triaminic Cold Medicine
Triaminic Cold, Allergy, Sinus
Medicine

Triaminic Multi-Symptom Cold
and Cough Medicine
Triaminic-12 Maximum Strength
12 Hour Relief
Tylenol Allergy Sinus Medication
Maximum Strength
Tylenol Cold & Flu Hot
Medication
Tylenol Cold Medication,
Effervescent
Vicks DayQuil
Vicks Formula 44D Cough &
Decongestant Medicine
Vicks Formula 44E Cough &
Expectorant Medicine
Vicks Formula 44M Multi-
Symptom Cough & Cold
Medicine
Vicks NyQuil Nighttime Cold/
Flu Medicine

Laxatives, Diuretics, and Digoxin

People love laxatives. Goodness only knows why we are so obsessed with bowel function and regularity. Perhaps it's because commercials on television reinforce the notion that we need to make a daily bathroom pit stop to be healthy. Or it may stem from old folk beliefs that one has to rid the body of toxic by-products. A hundred years ago we didn't have very many effective medicines. Most remedies relied on placebo power. But doctors could prescribe a purgative or cathartic and produce a pretty impressive outhouse experience. Patients knew something important was going on and that might have inspired them to believe they were getting better.

Whatever the reason, we are fixated on our bowels. We spend millions of dollars on products such as **Black Draught**, **Dialose Plus**, **Doxidan**, **Dulcolax**, **Evac-Q-Kwik**, **Ex-Lax Maximum Relief Formula**, **Feen-a-mint**, **Fleet Laxative Tablets**, **Modane Plus**, **Nature's Remedy**, and **Senolax**. The occasional use of such stimulant laxatives probably doesn't cause any trouble, though high-fiber foods (such as bran), liquid, and exercise are generally a safer and better solution to constipation.

The real problem occurs when people develop a laxative habit. Regular use of strong laxatives can lead to diarrhea, fluid loss, and serious changes in electrolytes (minerals such as potassium and sodium). A reader of our syndicated newspaper column shared the following story:

> My husband is 73 years old. For the past 3 or 4 years he has had problems with his bowels. Either he's constipated or he's taking epsom salts or Ex-Lax. Then he seems to have diarrhea due to his medicating himself. His bowels are so bad, he can't control them. There are splatters and messes in his clothes, and the bathroom is a mess! When we travel I've had to rinse his clothes and head for a laundromat. Then he takes Kaopectate or Pepto-Bismol for the diarrhea, but it doesn't seem to work well. I wish he would go to a doctor but he's embarrassed.

A surprising number of people develop a dependency on laxatives. And we're not just talking about older folks. Young women who are concerned about their weight may get trapped into this kind of regimen.

They may also take diuretics to rid themselves of fluid so they can lose a few extra pounds.

Laxative abusers are often afraid to talk to a physician for fear of criticism. But such practices lead to a vicious cycle and can create dangerously low levels of potassium. This can be especially hazardous for people taking certain prescription medications. Diuretics such as **Bumex**, **HydroDIURIL**, **Lasix**, and **Lozol** also deplete potassium from the body. This combination (laxatives and diuretics) could lead to a serious imbalance that could be life threatening, especially if a person were also taking a digitalis-type heart medicine such as **Lanoxin** (see page 370). Irregular heart rhythms or cardiac arrest are real dangers. Bottom line: Avoid regular use of stimulant laxatives if at all possible. And monitor your potassium levels if you also take diuretics (normal values are 3.5 to 5.0 mEq/L).

Laxatives may also alter the absorption and effectiveness of other medications. There is, unfortunately, very little research on this kind of interaction. High-powered investigators probably don't get a whole lot of respect from their colleagues by focusing on laxative complications. But the issues are important because so many people are affected. Some years ago questions were raised about laxatives and oral contraceptives, the fear being that cathartics or harsh laxatives might cause diarrhea, reduce absorption, diminish effectiveness, and increase the risk of an unplanned pregnancy. We have been unable to confirm this rumor, however, and so this is one possible interaction that remains mysterious.

One study has shown that the laxative lactulose (**Cephulac**, **Cholac**, **Chronulac**, **Constilac**, **Constulose**,

Duphalac, and **Enulose**) could interfere with blood pressure drugs such as **Tenormin** (atenolol) and **HydroDIURIL** (hydrochlorothiazide).[3] Other research has shown that the popular laxative bisacodyl (**Carter's Laxative**, **Dulcogen**, **Dulcolax**, **Fleet Laxative**, etc.) can reduce absorption of the heart medicine **Lanoxin** (digoxin).[4] By the way, bisacodyl should not be swallowed with milk or dairy products. Such food could cause the drug to dissolve in the stomach instead of the small intestine, resulting in a very bad bellyache.

Antacids, Pepto-Bismol, and Broad-Spectrum Antibiotics

People are hard on their stomachs. We vacillate between being dietarily correct—bran, beans, and broccoli—and devilishly decadent—coffee, cookies, and chocolate. No wonder we swallow tons of antacids.

Many people don't think of these products as drugs. One friend won't go anywhere without his roll of **Rolaids**. He pops them down almost out of habit—as if they were candy. And now that calcium is the hottest nutritional supplement, millions of people are relying on antacids such as **Tums** to supply cheap calcium. Some women swallow these OTC remedies religiously and think of them as the nutritional equivalent of a glass of milk or a container of yogurt.

The trouble is that antacids interact with a variety of medications. Broad-spectrum antibiotics called quinolones have become very popular in recent years. They include compounds such as **Cipro** (ciprofloxacin), **Floxin** (ofloxacin), **Maxaquin** (lomefloxacin), **Noroxin** (norfloxacin), and **Penetrex** (enoxacin). These drugs are prescribed for a variety of infections including pneumonia, bronchitis, sinusitis, prostatitis, cervicitis, otitis media, urethritis, pelvic inflammatory disease, and more.

Antacids that contain aluminum, calcium, or magnesium can dramatically interfere with the absorption of these antibiotics. Researchers have demonstrated, for example, that there was a 17-fold reduction in **Cipro** levels in the blood after patients took antacids containing aluminum and magnesium.[5] It would almost be like not taking any medicine. Infections may not be cured if blood levels of antibiotics are inadequate.

Tetracycline is another broad-spectrum antibiotic that is widely prescribed. Dermatologists rely on it as a mainstay in the treatment of acne. It is the drug of choice against *Chlamydia* infection, the most common sexually transmitted disease in women, and deadly Rocky Mountain spotted fever. There are a variety of tetracycline-type antibiotics on the market, including **Achromycin V**, **Declomycin**, **Minocin**, **Panmycin**, **Sumycin**, **Terramycin**, and **Vibramycin**.

Antacids can reduce absorption of such drugs by more than 90 percent. Not only would you be wasting your money on expensive antibiotic therapy, but serious infections might not be cured. (For more details on the interaction between tetracycline and calcium, see pages 99-100.)

So why would anyone even contemplate combining antacids with antibiotics? Clearly no one would ever intentionally sabotage antibiotic therapy. But such antibiotics can cause upset stomach, indigestion, nausea, abdominal pain, and general digestive tract discomfort. Many folks might reach for an antacid without even thinking.

Another easily overlooked problem is **Pepto-Bismol** (bismuth subsalicylate). Because it is not officially an antacid, many people may not realize that this common stomach medicine can also interact with tetracyclines. Since such antibiotics often produce diarrhea and stomach upset, you can imagine how tempted someone might be to reach for the **Pepto** to relieve discomfort. Doing so, however, can reduce absorption of the antibiotic by one third. Levels of tetracycline-like drugs such as **Vibramycin** (doxycycline) can be reduced by over 50 percent—enough to decrease effectiveness.

Antacids That Affect Antibiotics

aluminum hydroxide gel	Mylanta II
Amitone	Phillips' Milk of Magnesia
Calcium Carbonate	Riopan
Chooz	Riopan Plus Di-Gel
Dicarbosil	Rolaids
Di-Gel Advanced Formula	Rolaids Calcium Rich/
Gas-X	Sodium Free
Gaviscon	Rulox
Gaviscon Cool Mint Flavor	Rulox Plus
Gaviscon ESR	Simaal 2 Gel
Gaviscon-2	Titralac
Gelusil	Titralac Plus
Kudrox	Tums
Maalox HRF	Tums Anti-gas
milk of magnesia	Tums E-X Extra Strength
Mylanta Double Strength	WinGel

The take-home message is DO NOT take antacids if your physician prescribes tetracycline or quinolone antibiotics. If you absolutely, positively must seek such stomach relief, do so only with your doctor's awareness. The antacid should be taken at least six hours before or three to four hours after the antibiotic.

Antacids may also interfere with proper absorption of the heart and blood pressure medications **Capoten** (captopril), **Inderal** (propranolol), and **Tenormin** (atenolol); the heart drug **Lanoxin** (digoxin); the ulcer drugs **Zantac** (ranitidine) and **Tagamet** (cimetidine); the antifungal agent **Nizoral** (ketoconazole); the antibacterial **Macrodantin** (nitrofurantoin); the seizure medicine **Dilantin** (phenytoin); and the antistroke compound **Ticlid** (ticlopidine). Although the clinical significance of such interactions remains murky, it only makes sense to avoid such antacids unless they are absolutely essential for health.[6]

The thyroid medicine **Synthroid** (levothyroxine) may also be affected by aluminum-containing antacids. Although this interaction needs better documentation, it would be wise either to stay away from such antacids or to monitor TSH (thyroid-stimulating hormone) levels carefully before and after exposure to antacids.

Activated Charcoal (the Gas-Busters)

It is not a topic for polite company, but flatulence is a fact of life. Everyone passes gas, some more than others. A few of the products sold in pharmacies to fight excess gas contain activated charcoal, the same material found in gas masks and water filters. Charcoal adsorbs all sorts of noxious stuff and is used as an antidote in cases of overdose or poisoning. There is also some research that suggests activated charcoal capsules reduce gaseous emissions. Products that contain activated charcoal include **Charcocaps**, **Charcoal Plus**, and **Flatulex**.

Drugs Affected by Activated Charcoal

Acetaminophen (**Anacin-3**, **Panadol**, **Tylenol**, etc.)
Antidepressants (tricyclic) (**Elavil**, **Pertofrane**, etc.)
Aspirin (**Alka-Seltzer**, **Anacin**, **Ascriptin**, etc.)
Barbiturates (**Fiorinal**, **Nembutal**, etc.)
Carbamazepine (**Tegretol**)
Diabetes drugs (**Diabinese**, **Tolinase**, etc.)
Digoxin (**Lanoxin**)
Furosemide (**Lasix**)
Methotrexate (**Rheumatrex**)
Nizatidine (**Axid**)
Phenothiazines (**Thorazine**, **Mellaril**, etc.)
Phenytoin (**Dilantin**)
Propoxyphene (**Darvon**, **Darvocet-N**, etc.)
Tetracycline (**Achromycin V**, **Sumycin**, etc.)
Theophylline (**Slo-bid**, **Theo-Dur**, etc.)
Valproic acid (**Depakene**, **Depakote**)

As good as activated charcoal can be at saving
people from drug overdoses or sparing them from flatulence, it can also prevent the absorption of medicine.
This could reduce effectiveness. Someone who is
using a product like **Charcocaps** or **Flatulex** should
avoid taking it at least several hours before and after
taking medicine.

Antihistamines

It is almost impossible to find a cold, allergy, cough, or
flu remedy these days that doesn't contain an antihistamine as a main ingredient. Check the label on your
favorite brand and you are likely to find compounds
such as brompheniramine, carbinoxamine, chlor-
pheniramine, clemastine, diphenhydramine, doxylamine, pyrilamine, tripelennamine, and triprolidine.

But these are tongue twisters and most people can't remember such terms.

Brand names are easier to pronounce and recall. Almost everyone has heard of products such as **Actifed**, **Benadryl**, **Benylin**, **Chlor-Trimeton**, **Comtrex**, **Contac 12 Hour**, **Dimetane**, **Dimetapp**, **Nyquil**, **PBZ**, **Sudafed Plus**, **Tavist**, and **TheraFlu Flu Cold & Cough Powder**.

Most over-the-counter antihistamines can make people drowsy, cloudy, fuzzy, or spacey. Many people find these drugs just plain put them to sleep. In fact, ingredients such as diphenhydramine and doxylamine are found in nonprescription sleeping products, including **Compoz**, **Excedrin P.M.**, **Nytol**, **Sleep-Eze 3**, **Sominex**, **Tylenol Extra Strength PM**, and **Unisom Nighttime Sleep Aid**.

It should come as no surprise that such antihistamines interact badly with prescription drugs that also have a sedating potential. People taking anti-anxiety agents such as **Ativan**, **Librium**, **Tranxene**, **Valium**, and **Xanax** should not combine OTC cough, cold, or allergy remedies with their nerve pills. The two drugs could make you a zombie. So could the tension headache pill **Fiorinal**, which contains the barbiturate butalbital. And watch out for traditional tricyclic antidepressants. They too could be a problem. Anticonvulsants, anti-Parkinson's disease drugs, alcohol, prescription pain relievers, and muscle relaxants can also add to the sedative effect. Before taking any antihistamine with a prescription medicine, check with a pharmacist to make sure it won't cause complications. Do not drive if you take antihistamines, even if you think you are unaffected. Reflexes and coordination could be affected.

Pain Relievers

The numbers are mind boggling. Americans toss down almost 30 billion aspirin pills annually. We swallow aspirin to relieve headaches, backaches, muscle sprains and strains, and arthritis. Millions more take a little aspirin every other day to prevent heart attacks and strokes. If preliminary research holds up, lots more will be taking aspirin to prevent a number of common cancers (stomach, colon, rectal, etc.). Now add millions more who casually pop acetaminophen (**Anacin-3, APAP, Bayer Select Maximum Strength Headache, Panadol, Tylenol,** etc.) and ibuprofen (**Advil, Bayer Select Ibuprofen Pain Reliever/Fever Reducer, Excedrin IB, Midol IB, Motrin IB, Nuprin,** etc.) to relieve minor aches and pains.

Analgesics are clearly the most popular pills in the medicine chest. We rely on them so routinely that we hardly think of such products as drugs. And yet aspirin, acetaminophen, and ibuprofen can all interact with a large number of other medications.

Aspirin Versus Capoten and Vasotec

One of the most controversial interactions in this entire book has to do with the combination of aspirin and **Capoten** (captopril) or **Vasotec** (enalapril). Millions of people take these prescription heart and blood pressure medicines. At last count, **Vasotec** was number 8 and **Capoten** was number 13 on the doctor's hit parade of most prescribed drugs.[7] These medications belong to a class referred to as ACE (angiotensin-converting enzyme) inhibitors. Without going into detail, such compounds lower blood pressure and protect against congestive heart failure with relatively few side effects—hence their extraordinary popularity.

It is not surprising that many of the same people who have hypertension or heart problems would also be taking aspirin. After all, this wonder drug saves tens of thousands of lives each year by preventing blood clots. (See *The Aspirin Handbook*, Bantam Books, New York, 1993, by Joe Graedon, Teresa Graedon, and Tom Ferguson, for everything you ever wanted to know about aspirin.)

When we first discovered the possibility that aspirin might partially compromise the effectiveness of ACE inhibitors, we tentatively wrote about it in our newspaper column. We were chastised by the company that makes **Vasotec** for shooting from the lip without adequate documentation. But subsequently we received a fascinating letter:

> A friend told me that you recently had an article in the paper regarding the side effects of aspirin and Vasotec. In December I took four 325 mg Ecotrins a day for three days for back pain. I was on either 5 or 10 mg of Vasotec twice a day when my blood pressure went up to 210/90 and my nose bled profusely.

At this time it is impossible to say whether this increase in blood pressure was caused by the aspirin in **Ecotrin**. But an extraordinary article in the *Journal of the American College of Cardiology* suggests that as little as one aspirin tablet can modify the benefit of **Vasotec** in controlling severe heart failure. These investigators concluded: "Our results indicate that enalapril works better when given without aspirin."[8]

The company that makes **Vasotec** does not specifically warn physicians about this interaction.[9] It may not be cause for concern. Nevertheless, if heart failure is not controlled adequately, this serious health condition could become life threatening. This is the kind of interaction that might sneak up in such a subtle way that no one would even realize that the anticipated benefits of **Vasotec** were not forthcoming. We encourage all physicians who prescribe **Vasotec** and aspirin together to treat heart failure to read Dr. Donald Hall's article in the *Journal of the American College of Cardiology* 1992; 20:1549–1555. Until more research is conducted, caution and vigilance are appropriate watchwords.

What should people with high blood pressure do? Well, they should definitely not stop taking aspirin, especially if it has been prescribed by a physician. Aspirin prevents heart attacks and strokes. But pharmacologist Morton J. Rodman warns that aspirin may partially counteract the blood-pressure-lowering effect of **Capoten**.[10] It may also impact **Vasotec** and other ACE inhibitors.

The answer to this dilemma is to monitor blood pressure carefully before someone starts taking such medicine to get a good baseline. When the ACE inhibitors are started, blood pressure should be recorded before aspirin is introduced. Then blood pressure should be checked once aspirin is added. A careful daily diary should reveal whether aspirin is blunting the benefits of these important medications. If it is, the physician can tailor a program that takes this effect into account. People with hypertension should definitely invest in a home blood pressure monitor so they can track these readings themselves, record them in a diary, and show them to the doctor for supervision.

We have detailed the interactions of ibuprofen

together with other arthritis medicines in the Guides to Dangerous Drug Interactions (see pages 304–312). On pages 143–152 you will find a table that lists the most common and serious aspirin and acetaminophen interactions. Please refer to this reference material if you rely on any of these pain relievers.

Drugs That Interact with Aspirin

DRUG	INTERACTION WITH ASPIRIN

ACE Blood Pressure Drugs
   Accupril
   Altace
   Capoten
   Captopril
   Lotensin
   Monopril
   Prinivil
   Vasotec
   Zestril
	The ACE inhibitor drugs, especially **Capoten** (captopril) and **Vasotec** (enalapril), are very widely used, not only to control blood pressure, but also to help ward off congestive heart failure. Current indications suggest they may also delay deterioration of kidney function in diabetics. Aspirin appears capable of interfering with the effectiveness of **Capoten** in lowering blood pressure, although there is little research to document this. It can also reduce the benefit of **Vasotec** in treating congestive heart failure.
	
	 If you are currently taking aspirin and one of these drugs, *do not stop taking either one.* Aspirin may be essential to your health. Keep track of your blood pressure and check with your doctor on whether you are getting the expected benefit from your blood pressure medicine. The interaction summary in the Guides to Dangerous Drug Interactions on page 378 and the discussion on pages 140–142 have more details.

Activated Charcoal	Activated charcoal, sometimes taken for flatulence, can attach to and re-

DRUG	INTERACTION WITH ASPIRIN
	duce the effect of many other drugs, aspirin among them.
Alcohol	Taking aspirin together with an alcoholic drink could easily aggravate stomach irritation. There is also a possibility that blood alcohol levels might end up higher than expected after just one and a half drinks if aspirin is taken an hour beforehand. There is disagreement about the clinical and legal implications of this interaction.
Antacids **Advanced Formula** **Di-Gel** **Gelusil** **Maalox** **Milk of magnesia** **Tums** **and others**	Using antacids regularly can reduce the amount of aspirin circulating in the body. People using anti-inflammatory doses of aspirin should be monitored if they start or stop taking antacids daily.
Anticoagulants **Coumadin** (warfarin) Dicumarol Heparin **Miradon** (anisindione)	Because aspirin also has anticlotting action, any of these prescription blood thinners (including heparin) might work too well in combination with aspirin. The potential exists for dangerous excessive bleeding. Careful monitoring is crucial.
Arthritis Drugs **Advil** (ibuprofen) **Clinoril** (sulindac) **Feldene** (piroxicam)	Although this interaction is not well established, some people find that these drugs for arthritis, bursitis, tendinitis, and other problems are less

DRUG	INTERACTION WITH ASPIRIN
Motrin (ibuprofen) **Naprosyn** (naproxen) and others	effective in combination with aspirin. In addition, stomach irritation may become worse.
Ascorbic Acid Vitamin C	People who take aspirin on a regular basis may have lower levels of this vitamin inside certain cells. It's not clear, though, whether there are any medically significant consequences. The interaction between aspirin and vitamin C is complicated and seems to differ with dietary levels of the vitamin. In one study, aspirin reduced urinary excretion of ascorbic acid when the vitamin was in ample supply; paradoxically, when dietary levels were low, aspirin led to greater excretion of vitamin C. Questions have been raised about whether large doses of vitamin C could make high doses of aspirin more toxic.
Baking Soda	This home remedy for indigestion could make urine alkaline. The result would be more rapid elimination of aspirin from the system.
Beta-Blockers **Blocadren** (timolol) **Cartrol** (carteolol) **Corgard** (nadolol) **Inderal** (propranolol) **Lopressor** (metoprolol) **Sectral** (acebutolol)	These medicines used to treat high blood pressure and heart disease may not work as effectively in the presence of aspirin. Research on this issue is not solid, but if you must take aspirin as well as one of the beta-blockers, you and your doctor should monitor your blood pressure

DRUG	INTERACTION WITH ASPIRIN
Tenormin (atenolol) **Visken** (pindolol) and others	response carefully. See the interaction summary on page 388.

Corticosteroids
 Cortef
   (hydrocortisone)
 Decadron
   (dexamethasone)
 Deltasone
   (prednisone)
 Medrol
   (methylprednisolone)
	Aspirin is eliminated more rapidly in the presence of these strong prescription steroids. Physicians should monitor dosing carefully, especially if anti-inflammatory effects are desired.

Diabetes Drugs **DiaBeta** (glyburide) **Diabinese** (chlorpropamide) **Glucotrol** (glipizide) **Micronase** (glyburide) and others Insulin	Type II diabetics should take aspirin only under a doctor's supervision, with careful blood sugar monitoring. Otherwise, blood glucose might drop too low unexpectedly. See the interaction summary on page 338 in the Diabetes Drugs section.
Diuretics **Bumex** (bumetanide) **Edecrin** (ethacrynic acid) **Lasix** (furosemide)	Aspirin can counteract the effectiveness of these strong "loop" diuretics in people with kidney or liver problems, especially if there is fluid buildup in the abdomen (ascites). This could have serious consequences; consult your physician.
Epilepsy Drugs **Depakene** (valproic acid)	These important anticonvulsant drugs could become more toxic in the presence of aspirin. A person who

DRUG	INTERACTION WITH ASPIRIN
Dilantin (phenytoin)	must take aspirin should be monitored closely for adverse reactions and blood levels of these medicines.
Glaucoma Drugs **Daranide** (dichlorphenamide) **Diamox** (acetazolamide) **Neptazane** (methazolamide)	Aspirin might increase blood levels of these glaucoma medicines to potentially toxic amounts. Elderly patients and people with kidney trouble are at particular risk. Check with your ophthalmologist before adding aspirin. **Diamox** is also sometimes used to treat mountain sickness in people traveling to high altitudes. Caution should be exercised in mixing this drug with aspirin.
Gout Medicine **Anturane** (sulfinpyrazone) **Benemid** (probenecid)	Taking aspirin with either of these gout medicines may keep them from controlling the uric acid buildup. In addition, aspirin won't be able to work against gout, either. It takes no more than 700 mg of aspirin to block **Anturane** almost totally.
Methotrexate **Folex** **Methotrate** **Mexate** **Rheumatrex,** and others	This medication, used to treat psoriasis, rheumatoid arthritis, and cancer, could reach surprisingly high levels in the body when combined with aspirin. This is a double-edged action, potentially increasing the power of the drug, but also its toxicity. Don't take any chances. Check with your doctor before taking any aspirin while you are also taking methotrexate.

DRUG	INTERACTION WITH ASPIRIN
Nitroglycerin	In one study, patients who took 1 gram of aspirin (two extra-strength tablets) along with nitroglycerin had lower blood pressure and a faster heart rate than those who took nitroglycerin alone. This could be a beneficial interaction, but it might also result in more nitroglycerin side effects such as headache or dizziness.
Oral Contraceptives	Women using oral contraceptives seem to metabolize aspirin more rapidly and may not get the same effectiveness. If aspirin is being used for minor pain, this is an inconvenience. If it is being used as an anti-inflammatory agent, this interaction might be more of a problem.
Penicillin	In the presence of aspirin, penicillin reaches higher concentrations in the blood and may last longer in the body. No studies have shown whether this makes any practical difference in fighting infection.
Spironolactone **Aldactazide** **Aldactone**	Spironolactone is a potassium-sparing diuretic that helps the body rid itself of sodium. Aspirin can interfere with the sodium-shedding effect, although potassium conservation and blood pressure do not seem to suffer.

Drugs That Interact with Acetaminophen

DRUG	INTERACTION WITH ACETAMINOPHEN
Activated Charcoal	Activated charcoal is sometimes taken for flatulence or other digestive problems. This is also the substance found in gas masks, because it is very efficient at grabbing other chemicals and hanging on to them. It can adsorb acetaminophen and reduce its effectiveness.
Alcohol	Although people often take **Anacin-3**, **Panadol**, or **Tylenol** to treat a hangover, alcohol and acetaminophen is a combination that worries us. Regular drinkers have a much greater risk of liver damage from overuse or overdose of acetaminophen. The danger is greater when a person is not eating much and taking large amounts of either alcohol or the painkiller. Deaths have been reported. Be aware that some medicines, especially cold remedies, contain both ingredients and should not be taken on a regular basis.
Anticoagulants **Coumadin** **Panwarfin** **Warfarin**	There is concern that regular use of acetaminophen for more than a few days could increase prothrombin time (PT) and increase the risk of unwanted bleeding. Ask the doctor to monitor PT and INR if you will need to start taking significant doses of acetaminophen.

DRUG	INTERACTION WITH ACETAMINOPHEN

Anticonvulsants
Dilantin (phenytoin)
Mesantoin
   (mephenytoin)
Peganone (ethotoin)
Phenobarbital
Tegretol
   (carbamazepine)
	Any of these seizure medicines may reduce the effectiveness of acetaminophen, so that pain relief might be harder to achieve. Don't be tempted to increase the dose of the pain medicine, though; the seizure drugs also make the liver more susceptible to damage from high doses or long-term use of acetaminophen. Please note that any barbiturate taken on a regular basis could interact with this nonprescription pain reliever in a similar way. The headache remedies **Fiorinal** and **Fioricet** both contain a barbiturate, butalbital.

AZT **Retrovir** (zidovudine)	Anyone taking the anti-AIDS drug AZT should consult the doctor before swallowing **Tylenol** or any other acetaminophen pain pill. Acetaminophen speeds elimination of AZT. Just one week of taking 650 mg acetaminophen (two regular-strength pills) with each AZT dose reduced AZT in the body by 33 percent. The clinical significance is unknown, but because **Retrovir** is used for a serious condition, it is probably unwise to interfere with it.
Beta-Blockers **Inderal** (propranolol) **Lopressor** (metoprolol) **Tenormin** (atenolol) and others	This interaction is probably no big deal. **Inderal** slows the elimination of acetaminophen slightly, which could lead to higher levels or longer action of the pain reliever. Unless you are taking frequent high doses of acetaminophen, that shouldn't be a

DRUG	INTERACTION WITH ACETAMINOPHEN
	problem. Some other beta-blockers may also interact in a similar fashion.
Gout Medicine **Anturane** (sulfinpyrazone)	When **Anturane** is taken on a regular basis, as it normally is in the treatment of gout, it can make the liver more vulnerable to damage. High doses of acetaminophen should be avoided.
Oral Contraceptives **Loestrin** **Lo/Ovral** **Ortho-Novum** and others	Acetaminophen may take a little longer to kick in, and the pain relief may fade a little sooner in women on birth control pills. Overall, however, pain relief shouldn't be much affected. This is not a dangerous interaction.
Parkinson's Disease Drugs **Artane** (trihexyphenidyl) **Cogentin** (benztropine)	These two medications for Parkinson's disease may slow the onset of acetaminophen's action. Overall pain relief should not be greatly affected, however.
Stomach Medicine **Banthine** (methantheline) Belladonna **Bentyl** (dicyclomine) **Pro-Banthine** (propantheline) **Robinul** (glycopyrrolate)	These medications for ulcers and other digestive disorders can delay the onset of pain relief from acetaminophen. The effectiveness is not reduced, however, so patience is in order.

DRUG	INTERACTION WITH ACETAMINOPHEN
Tuberculosis Drugs **INH** (isoniazid) **Laniazid** (isoniazid) **Nydrazid** (isoniazid)	The tuberculosis drug isoniazid makes the liver more susceptible to potential damage from acetaminophen. High doses or long-term use of the over-the-counter pain reliever should be avoided if at all possible. Discuss this issue with the physician.
Tuberculosis Drugs **Rifadin** (rifampin) **Rimactane** (rifampin)	The tuberculosis medicine rifampin can lower the effectiveness of acetaminophen somewhat. It would, however, be a serious error to increase the dose in a search for better pain relief, because acetaminophen in high doses or over the long term can make the liver more vulnerable to damage from rifampin. Check with the doctor.

Caffeine

Caffeine hardly seems like a drug. After all, many of us rely on that morning cup of coffee to get the day started, not to mention for a midday pick-me-up. Caffeine is a mainstay in many soft drinks including Coke, Pepsi, and Mountain Dew. You will also find caffeine in a surprising number of medications, from pain relievers to daytime stimulants.

Few physicians think to warn their patients about caffeine/drug interactions. Yet a number of prescription medications can boost caffeine levels to the point that someone could be wired for hours. Barry is a photojournalist for a major news magazine. When he developed an ear infection the doctor prescribed **Cipro** (ciprofloxacin). Not a word was mentioned about possible interactions. When Barry had his usual double cappuccino, his nervous system went into overdrive. He was jittery and unable to hold the camera steady. The effect lasted far longer than one might have expected from a strong cup of coffee. Barry had no idea why his normal caffeine hit had left him so uptight.

Products That Contain Caffeine

Anacin	Excedrin Extra-Strength
Aqua-Ban Plus	No-Doz
Bayer Select Maximum Headache Capsules	Quick Pep
	Tirend
BC Headache Powders	Vanquish
Caffedrine	Vivarin

Cipro, **Noroxin** (norfloxacin), and **Penetrex** (enoxacin) are quinolone antibiotics that can all affect metabolism of caffeine and give it a longer ride in the body. So can the ulcer drug **Tagamet** (cimetidine) and even birth control pills.[11] Women on the Pill may find that they get a bigger jolt from that cup of coffee.

Although these interactions are probably not hazardous for most people, the extra caffeine effect can come as a shock to some. Barry certainly wasn't prepared to be wired for hours. Some people may develop serious insomnia from what they think is a modest amount of coffee early in the day. Don't risk it—skip the java.

People with asthma often take theophylline (**Bronkaid Tablets, Bronkodyl, Bronkotabs, Elixophyllin, Primatene Tablets, Slo-bid, Slo-Phyllin, Sustaire, Theo-24, Theobid, Theo-Dur, Theolair, Uniphyl**, etc.). Theophylline can interact with a large number of other medications (see page 313). The chemical structure and pharmacological action of theophylline is very similar to that of caffeine. In fact, if someone were to be caught without his theophylline, and mild symptoms of asthma began to be a problem, several cups of caffeinated coffee might bring relief. But if one were to take theophylline and also drink regular coffee, it would be like getting an overdose of caffeine. That also goes for soft drinks and over-the-counter products that contain this ubiquitous stimulant.

Herbal Remedies

If it is rare for a physician to warn people about interactions between drugs such as caffeine and **Tagamet**, you can imagine how unlikely it would be to get a precaution about herbal products that can interact with drugs. For one thing, few patients are likely even to share with their doctors the fact that they use herbal products. Such products are, after all, considered somewhat flaky by the medical establishment. Yet in recent years alternative remedies—including herbal products available in health food stores and through the mail—have become increasingly popular.

There is, sad to say, very little research on the potential for herbal products to interact with other medications. You won't find many references to such problems in standard interaction references or data bases. That interactions can occur, however, is unquestioned.

Guarana

Guarana is a popular herbal ingredient found in a number of so-called natural products. It has been used as a diet aid and stimulant. One brand name remedy is aptly called **Zoom**. Guarana comes from Central and South America. It is especially popular in Brazil, where natives have used this herb as a treatment for malaria and dysentery. Not surprisingly, they also drink it as a hot beverage, much as we do tea or coffee. Guarana contains a whopping dose of caffeine—3 to 5 percent by dry weight, compared to 1 to 2 percent in coffee beans, by dry weight. Therefore the same warnings that apply to caffeine would also apply to guarana.

Licorice

Many herbal preparations contain licorice (glycyrrhiza). This natural product has been used for centuries in cough and cold remedies and as a digestive aid. It is also employed as a flavoring agent in many natural remedies. But too much licorice (in candy or an herbal product) can deplete the body of potassium. People taking diuretics or digoxin (**Lanoxin**) can get themselves into serious trouble if they also gorge on licorice (see pages 55 and 56 for more details).

Garlic

Garlic, variously nicknamed "stinking rose" and "nectar of the gods," has been used medicinally for thousands of years. Currently garlic extracts are sold in health food stores and pharmacies as a general tonic, but also with the idea that garlic may reduce blood sugar levels, lower blood cholesterol, and help prevent the formation of blood clots that could trigger heart attacks. It may also prove helpful, upon further research, in some intestinal disorders. Experts worry that garlic might interact with diabetes medicines or a blood thinner such as **Coumadin** to increase their activity unexpectedly. No studies have been conducted yet to confirm or refute this possibility of troublesome interactions.

Glucomannan

Also known as konjac, glucomannan is similar in its actions to guar gum, a dietary fiber that is used as a thickening agent in lots of processed foods and pharmaceuticals. Glucomannan is employed as a gentle laxative and has been used in weight loss products to produce a "full feeling." It has also been found to help lower cholesterol levels.

Glucomannan and guar gum can have a major impact on blood sugar. They may lower glucose levels and change insulin requirements. This means that patients with diabetes will have to be especially vigilant about monitoring blood glucose if they take an herbal remedy containing glucomannan or guar gum.

Dosage modifications may become necessary for insulin injections or for oral diabetes medicines such as **DiaBeta, Diabinese, Dymelor, Glucotrol, Glynase, Micronase, Orinase, Tolamide**, and **Tolinase**. Any diabetic considering an herbal remedy containing glucomannon or guar gum must stay in close touch with a physician.

Goldenseal

This plant is found from Arkansas to Vermont. It is also known as yellow root, turmeric root, or orange root. People use it for coughs, menstrual problems, arthritis, and stomach upset. One of the active components in goldenseal, hydrastine, can constrict blood vessels. Although there is little research on drug interactions with goldenseal, we fear that this pharmacological action might raise blood pressure. This could complicate treatment for people taking antihypertensive medication, especially beta-blockers such as **Corgard** (nadolol), **Inderal** (propranolol), **Lopressor** (metoprolol), and **Tenormin** (atenolol).

Feverfew

Feverfew is a European herbal medicine from the Greek tradition. Like many other medicinal herbs, it has recently enjoyed a strong revival of interest. Some people recommend it for the prevention of migraine headaches, and there is research to indicate it is more effective for this purpose than a placebo.[12] There are worrisome reports of a rebound syndrome in those who stop feverfew suddenly, however, and an interaction with anticoagulants such as **Coumadin** is suspected, although it hasn't been studied.

Ubiquinone (Coenzyme Q₁₀)

CoQ_{10}, as it is sometimes called, is not an herb, but it is sold in health food stores as a nutrient. It is a very popular alternative treatment for everything from heart failure and gum disease to lowered immunity and lack of energy. Ubiquinone is a natural substance made by the body and is important to many biochemical reactions. While this substance appears to be relatively nontoxic by itself, it may interact in a dangerous way with **Coumadin** (warfarin). Preliminary research suggests that CoQ_{10} may reduce the effectiveness of this anticoagulant and increase the risk of blood clots.[13]

Anyone taking coenzyme Q_{10} must alert a physician and make sure to have frequent blood tests if **Coumadin** is part of the program. In fact, it is probably not a good idea to combine CoQ_{10} and **Coumadin** unless advised to do so by a doctor who is monitoring the situation very carefully.

Chamomile

Chamomile tea is a traditional remedy for stomach upset in many parts of the world. Scientific research backs up this tradition to some extent, suggesting that the principal component of chamomile, bisabolol, may calm intestinal spasms and helps prevent the development of gastric ulcers in rats given ulcer-causing compounds such as indomethacin (a potent arthritis medicine) or alcohol.[14] While this protective effect might potentially be useful for someone who has to take arthritis medicine on a regular basis, the editors of *The Lawrence Review of Natural Products* also warn that chamomile may delay the absorption of medications taken at the same time.[15]

Yohimbine

The bark from the yohimbe tree was a favorite impotence remedy of West African traditional healers, and the compound derived from that bark is being used by many American men for the same purpose. Like many natural remedies, though, yohimbine does have some side effects. It can cause dizziness and a fall in blood pressure. Medical supervision is essential. This compound also appears to block the enzyme monoamine oxidase (MAO) and therefore it should not be taken with a variety of prescription and over-the-counter medications. See pages 59 and 129–131 for lists of foods and drugs that should be avoided.

Valerian

This herb has become very popular as a calming agent. In other words, it may help people relieve minor anxiety and perhaps even get to sleep. Be aware, however, that valerian might interact with alcohol or other tranquilizers or sedatives. This means that someone taking **Valium** (diazepam), **Xanax** (alprazolam), or an antidepressant such as **Elavil** (amitriptyline) that may cause drowsiness should be very cautious about adding valerian.

Herbs are popular these days. People like to think of such remedies as natural and organic, with no side effects or complications. If an over-the-counter remedy or prescription drug doesn't live up to expectations, some folks may decide to self-medicate with an herbal product. Such combinations might lead to serious reactions, however. Caution is called for since your pharmacist may not be able to determine the potential for dangerous interactions.

Conclusion

Over-the-counter medications are not wimpy drugs, and herbal remedies are not necessarily harmless. These products can have side effects and may interact with a wide variety of other compounds. A sensible consumer will learn which precautions apply. As more and more medicines jump the counter (**Aleve**, **Pepcid AC**, and **Tagamet HB** are examples, with **Carafate**, **Feldene**, and **Zantac** under review), you will have greater need than ever to check for interaction potential. The labels on OTC bottles and herbal remedies will likely remain woefully inadequate, so it will be up to you to learn the rules to use such products safely.

References

1. Harrison, W., et al. "MAOIs and Hypertensive Crisis: The Role of OTC Drugs." *J. Clin. Psychiatry* 1989; 50:64.

2. Rivers, N., et al. "Possible Lethal Reaction Between Nardil and Dextromethorphan." *Can. Med. Assoc. J.* 1970; 103:85.

3. Riley, S.A., et al. "Effects of a Non-Absorbable Osmotic Load on Drug Absorption in Healthy Volunteers." *Br. J. Clin. Pharmacol.* 1992; 34:40–46.

4. Wang, D.J. "Drug Interaction Between Digoxin and Bisacodyl." *Taiwan I. Hsueh. Hui. Tsa. Chih.* 1990; 89:915–919.

5. Lomaestro, B.M., et al. "Quinolone-Cation Interactions: A Review." *DICP Ann Pharmacother.* 1991; 25:1249–1258.

6. Holden, Mark D. "Over-the-Counter Medications: Do You Know What Your Patients Are Taking?" *Postgraduate Medicine* 1992; 91(8):191–200.

7. Simonsen, Laura La Piana. "What Are Pharmacists Dispensing Most Often?" *Pharmacy Times* 1993; April: 29–44.

8. Hall, Donald, et al. "Counteraction of the Vasodilator Effects of Enalapril by Aspirin in Severe Heart Failure." *J. Am. Coll. Cardiol.* 1992; 20:1549–1555.

9. Hopkins, Martha, Professional Services. Personal communication, December 21, 1993.

10. Rodman, Morton J. "OTC Interactions: Analgesics and Anti-Inflammatories." *RN* 1993; January: 54–60.

11. Myers, Martin G. "Caffeine, Oral Contraceptives, and Over-the-Counter Drugs." *Arch. Int. Med.* 1989; 149:1217–1222.

12. Murphy, J. J., et al. "Randomised double-blind placebo-controlled trial of feverfew in migraine prevention." *Lancet* 1988; 2:189.

13. Spigset, Olav. "Reduced effect of warfarin caused by ubidecarenone." *Lancet* 1994; 344:1372–1373.
14. Szelenyi, I., et al. "Pharmacological experiments with compounds of chamomile. III. Experimental studies of the ulcer protective effects of chamomile." *Planta Medica* 1979; 35:218.
15. "Chamomile." *Lawrence Review of Natural Products*. St. Louis: Facts & Comparisons, 1991.

References for Aspirin and Acetaminophen Interaction Tables

Graedon, J., et al. *The Aspirin Handbook: A User's Guide to the Breakthrough Drug of the '90s*. New York: Bantam Books, 1993.

Hall, D., et al. "Counteraction of the Vasodilator Effects of Enalapril by Aspirin in Severe Heart Failure." *J. Am. Coll. Cardiol.* 1992; 20:1549–1555.

Holden, M. D. "Over-the-counter Medications." *Postgraduate Medicine* 1992; 91:191–200.

Johansson, U., and B. Akesson. "Interaction Between Ascorbic Acid and Acetylsalicylic Acid and Their Effects on Nutritional Status in Man." *Int. J. Vitam. Nutr. Res.* 1985; 55(2):197–204.

Olin, B.R., editor-in-chief. *Drug Facts and Comparisons*. St. Louis: Facts & Comparisons (A Wolters-Kluwer Company), 1993.

Rodman, M.J. "Analgesics and Anti-inflammatories." *RN* 1993; January: 54–60.

Roine, R., et al. "Aspirin Increases Blood Alcohol Concentrations in Humans after Ingestion of Ethanol." *JAMA* 1990: 264:2406–2408.

Tatro, D. S., ed. *Drug Interaction Facts*. St. Louis: Facts & Comparisons (A Wolters-Kluwer Company), 1993.

chapter seven

Drug Interactions That Affect Women, Children, and Older People

Drug Interactions That Affect Women

For centuries women have gotten the short end of the stick. Although they are often called upon to be Dr. Mom, caring for sick children, older parents, and ailing spouses, their own health has often been ignored by medical researchers. Nowhere is this problem more acute than in the world of pharmaceuticals.

There are so many unanswered questions about the relationship between drugs and women's health that it leaves us dazed. For example, estrogen hormones are supposed to help protect women against osteoporosis, heart disease, and ovarian cancer. But they increase the incidence of uterine (endometrial) cancer and possibly even breast cancer (a disease that now strikes one in eight women). Because the research to resolve such an important issue as breast cancer has been delayed for decades, it will be many years before women know if they are trading some benefits for other serious risks.

Investigators running drug studies have traditionally focused their attention on healthy young men. Testing relied on subjects who couldn't become pregnant, didn't suffer from chronic diseases, weren't taking any other medicines, and didn't reflect the real world. Women, children, and older people were pretty much ignored by pharmaceutical researchers.

As a result, we don't really know if women benefit from drug-induced cholesterol reduction. There are unresolved questions about blood pressure treatment in women. We cannot assume that women always react the same way that men do. For example, women appear to lack the enzyme alcohol dehydrogenase in the stomach. There is some preliminary information that suggests this enzyme is responsible for early metabolism of alcohol. Perhaps this explains why some men can seemingly drink more than some women without getting as drunk.

Birth Control Pills

The problem is that there has been little motivation to address many of the health issues that really concern women. Take the Pill. More than ten million women rely on this form of contraception to prevent pregnancy. They have been reassured that this is about as good as it gets, next to sterilization. Many people believe that birth control pills are just about perfect. Yet experts have confided to us that there may be as many as "250,000 pregnancies per year in the U.S. attributed to incorrect use of OCs (oral contraceptives), according to research by the National Academy of Science."[1]

Many of these contraceptive failures are undoubtedly due to mistakes. Instructions are surprisingly confusing. There are now roughly 60 different brands of oral contraceptives on the market. There is an amazing variability in dose and type. And there is conflicting information on the proper use of these pills and what to do if one dose is missed. Since many oral contraceptives now have much lower amounts of estrogen and progestin than they did 30 years ago, there is less room for error. Experts tell us that "being just a few hours late may increase risk for pregnancy."[2]

Drug interactions may also contribute to some of those unwanted pregnancies. Many medications can interfere with the effectiveness of the Pill. Today's low-dose contraceptives are less likely to cause side effects, but they seem more vulnerable to inactivation. Although the package insert on a number of brands mentions drug interaction precautions, this crucial information may be buried amidst the fine print. Anyone who has ever looked at one of these inserts knows that your eyes glaze over pretty fast. We wonder whether physicians read, appreciate, and warn patients about the precaution:

> Reduced efficacy and increased incidence of breakthrough bleeding and menstrual irregularities have been associated with concomitant use of rifampin. A similar association, though less marked, has been suggested with barbiturates, phenylbutazone, phenytoin sodium, and possibly with griseofulvin, ampicillin, and tetracyclines.

The Effect of Barbiturates on Birth Control Pills

The real problem is that good research is lacking. Several years ago the manufacturer of the popular tension headache reliever **Fiorinal** (aspirin, butalbital, caffeine) disputed our warning to women that its product might reduce the effectiveness of the Pill. Our concern seemed justified since the barbiturate butalbital is listed in standard reference books as having the potential to reduce contraceptive effectiveness.[3, 4]

A similar barbiturate comes with the warning "Pretreatment with or concurrent administration of phenobarbital may decrease estradiol by increasing its

metabolism. There have been reports of patients treated with antiepileptic drugs (e.g., phenobarbital) who
become pregnant while taking oral contraceptives. An
alternate contraceptive method might be suggested to
women taking phenobarbital."

The company maintained that since they had
never heard of accidental pregnancies associated with
Fiorinal or **Fioricet** (acetaminophen, butalbital, caffeine) and birth control pills, the problem did not exist.
Of course, there is no mention of an interaction in the
package insert, and many women don't even realize
that their headache remedy contains a barbiturate. If
they got pregnant it is entirely possible that neither
they nor their physicians would make such a connection or report it to the company or the FDA.

There is no good answer to this dilemma. Epidemi-
ological studies are sorely lacking. And don't expect
anyone to do quality research anytime soon. There is
no incentive for drug companies to look for what they
perceive as bad news. As we have stated earlier in this
book, there is no scientific system to track, report, or
warn about dangerous drug interactions. And make no
mistake, an unwanted pregnancy can be dangerous.
For some women it is intolerable for health reasons,
while for others it may be psychologically devastating.
Furthermore, barbiturates themselves may cause birth
defects.

We suspect that if there were an effective male
contraceptive that could be altered by other medications, a solution would be found swiftly.
Unfortunately, the medical establishment is playing
catch-up on women's health and many unresolved
questions may never be answered.

What we can say with certainty is that there are

cases of unintended pregnancy associated with the use of barbiturates and birth control pills. We suggest that common sense would encourage extra contraceptive protection if such an interaction were to occur.

Products Containing Barbiturates

Alurate (aprobarbital)	**Gemonil** (metharbital)
Amytal (amobarbital)	**Isobutal** (butalbital)
Anaphen (butalbital)	**Isocet** (butalbital)
Anoquan (butalbital)	**Isolin** (butalbital)
Axotal (butalbital)	**Isollyl** (butalbital)
Bancap (butalbital)	**Isopap** (butalbital)
Barbased (butabarbital)	**Laniroif** (butalbital)
Bucet (butalbital)	**Lanorinal** (butalbital)
Butace (butalbital)	**Lotusate** (talbutal)
Buticaps (butabarbital)	**Marnal** (butalbital)
Butisol (butabarbital)	**Mebaral** (mephobarbital)
Conten (butalbital)	**Medigesic** (butalbital)
Dolmar (butalbital)	**Mysoline** (primidone)
Esgic (butalbital)	**Nembutal** (pentobarbital)
Ezol (butalbital)	**Pharmagesic** (butalbital)
Femcet (butalbital)	Phenobarbital
Fiorgen (butalbital)	**Phrenilin** (butalbital)
Fioricet (butalbital)	**Sarisol No. 2** (butabarbital)
Fiorinal (butalbital)	**Seconal** (secobarbital)
Fiorinal with Codeine (butalbital)	**Tri-Barbs** (phenobarbital, butabarbital, secobarbital)
Fiormor (butalbital)	**Tuinal** (amobarbital, secobarbital)
Fortabs (butalbital)	

The Effect of Antibiotics on Birth Control Pills

Perhaps even more controversial than barbiturate complications is the question of antibiotic interaction with birth control pills. Researchers have been debating the significance of this combination for years. You can understand why. It is not uncommon for a woman to get a urinary tract infection, an ear infection, a reproductive tract infection, or just a common case of acne. The doctor is likely to prescribe an antibiotic for each of these problems.

Check the package insert that comes with oral contraceptives and you will find mention of interaction potential with tetracycline and ampicillin, two of the most commonly prescribed antibiotics. Experts also warn that other penicillin-type antibiotics such as **Amoxil** (amoxicillin), **Prostaphlin** (oxacillin), and **Beepen-VK** (penicillin V) may diminish contraceptive power.[5]

The theory is that these broad-spectrum antibiotics kill bacteria in the digestive tract that play an important role in maintaining adequate blood levels of contraceptive hormones. Researchers have been fighting about the clinical significance of this interaction for years. That there are cases of unintended pregnancy associated with antibiotics and birth control pills seems unequivocal.[6,7] How common this is and what other factors may play a role remain highly controversial.[8,9,10,11,12,13,14] Even the most outspoken British critics of an interaction between antibiotics and birth control pills warn that "practitioners are advised to recommend the use of alternative contraceptive precautions for women receiving broad-spectrum antibiotics concurrently with their OCs [oral contraceptives] preparation."[15] Such advice seems only prudent.

The Effect of Anticonvulsants on Birth Control Pills

There is little doubt that seizure medicine represents a real threat to contraceptive effectiveness. There is

Antibiotics That May Affect Birth Control Pills

Achromycin V (tetracycline)
Ala-Tet (tetracycline)
Amcill (ampicillin)
Amoxil (amoxicillin)
Augmentin (amoxicillin, potassium clavulanate)
Azlin (azlocillin)
Bactocill (oxacillin)
Beepen-VK (penicillin V)
Betapen-VK (penicillin V)
Bikomox (amoxicillin)
Biomox (amoxicillin)
Cloxapen (cloxacillin)
Coactin (aminocillin)
Declomycin (demeclocycline)
Doryx (doxycycline)
Doxy-Caps (doxycycline)
Doxychel (doxycycline)
Dycill (dicloxacillin)
Dynacin (minocycline)
Dynapen (dicloxacillin)
Geocillin (carbenicillin)
Geopen (carbenicillin)
Ledercillin VK (penicillin V)
Minocin (minocycline)
Monodox (doxycycline)
Nallpen (nafcillin)
Omnipen (ampicillin)

Panmycin (tetracycline)
Pathocil (dicloxacillin)
Pentids (penicillin G)
Pen-V (penicillin V)
Pen-Vee K (penicillin V)
Polycillin (ampicillin)
Polymox (amoxicillin)
Principen (ampicillin)
Prostaphlin (oxacillin)
Robicillin VK (penicillin V)
Robitet (tetracycline)
Spectrobid (bacampicillin)
Staphcillin (methicillin)
Sumycin (tetracycline)
Tegopen (cloxacillin)
Terramycin (oxytetracycline)
Tetracap (tetracycline)
Tetracyn (tetracycline)
Tetralan (tetracycline)
Totacillin (ampicillin)
Trimox (amoxicillin)
Unipen (nafcillin)
Uri-Tet (oxytetracycline)
V-Cillin K (penicillin V)
Veetids (penicillin V)
Vibramycin (doxycycline)
Vibra-Tabs (doxycycline)
Wymox (amoxicillin)

near unanimity that epilepsy drugs such as **Dilantin** (phenytoin), **Mesantoin** (mephenytoin), **Mysoline** (primidone), **Peganone** (ethotoin), phenobarbital, and **Tegretol** (carbamazepine) affect the metabolism of birth control pills. According to one source, "In a retrospective analysis of 82 women with seizure disorders receiving oral contraceptives, the risk of pregnancy was 25 times greater in those patients also receiving anticonvulsants than in those patients who were not."[16]

What is so serious about this interaction is that many of these very same drugs may cause birth defects. So a woman with a seizure disorder might well be told by her physician to use a reliable method of contraception while on a drug such as **Dilantin** or phenobarbital. Most women would then conclude that oral contraceptives are the best choice. But, as we have just described, reliability may be far less than anticipated when BC pills are combined with such drugs.

There is one anticonvulsant that does not appear to interact with oral contraceptives. Valproic acid (**Depakene**), and the similar divalproex sodium (**Depakote**) won't change metabolism and shouldn't interfere with effectiveness. There are also new seizure medications coming on line, such as **Neurontin** (gabapentin) and **Lamictal** (lamotrigine), that have fewer side effects than traditional anticonvulsants and do not appear to interact with birth control pills.[17,18] Women need to ask lots of questions and take extra precautions to avoid pregnancy no matter which seizure medicine is prescribed.

The Effect of Antifungals and TB Medicines on Birth Control Pills

Women who rely on oral contraceptives have to watch out for several other kinds of medicine. Drugs that fight fungal infections, such as griseofulvin (**Fulvicin**, **Grifulvin**, **Gris-PEG**, **Grisactin**), may reduce the effectiveness of the Pill. Unintended pregnancies have been reported after this combination. There are alternate antifungal medications on the market that have not been reported to have this interaction potential.

Tuberculosis is back. The current TB epidemic appears to be gaining victims at a rapid pace. The infections are more virulent and harder to treat. It is likely that more and more people will become infected, even some who have otherwise healthy immune systems.

One of the main drugs in the treatment of TB is rifampin (**Rifadin**, **Rifamate**, **Rimactane**). This drug increases the metabolism, lowers blood levels, and reduces the effectiveness of contraceptive hormones. Breakthrough bleeding and menstrual disturbances are common consequences of this interaction. It has been estimated that 6 percent of women on such a combination could become pregnant.

The Effect of Vitamin C on Birth Control Pills

A few other interactions with birth control pills concern us. Vitamin C can boost estrogen levels. This obviously won't reduce contraceptive protection but could make the Pill more potent.

In essence this interaction converts a low-dose Pill into a high-dose contraceptive. That could increase the possibility of estrogen side effects, including gallbladder disease, vaginal yeast infections, breast tenderness and enlargement, bloating, nausea, vomiting, cramps, facial skin darkening, hair loss, headaches, migraines, depression, increases in blood sugar, and changes in libido (usually reduction).

Vitamin C may have a similar impact on estrogen replacement therapy. Drugs such as **Estinyl**, **Estrace**,

Estratab, **Estratest**, **Estrovis**, **Menest**, **Ogen**, **Ovest**, and **Premarin** could also be affected by this common nutrient. What is unclear is the dose of ascorbic acid necessary to produce such an effect. One study found that 1,000 mg could increase estrogen (ethinyl estradiol) levels by almost 50 percent. Whether lower doses (say in the 50- to 100-mg range) have an impact is unknown.

One caution should be noted about stopping vitamin C suddenly. Concern has been expressed that estrogen levels might drop precipitously if this vitamin were discontinued too abruptly. Whether this might cause contraceptive failure has not been researched.

The Effect of Birth Control Pills on Anxiety Drugs and Antidepressants

Benzodiazepines are among the most frequently prescribed medicines for anxiety, panic, agoraphobia, and a host of other conditions that create fear and nervousness. We are talking about drugs such as **Dalmane** (flurazepam), **Doral** (quazepam), **Halcion** (triazolam), **Klonopin** (clonazepam), **Tranxene** (clorazepate), **Valium** (diazepam), and **Xanax** (alprazolam).

Oral contraceptives have been reported to increase blood levels of these medications. Likewise, the Pill appears to boost blood levels of antidepressants such as **Elavil** (amitriptyline). There is confusion about the significance of these interactions. Perhaps someone used to a certain amount of **Valium** or **Xanax** in her system might suddenly experience a greater impact from these anti-anxiety agents if she starts birth control pills. There have been reports of greater "psychomotor impairment" from this kind of combination. That could mean driving or operating machinery would be a greater hazard.

The Effect of Birth Control Pills on Asthma Medicine

Here is another controversial interaction. The data are hard to interpret. Some studies have shown that oral contraceptives prolong the effects of theophylline in the body. If true, this could lead to symptoms of toxicity, such as nausea, vomiting, stomach pain, diarrhea, nervousness, irritability, muscle twitching, and palpitations. Blood levels of theophylline can be monitored to assess the possibility of an interaction. Be alert for signs of overdose if birth control pills are added to this asthma medication.

Medicine Containing Theophylline	
Accurbron	Sustaire
Aerolate	Theo-Dur
Aquaphyllin	Theobid
Asmalix	Theochron
Bronkodyl	Theoclear
Constant-T	Theolair
Elixomin	Theospan
Elixophyllin	Theostat 80
Lanophyllin	Theo-24
Quibron-T	Theovent
Respbid	T-Phyl
Slo-bid	Uniphyl
Slo-Phyllin	

The Effect of Birth Control Pills on Caffeine

Don't forget to watch out for caffeine. It is pharmacologically similar to theophylline (see page 66). Someone on oral contraceptives could get an extra jolt from her java. Studies have shown that the effects of caffeine are prolonged and possibly even intensified. This could lead to nervousness, insomnia, and a generally wired feeling. Women on the Pill should probably be moderate in caffeine intake, especially late in the day, until they find out if they are affected by such an interaction.

The Effect of Smoking on Birth Control Pills

We have saved the scariest interaction for last. This one is definitely verboten. DON'T DO IT. Smoking and oral contraceptives just plain do not mix. The package insert has a bold, boxed warning that says:

> Cigarette smoking increases the risk of serious cardiovascular side effects from oral contraceptive use. This risk increases with age and with heavy smoking (15 or more cigarettes per day) and is quite marked in women over 35 years of age. Women who use oral contraceptives should be strongly advised not to smoke.

This combination increases the possibility of stroke, heart attack, pulmonary embolism (blood clots in the lungs), and other vascular problems. Women can die from this interaction.

Drug Interactions That Affect Children

Nothing is harder on a parent than a sick child. We feel so inadequate when that vulnerable person we love comes down with a high fever, a terrible cough, or an asthma attack. Giving medicine seems like such a caring thing to do. But watch out: There are thousands of products on drugstore shelves that are inappropriate and possibly even dangerous for children.

Children are not just smaller versions of adults. They react differently to medicine than adults because their nervous systems are not yet fully developed, their metabolism is different, and they are far smaller. That makes them far more susceptible to drug dangers. When a well-meaning adult tells a trusting toddler to swallow an irrational mixture of ingredients, we get angry. And believe us when we tell you that there are illogical products in pharmacies these days.

Cold and Cough Remedies

Let's start with cold remedies. When a child starts sniffling and sneezing, most parents go on alert. A runny nose and a horrible hack really get their attention. With so many products advertising instant relief, the temptation is great to start pumping medicine. And because so many products come in liquid formulas, it's tempting to reach for whatever is lurking in the medicine chest.

Don't do it, Dr. Mom. First, be especially wary of antihistamines. They are everywhere. In fact, it is hard to find a remedy that *doesn't* have an antihistamine on board. Although there is real doubt that they do anything for colds even in adults (they do provide some relief for allergies), in children they may cause more harm than good. See page 138 for a list of antihistamines common in over-the-counter cough and cold remedies.

Adults know that antihistamines make them drowsy. They assume the same thing happens to kids. Wrong! For reasons that are not entirely clear, many children react paradoxically to antihistamines. Such drugs can cause irritability, jitteriness, and insomnia.

Imagine the following scenario. Little Jimmy is snuffling and sneezing and has a nasty cough. It's bedtime and dear old dad thinks that a little of that leftover **NyQuil Adult Nighttime Cold/Flu Medicine, Cherry Flavor** would be just the thing. Big mistake. The antihistamine could have Jimmy wired for hours. Not only that, here is a remedy that also contains a decongestant (pseudoephedrine) that may also produce hyperactivity. There are even reports that some children have experienced terrifying visual hallucina-

tions—most of which involved insects or spiders—
after having taken a cold medicine containing both an
antihistamine and a decongestant. **NyQuil** also contains 25 percent alcohol (50 proof). What parent would
intentionally give a child a shot of booze? But that is
about what happens when you administer adult-for-
mula **Nyquil**. (See page 203 for other medications that
contain alcohol.)

The problem parents face is that many of these
over-the-counter products come with a drug interaction potential built in. These multi-symptom remedies
often contain three, four, or five ingredients. It's like
the proverbial kitchen sink. Even so-called pediatric
formulas may have antihistamines and decongestants
that could make a sick child feel worse.

The American Academy of Pediatrics has recommended single-ingredient cough preparations if your
child has a hack that keeps her awake. Small doses of
codeine are extremely effective. Dextromethorphan is
also helpful. Look for **Robitussin Pediatric Cough
Suppressant** or **St. Joseph Cough Suppressant for
Children**.

Antibiotics

Ask pediatricians what kind of prescriptions they
write most often and the answer will be antibiotics.
Children come down with all sorts of bugs—from
strep throat and ear infections to bronchitis and cysti-
tis. Out comes a prescription for **Amoxil** (amoxicillin), **Augmentin** (amoxicillin plus potassium clavulanate), **Bactrim** or **Septra** (co-trimoxazole), **Ceclor**
(cefaclor), **Ceftin** (cefuroxime), **Cefzil** (cefprozil),
Duricef (cefadroxil), **Lorabid** (loracarbef), **Pediazole**

(erythromycin ethylsuccinate and sulfisoxazole), **Polycillin** (ampicillin), or **Suprax** (cefixime).

Although some of these medicines can interact with other prescription drugs, the good news is that children are unlikely to be taking many other conflicting compounds. Anticoagulants, for example, are usually taken only by older people at risk for blood clots. Oral contraceptives are not likely to be an issue, except for some female adolescents.

The one interaction that we really do worry about, though, has to do with the antibiotic erythromycin. It is found in various formulations including **E.E.S.**, **ERYC**, **E-Mycin**, **EryPed**, **Ery-Tab**, **Eryzole**, **Ilosone**, **PCE**, and **Pediazole**. The nonsedating antihistamines **Seldane** and **Hismanal** may interact with erythromycin to produce life-threatening irregular heart rhythms.

This combination could be especially problematic for children, since a dermatologist could prescribe the antibiotic for acne, and an allergist could write a prescription for the antihistamine to relieve congestion. Neither might realize what the other had done. Such a combination could be a disaster. Please see pages 39–41 for other important erythromycin interactions, and talk to the pediatrician about these issues if she prescribes this common medicine.

Ritalin (methylphenidate)

This is probably the single most controversial medicine for children. These days it seems as if every fifth kid is on this drug for ADHD (attention deficit hyperactivity disorder). Children with ADHD have a hard time focusing or concentrating. Some also have a hard time sitting still and can become behavior problems as well.

We won't enter the battle of whether **Ritalin** is a good drug or a bad drug. No one really understands exactly how it works to help children stay on task. It is a stimulant, pharmacologically similar to amphetamine. Such drugs can make an adult hyper, but they tend to calm overactive children and allow them to focus. Some physicians and parents think **Ritalin** is evil incarnate. Others believe it is heaven-sent. No matter what your philosophy, **Ritalin** should be used only as part of a total treatment program, with behavioral modification and lots of support.

Ritalin has the potential to cause side effects such as irritability, jitteriness, skin rash, loss of appetite, stomach pain, weight loss, palpitations, mood swings, insomnia, and growth delay. Most children, however, do not experience such problems, especially if the dose is kept under control and the last pill is not taken late in the day. What concerns us more is the potential for dangerous interactions with drugs such as clonidine, **Tofranil,** and **Dilantin**.

Although we find it hard to understand, some physicians prescribe tricyclic antidepressants to children who have problems with bed-wetting. **Tofranil** (imipramine) and other drugs in this class have side effects such as urinary retention and delayed urination. Physicians have tried to employ this adverse reaction to prevent the condition they call enuresis (bed-wetting). While it may help some children, we find this to be a heavy-duty drug with a number of worrisome side effects including nervousness, tiredness, sleep problems, digestive upset, constipation, palpitations, and emotional instability. In overdose, tricyclic antidepressants can kill.

The problem occurs when you combine **Ritalin** and drugs such as **Tofranil**. This interaction may lead to increased levels of the tricyclic antidepressant in the bloodstream. There is a report that two adolescents developed dysfunctional behavior (including violence) and depression when put on this combination. While cause and effect has not been clearly established, we think the potential for such an interaction is strong enough to demand great caution.

The other interaction with **Ritalin** that concerns us involves the anticonvulsant drug **Dilantin** (phenytoin). Children with seizure disorders are frequently prescribed this medication. But anecdotal reports suggest that **Ritalin** could increase blood levels of **Dilantin** and possibly produce side effects such as dizziness, nausea, and headaches. If such a drug combination is contemplated, blood levels of phenytoin should be monitored very carefully. Side effects of **Dilantin** to watch out for include incoordination, confusion, dizziness, slurred speech, difficulty sleeping, muscle twitches, double vision, tiredness, tremor, nervousness, depression, bellyaches, headaches, diarrhea, and rashes.

How to Protect Your Children from Drug Interactions

Whenever you receive a prescription for a child, ask some important questions. First, always find out exactly what the medicine is, why it is being prescribed, how it should be taken (with food or on an empty stomach), and what side effects to watch out for. We will never forget the tragic story we heard from a grandmother who lost her grandchild because of a terrible skin side effect (Stevens-Johnson syndrome) brought on by an antibiotic. Neither the parents nor the physician realized this adverse reaction was caused by the medicine until it was too late. And always ask about interaction precautions. While children rarely receive more than one medicine at a time, it is better to be informed than ignorant.

Finally, be supercautious about giving children over-the-counter remedies. Never administer an adult drug to a child, and always check with your pediatrician to make sure what you are doing is appropriate. Children cannot defend themselves against adult ignorance. They trust us when we insist that the medicine is good for them. Such faith may be unwarranted. We all want our children to get better as quickly as possible, but don't let the cure become worse than the disease.

Drug Interactions That Affect Older People

In a very real sense this book is dedicated to people over 50. Just like a car that has accumulated more than 100,000 miles and may need some extra love and attention, an older person deserves admiration, support, and respect for surviving in what is often a cruel world.

Nowhere is the environment fraught with greater danger than in this crazy world of drug interactions. Here is a place where, as Lewis Carroll once wrote,

> "The time has come," the Walrus said,
> "To talk of many things:
> Of shoes—and ships—and sealing wax—
> Of cabbages—and kings—
> And why the sea is boiling hot—
> And whether pigs have wings."

Standard rules fall apart in this pharmacological wonderland. Because older people often see so many different kinds of physicians for a variety of ills, they are the ones most likely to suffer interaction misadventures. The rheumatologist may prescribe an arthritis medicine, the cardiologist could add a high blood pressure pill, something for heart palpitations, and aspirin to prevent blood clots. The gastroenterologist must deal with the stomach upset and possible ulceration so he adds several more prescriptions to the mix. A case of seborrheic dermatitis could send this patient to the dermatologist for more medicine. Oh, and let's not forget the urologist. As we age the plumbing tends to break down too.

As you can see, older people are the most likely targets for dangerous or deadly drug interactions. The nervous system can become more sensitive to a variety of medications, making us vulnerable to dizziness, drowsiness, or slowed reflexes. Now add to this the fact that liver and kidney function may gradually diminish as we age and you have a volatile mixture.

There is only one answer—vigilance. Become an active participant in your own health care. Ask questions and demand answers. Do not try to be a "good" patient if that means passivity. The meek may inherit the earth, but they may also die prematurely from deadly drug interactions. Ask your physician and pharmacist to check periodically on the compatibility of all your medicines, including over-the-counter remedies and even vitamins and minerals.

Look out for your friends, neighbors, and loved ones; they may not always be able to protect themselves. Why not loan them this book so they can do some checking of their own? Remember, good health is your most valuable possession. Fame and fortune fade very quickly in the face of illness and death.

References

1. Reid, Dee, Managing Editor, Publications, Family Health International. Personal letter, November 14, 1990.

2. Ibid.

3. *The Johns Hopkins Handbook of Drugs*. Margolis, Simeon, ed. New York: Rebus (Distributed by Random House), 1993.

4. *Drug Interaction Facts*. Tatro, David S., ed. St. Louis: Facts and Comparisons (A Wolters Kluwer Company), 1995.

5. Ibid.

6. Fleissig, A. "Unintended Pregnancies and the Use of Contraception: Changes from 1984 to 1989." *British Med. J.* 1991; 302:147

7. Orme, Michael L.E., and David J. Black, "Pharmacokinetics of Oral Contraceptive Steroids and Drug Interactions: Factors Affecting the Enterohepatic Circulation of Oral Contraceptive Steroids." *Am. J. Obs. Gyn.* 1990; 163(6S):2146–2152.

8. Orme, Michael, and David J. Black. "Unintended Pregnancies and Contraceptive Use." *British Med. J.* 1991; 302:789.

9. Guengerich, F. Peter. "Pharmacokinetics of Oral Contraceptive Steroids and Drug Interaction: Inhibition of Oral Contraceptive Steroid-Metabolizing Enzymes by Steroids and Drugs." *Am. J. Obs. Gyn.* 1990; 163(6S):2159–2163.

10. Fotherby, Kenneth. "Pharmacokinetics of Oral Contraceptive Steroids and Drug Interaction: Interactions with Oral Contraceptives." *Am. J. Obs. Gyn.* 1990; 163(6S):2153–2159.

11. Zachariasen, R.D. "Effect of Antibiotics on Oral Contraceptive Efficacy." *J. Dent. Hyg.* 1991; 65:334–338.

12. Fazio, A. "Oral Contraceptive Drug Interactions: Important Considerations." *South. Med. J.* 1991; 84:997–1002.

13. Shenfikeld, G.M., and J.M. Griffin. "Clinical Pharmacokinetics of Contraceptive Steroids. An Update." *Clin. Pharmacokinet.* 1991; 20:15–37.

14. Willis, Judith. "'The Pill' May Not Mix Well with Other Drugs." *FDA Consumer* 1987; 21(March):26.

15. Orme, Michael, and David J. Black. "Oral Contraceptive Steroids—Pharmacological Issues of Interest to the Prescribing Physician." *Adv. Contracept.* 1991; 7:325–331.

16. *Drug Interaction Facts.* Tatro, David S., ed. St. Louis: Facts & Comparisons (A Wolters Kluwer Company), 1995.

17. Welling, Peter, Parke-Davis/Warner Lambert. Personal Communication, December 22, 1993.

18. Brodie, Martin J. "Lamotrigine (Drug Profiles)" *Lancet* 1992; 339:1397–1401.

chapter eight

Drug/Alcohol Interactions

Alcohol is so much a part of our daily lives that most of us don't think of it as a drug. We have a glass of wine at lunch, a beer at the ball park, or a cocktail before dinner without a moment's hesitation; yet alcohol was one of the first drugs discovered by humans. Use of fermented beverages probably dates back to earliest civilization. If you can make bread, you can make beer.

Putting aside issues of alcohol abuse, we are most concerned with the very serious potential for this substance that is so much a part of our behavior to interact with other medications we may take. People rarely volunteer to their physicians that they occasionally indulge in a nightcap. It may seem too trivial a detail. And yet an amazing number of drugs can create unexpected and hazardous combinations with alcohol.

As we described in the introduction, sailors were among the first guinea pigs of drug and alcohol interaction. Captains of sailing ships often needed extra crew members at the last minute. Knowing that it might be hard to round up voluntary recruits, they sometimes made a deal with scurrilous bartenders. A likely prospect would be slipped some chloral hydrate (a tranquilizer that was a forerunner of barbiturates) in the rum or grog. The chloral hydrate produced a supra-additive effect. By delaying and modifying alcohol metabolism and adding a sedative action all its own, the drug would knock the sailor out cold. By the time he awoke, he could be far out at sea.

Many medicines can add to alcohol's wallop. Anti-anxiety agents such as **Librium**, **Tranxene**, **Valium**, or **Xanax** should never be combined with alcohol (even a beer) since reflexes can be slowed and mental function impaired at very low doses.

Antidepressants are a no-no for the same reason. Even a tension headache reliever such as **Fiorinal** or **Fioricet** (which contain the barbiturate butalbital) could get people into trouble if they also drink. Antihistamines are another danger. They are found in hundreds of allergy, cold, cough, and flu remedies. Always read labels, ask the pharmacist, and be cautious with OTC remedies.

Ulcer Drug/Alcohol Interactions

The most controversial drug/alcohol interactions involve drugs that may raise blood alcohol levels. Researchers have been fighting over this one for years, and the Food and Drug Administration has tried to make sense out of confusion. Because profits are at stake, pharmaceutical manufacturers have been battling to prove there is no problem. We are still undecided and await further research.

The controversy erupted when one of this country's leading alcohol investigators, Dr. Charles Lieber, reported that a number of common drugs could boost blood alcohol levels unexpectedly. What Dr. Lieber discovered was an enzyme in the stomach called alcohol dehydrogenase (ADH). According to his team of researchers, this enzyme breaks down some of the alcohol from a drink even before it is absorbed into the blood stream.[1, 2] ADH in the stomach diminishes with age and regular alcohol intake, and is present only at low levels in women. Perhaps this is why it is believed that some women seem to get drunk more easily than men after less alcohol.[3]

This esoteric enzyme would be of interest only to a few scientists except for one thing: a number of medicines can deactivate it. Dr. Lieber believes that these drugs could lead to higher blood alcohol levels and a longer period of elevated alcohol concentrations. His work has shown that aspirin (two extra-strength tablets) taken an hour before drinking interferes with ADH activity enough to cause a measurable increase of alcohol in the bloodstream.[4] There is preliminary evidence that some other drugs may also affect this enzyme, including acetaminophen and propranolol.

What really got the drug companies' attention, though, was the report that ranitidine (**Zantac**) and cimetidine (**Tagamet**) could also affect blood alcohol.[5,6] **Zantac** is one of the most successful drugs in the history of the pharmaceutical industry. Last year alone it earned roughly three billion dollars. **Tagamet** is not far behind. These drugs are prescribed for ulcers and bad heartburn (reflex esophagitis). Since drinkers often tend to have stomach trouble, you can see that they might be prime candidates for these medications.

Dr. Lieber and his colleagues concluded:"Thus our study revealed that ranitidine and cimetidine (but not famotidine) lead to substantial increases in blood alcohol levels after consumption of an amount of ethanol that corresponds to common social drinking. The blood alcohol levels achieved have been clearly shown to impair tasks that require a high degree of attention and motor coordination. Therefore, the possibility exists that some patients who are receiving treatment with these H_2-receptor antagonists may suffer unexpected impairment . . . a warning may be appropriate when these drugs are prescribed, especially in social drinkers who may drive vehicles or operate other machinery that require a high degree of attention and/or coordination."[7]

The article in which these findings were reported, published in *The Journal of the American Medical Association*, created a firestorm of controversy. The companies complained that the conclusions were not justified, that the results were inaccurate, that the studies were conducted incorrectly, that there was no clinical significance to the reaction, and that no warning or label change was necessary. Additional research has shown that Dr. Lieber's results are still debatable. Dr. M. D. Levitt reviewed all available data and concluded "very little, if any, metabolism of ethanol is likely to occur in the gastric mucosa, and the interaction between H_2-antagonists and ethanol is clinically insignificant."[8]

An expert committee for the Food and Drug Administration concluded in 1993 that although blood alcohol levels do go up, "H_2 blockers' interaction with alcohol has not been shown to be clinically significant."[9] So why have we belabored this issue if there is no problem? We are not yet convinced the final chapter has been written on this fascinating and controversial interaction. There is still disagreement among researchers, and Dr. Lieber believes that caution is appropriate. The FDA committee has called for more data to determine if there could be an effect on coordination, reflexes, or behavior. Until that work is completed, we urge people who take such drugs and drink alcohol to take care to be moderate in consumption and be vigilant for unexpected impairment.

Verapamil (Calan, Isoptin, Verelan)/ Alcohol Interactions

This is one of the most popular heart and high blood pressure medications on the market. It is far less likely to cause side effects when compared to drugs that used to be prescribed for hypertension. Millions of people rely on these pills to prevent heart disease, stroke, irregular heart rhythm, and chest pain.

We can claim with some assurance that verapamil does not mix well with alcohol. This medicine raises blood alcohol levels and prolongs the effect in the body. The subjects of this experiment were young healthy men and they felt inebriated longer. Goodness knows how older people taking other multiple prescriptions would be affected. The investigators concluded: "The findings of our study suggest that verapamil significantly inhibits ethanol elimination, resulting in elevated blood ethanol concentrations that prolong the intoxicating effects of alcohol."[10]

Beta Carotene/Alcohol Interactions

Beta carotene is popular in health food stores. It is a precursor to vitamin A, and people are swallowing these little orange pills with great enthusiasm. You can get beta carotene from carrots, other orange fruits and vegetables, and green leafy vegetables such as spinach, chard, and kale.

The excitement about beta carotene surrounds its antioxidant properties. This pharmacological action may help prevent heart disease and even certain cancers. But heavy drinkers, beware. Researchers at the Bronx Veterans Administration Hospital have found that the combination of booze and beta carotene could be hard on the liver. The preliminary studies have been done only on baboons. What they found was that the combination of alcohol and beta carotene led to more liver damage than that produced by alcohol exposure alone.[11] Although this work needs to be confirmed with further research on humans, the warning flags are flying. People who drink regularly and use beta carotene should discuss this interaction with their physician. Maybe some liver enzyme tests would be in order.

Conclusion

Alcohol is a drug, one of the most widely used in the world. Like any chemical compound it can interact with other medications. Please protect yourself and those around you from a dangerous combination. Too many people die on our highways because of the effects of alcohol. Check the following table for detailed information on the most common and dangerous drug/alcohol interactions.

Drug/Alcohol Interactions

DRUG	INTERACTION WITH ALCOHOL
Acetaminophen	The risk that this over-the-counter pain reliever might cause higher blood alcohol levels from modest amounts of alcohol is still uncertain and may not turn out to be terribly important. The real trouble comes when someone uses both acetaminophen and alcohol on a regular basis. This can put quite a strain on the liver, which metabolizes both drugs. You don't have to be an "alcoholic" to get into trouble. If you have a drink every day, don't make a habit of using medicines containing acetaminophen. Not only might you risk serious liver damage, but also you might find that ordinary doses are less effective than expected and be tempted to take extra. Be alert for acetaminophen in many other products besides nonprescription pain relievers. It is an ingredient in many cold, allergy, or sinus formulas, menstrual cramp remedies, and even a number of prescription pain relievers (for example, **Darvocet-N** and **Tylox**). Be sure to read the label of any medication if you need to watch for this interaction.
Antabuse	This interaction is almost too obvious to mention. It can, however, be extremely hazardous. **Antabuse** (disulfiram) is prescribed for alcoholics who need chemical assistance to reinforce their resolve to abstain. In

DRUG	INTERACTION WITH ALCOHOL
	combination with alcohol, even the small amounts found in cough syrup or cold remedies, this medication produces violent illness. The symptoms are nausea, vomiting, stomach cramps, palpitations, flushing, low blood pressure, blurred vision, breathing problems, and headache. In some cases, the reaction could be lethal, so anyone on **Antabuse** really needs to watch out for alcohol.
Anticoagulants **Coumadin** warfarin	Moderate to heavy drinkers (at least two or three drinks daily) may metabolize blood thinners such as **Coumadin** (warfarin) more rapidly. This could be a problem if a person suddenly changed drinking habits dramatically. The dose of the medicine might need adjustment. For most people an occasional beer or cocktail is not likely to interfere with anticoagulant medication.
Antidepressants amitriptyline desipramine **Desyrel** doxepin **Elavil** **Endep** **Norpramin** **Pertofrane** **Sinequan** **Surmontil** **Tofranil** **Triavil**	Beware! Some antidepressants can make people feel drowsy or "spaced out." They may have trouble paying attention. Alcohol in addition could make matters worse and affect coordination. A drink or two can also slow metabolism of amitriptyline and possibly other antidepressants. Driving or operating machines may become far more dangerous with the double whammy of alcohol and medicine.

DRUG	INTERACTION WITH ALCOHOL
Antidepressants **Wellbutrin**	The antidepressant **Wellbutrin** (bupropion) can cause trouble when combined with alcohol. Susceptibility to seizures may increase when people change drinking patterns. Abstinence is recommended.
Antihistamines	Most antihistamines, except for **Claritin**, **Hismanal**, and **Seldane**, tend to make people feel groggy and less than completely alert. In fact, a person taking a sedating nonprescription antihistamine such as **Benadryl**, for example, might be just as dangerous behind the wheel as someone who is legally drunk. Alcohol can intensify this common reaction. Remember, cold medicines as well as allergy pills may contain antihistamines. Do not drive or do anything else requiring attention if you have had alcohol together with such medication. Reflexes and coordination could be seriously impaired.
Anxiety Pills **Ativan** diazepam **Klonopin** **Librium** meprobamate **Paxipam** **Serax** **Tranxene** **Valium** **Xanax**	We worry more about this drug alcohol interaction than most others because it is so common. People swallow tons of anti-anxiety agents and often seem to take these drugs for granted. But many of these compounds, both the popular benzodiazepines such as **Xanax** and the much older meprobamate (**Equanil** or **Miltown**), can alter reaction time and interfere with driving ability. Adding alcohol can lead to severe

DRUG	INTERACTION WITH ALCOHOL
	impairment of coordination and concentration, worse than with alcohol alone. Do not try to drive or engage in work that requires hand–eye coordination if you take one of these drugs and have anything to drink.
Aspirin and Salicylates **Alka-Seltzer** **Anacin** **Ascriptin** aspirin **Bayer Aspirin** **Bufferin** **Excedrin caplets** **Pepto-Bismol** and others	Many people pop a few aspirin tablets before going out for a big night on the town in the hope of heading off a hangover. New research suggests this might be a bad idea. Not only could it increase stomach irritation, but also it could make someone more impaired because of higher blood alcohol levels. One study found that aspirin taken an hour before drinking a modest amount of alcohol (one and a half drinks) raised levels in the bloodstream 26 percent. The authors caution that this could be enough to "impair some complex forms of human behavior." Be careful.
Barbiturates **Amytal** **Butisol** **Fiorinal** **Gemonil** **Mysoline** **Nembutal** phenobarbital **Seconal** **Tuinal** and others	Barbiturates don't mix well with alcohol at all. The interaction is actually rather complicated, because it differs if people are regular drinkers or go on a binge. Those who imbibe every day or several times a week metabolize these medicines more rapidly. The medicine may not work as it should. In some cases, that could lead to seizures. Both barbiturates and alcohol can put a strain on the liver.

DRUG	INTERACTION WITH ALCOHOL
Barbiturates cont'd	People who don't usually drink and then have a couple of stiff ones also get into big trouble. They may become incapable of doing complicated things such as driving, walking, or even breathing. If you are taking one of these medicines, play it safe and steer clear of alcohol in any guise, including medicines. See the list on page 203.
Beta-Blockers atenolol **Blocadren** **Cartrol** **Corgard** **Inderal** **Lopressor** propranolol **Tenormin** timolol and others	Heart and blood pressure medicines such as **Corgard**, **Inderal**, **Lopressor**, **Tenormin**, and others like them may be affected by alcohol. Beta-blockers like these can increase the impact alcohol has on reflexes and coordination. Current research suggests this is not usually a serious interaction unless you are driving, but you might want to be judicious in your alcohol intake.
Beta Carotene	Beta carotene, a building block for vitamin A, may help reduce the risk of heart disease or even some types of cancer. This supplement may be harmful, however, to people who are regular or heavy drinkers. In studies on baboons, the combination of alcohol and beta carotene led to more liver damage than that produced by alcohol exposure alone. This work needs to be confirmed with further research on humans. See page 188 for further details.

DRUG	INTERACTION WITH ALCOHOL
Cephalosporin Antibiotics Cefobid Cefotan Mandol Moxam	Some of these high-powered antibiotics for injection can trigger an **Antabuse**-like reaction. **Cefobid, Cefotan, Mandol,** and **Moxam** are all reported to cause flushing, wheezing and breathing difficulties, nausea and vomiting, sweating, and rapid heart beat after alcohol ingestion. These medicines would normally be given in the hospital, but the effect can last up to two or three days after stopping the antibiotic. Celebrating a hospital discharge prematurely could land you back there! **Monocid** or **Precef** might interact in a very similar way. It would be wise to avoid medicines containing alcohol. See the table on page 203.
Diabetes Drugs DiaBeta Diabinese Dymelor Glucotrol Micronase Orinase Tolinase	Oral diabetes medicines interact in peculiar ways with alcohol. People on **Glucotrol** may find that their blood sugar stays low longer after a drink or two, but drinkers on **Orinase** might discover that its effectiveness starts wearing off more quickly. In other words, more than a single drink from time to time could make blood sugar harder to control. **Diabinese** is reported to interact with alcohol much as **Antabuse** does, producing flushing, headache, nausea, a burning sensation, and rapid heart beat. This unpleasant experience is more likely with moderate or heavy alcohol intake. Even people on other diabetes pills, such as **DiaBeta, Dymelor, Micronase,** and **Tolinase,** would be wise to exercise caution.

DRUG	INTERACTION WITH ALCOHOL

Ibuprofen
  Advil
  Ibuprin
  Medipren
  Motrin IB
  Nuprin
  and others
	This popular pain reliever may interact with alcohol in several ways. For one thing, both ibuprofen and alcohol can have a negative effect on the digestive tract. Regular use could increase the risk of indigestion, heartburn, and even ulceration. There is also the possibility that ibuprofen may prolong the effects of alcohol within the system. Although this interaction is not yet well documented, it would be wise to use caution in drinking if you are relying on ibuprofen for pain relief.

Indomethacin
  Indocin
	Indomethacin and alcohol are both irritating to the digestive tract and should not be ingested together. Equally dangerous is their combined effect on the brain. **Indocin** can cause dizziness, drowsiness, and incoordination. Combined with alcohol, this complication could be aggravated.
	
	    Most other anti-inflammatory agents can cause stomach upset, and many can produce some degree of sedation. People taking **Anaprox**, **Ansaid**, **Clinoril**, **Feldene**, **Lodine**, **Meclomen**, **Motrin**, **Nalfon**, **Naprosyn**, **Orudis**, **Tolectin**, and **Voltaren** should also be prudent and avoid alcoholic beverages.

Ketoconazole **Nizoral**	**Nizoral** (ketoconazole) is a very effective antifungal drug. It can, however, cause liver toxicity and requires periodic monitoring with blood tests.

DRUG	INTERACTION WITH ALCOHOL

Regular drinking might increase the risk of liver problems.

There are also reports that some individuals may react to the combination of alcohol and **Nizoral** with symptoms of nausea, headache, flushing, and discomfort, apparently similar to an **Antabuse** reaction. Watch out for medicines that contain alcohol, page 203.

Major Tranquilizers
chlorpromazine
Compazine
Mellaril
Permitil
Phenergan
Prolixin
Serentil
Sparine
Stelazine
Temaril
Thorazine
Tindal
Trilafon
Vesprin

Many of the medicines used to treat serious mental disturbances can make people feel "spaced out" or interfere with their alertness. Add alcohol, and you have a situation in which dizziness, drowsiness, and lack of coordination could become downright dangerous. Muscle twitching and uncontrolled movements can be triggered with such a combination.

No one taking a major tranquilizer should be drinking. Driving is dangerous with these medicines all by themselves. If someone were foolish enough to add even one glass of wine, he could be a major hazard on the highways. Don't do it!

Methotrexate
Methotrate
Rheumatrex

Methotrexate is a potent medication used to treat cancer, severe arthritis, and psoriasis. It can cause liver toxicity and requires very careful monitoring. Since alcohol can also injure the liver, it is probably a good idea to avoid drinking alcoholic beverages while on methotrexate.

DRUG	INTERACTION WITH ALCOHOL
Metoclopramide **Reglan**	Few people would suspect that their medicine for heartburn can interact with a beer or cocktail. But **Reglan** can cause drowsiness, involuntary muscle movements, and dizziness. Alcohol could make such reactions worse. It would be prudent to avoid alcoholic beverages.

Metronidazole
  Femizole
  Flagyl
  Metizol
  Metryl
  Protostat
	This medication is useful for fighting a number of infections. It can cause dizziness, unsteadiness, and incoordination all by itself. These side effects may be aggravated by alcohol. In addition, some people experience nausea, vomiting, stomach cramps, flushing, and headaches when they consume alcohol together with metronidazole. Best to avoid drinking while on this drug.

Narcotics
  codeine
  Darvocet
  Darvon
  Demerol
  Empirin w/ Codeine
  Percocet
  Percodan
  propoxyphene
  Talwin
  Tylenol w/ Codeine
  Tylox
  Vicodin
	Heavy-duty pain relievers can themselves interfere with alertness and coordination. In combination with alcohol, any of them could make a person feel like a zombie. Driving or doing anything that requires concentration would be a big mistake. Medical examiners see far too many overdose deaths associated with this combination of drugs. Stay alive– don't imbibe.

DRUG	INTERACTION WITH ALCOHOL
Nitroglycerin **Nitro-Bid** **Nitro-Dur** **Nitrostat** **Transderm-Nitro,** and others	Nitroglycerin comes in many formulations. There are pills (**Nitro-Bid**, **Nitrong**, **Nitrostat**), ointments (**Nitrol**), and transdermal patches (**Minitran**, **Nitrodisc**, **Nitro-Dur**, and **Transderm-Nitro**). No matter how you use nitro, though, you should avoid alcohol, as it may lower your blood pressure and make you dizzy and vulnerable to fainting and falls.
Hormone Replacement Therapy *Oral Contraceptives*	Alcohol appears to boost circulating estrogen levels. Higher exposure to alcohol has been linked to breast cancer, so this may explain why women who drink are at greater risk of the disease.
Parlodel bromocriptine	**Parlodel** (bromocriptine) may produce more severe side effects if alcohol is taken at the same time. Watch out for nausea, stomach pain, and dizziness.
Sleeping Pills **Dalmane** **Doral** **Doriden** **Halcion** **ProSom** **Restoril**	This drug/alcohol interaction is, unfortunately, all too common. A lot of people take sleeping pills, and often take these drugs for granted. But many of these compounds can cause drowsiness, incoordination, and slow reaction time. In combination with a nightcap, coordination and concentration could be severely impaired. This is true of both the old-

DRUG	INTERACTION WITH ALCOHOL
Sleeping Pills *cont'd*	fashioned sleeping pills such as **Doriden** and the benzodiazepines. A long-acting sleeping pill such as **Dalmane** taken the night before can even interact badly with a drink or two the next afternoon. If you need sleeping pills, it is better to avoid alcohol.
Time Capsules **Compazine Spansule** **Dexedrine Spansule** **Isoclor Timesule** **Nicobid Tempule** **Ornade Spansule** **Tuss-Ornade** **Spansule**	This interaction is controversial, but if you use one of these timed-release medicines, you may want to keep it in mind. The fear is that alcohol might dissolve the protective coating that would normally slow absorption and spread it out over several hours. Once this coating is gone, the active ingredients can quickly end up in the bloodstream, and instead of 12-hour action you might end up getting too much medicine too fast. Play it safe and avoid alcohol when taking any slow-release time capsules.
Tuberculosis Drug **INH** **Laniazid** **Nydrazid**	Isoniazid, a medication often used in combination with others to treat tuberculosis, has the potential to be harmful to the liver. Regular intake of alcohol (drinking every day or several times a week) increases the risk of drug-induced hepatitis. This is a nasty possibility and is better avoided.

DRUG	INTERACTION WITH ALCOHOL
Ulcer Drugs **Tagamet** **Zantac**	There is controversy over the clinical significance of this interaction. Research has shown that **Tagamet**, **Zantac**, and possibly **Axid** can interfere with the activity of the stomach enzyme called alcohol dehydrogenase. Since some alcohol may be metabolized by this enzyme even before it gets into the bloodstream, drinking while on one of these ulcer medications could lead to higher blood alcohol levels. The manufacturers of **Zantac** and **Tagamet** insist that this interaction is unimportant in the real world, as investigations showed the biggest effect in men who drink modestly, just about one and a half or two drinks, after eating. Although in such a situation a man might be more impaired than he realized, he might not be legally drunk. We agree with the researchers, who concluded, "A warning may be appropriate when these drugs are prescribed, especially in social drinkers who may drive vehicles or operate other machinery that require a high degree of attention and/or coordination." [7]
Verapamil **Calan** **Isoptin** **Verelan**	A careful study has shown that a standard amount of alcohol results in higher blood alcohol levels that last longer in the body when a person is taking verapamil. This could interfere with the judgment and coordination

DRUG	INTERACTION WITH ALCOHOL
Verapamil cont'd	needed to drive or do other complex tasks. A person who had not been warned about this interaction might not realize how much more impaired he or she would become.
Vitamin C	Here's a twist. In one study, the volunteers who took 1 gram of ascorbic acid (vitamin C) every day for two weeks got the alcohol out of their bloodstream slightly more quickly. Perhaps they revved up their alcohol dehydrogenase this way; no one is quite sure. This doesn't offer license to go out and drink heavily, but it shows it's hard to go wrong with vitamin C.

Medicines Containing Alcohol

Alcohol is an ingredient in many over-the-counter and even some prescription medicines. The amounts are modest in most cases, but a few reach concentrations of 40 or 50 proof. Cough and cold elixirs are the most likely sources, but some vitamin "tonics" and laxatives also contain alcohol.

For most people, the amount of alcohol in a spoonful of cough syrup is negligible. Anyone taking a medicine that reacts with alcohol the same way **Antabuse** does need to be especially cautious. Some alcohol-containing medicines are listed below. Careful label reading is also advised.

Ambenyl-D
   Decongestant
Benadryl Plus Nighttime
Benylin Decongestant
Black-Draught
Cheracol Plus Head
   Cold/Cough Formula
Comtrex Liquid
Contac Nighttime Cold
   Medicine Liquid
Entex Liquid
Geravite Elixir
Geriplex-FS Liquid
Gevrabon Liquid
Hycotuss Expectorant
Lomotil Liquid
Medi-Flu Liquid
Novahistine Elixir
NyQuil Nighttime Cold
Peri-Colace
Pertussin PM Liquid
Phenergan VC Syrup
Senokot Syrup
Triaminic Expectorant
   with Codeine
Trind Liquid
Tussar SF Syrup
Tuss-Ornade Liquid
Tylenol Cold Night Time
Vicks Formula 44
   (D or M) Liquid
Vigortol Liquid
Vitamin B
   Complex Elixir
Zantac Syrup

References

1. Caballeria, J., et al. "The Contribution of the Stomach to Ethanol Oxidation in the Rat." *Life Sci.* 1987; 41:1021–1027.

2. Caballeria, J., et al. "Gastric Origin of the First-Pass Metabolism of Ethanol in Humans: Effects of Gastrectomy." *Gastroenterology* 1989; 97:1205–1209.

3. Frezza, C., et al. "High Blood Alcohol Levels in Women. The Role of Decreased Gastric Alcohol Dehydrogenase Activity and Blood Ethanol Levels. *N. Engl. J. Med.* 1990; 322:95–99.

4. Roine, Risto, et al. "Aspirin Increases Blood Alcohol Concentrations in Humans after Ingestion of Ethanol." *JAMA* 1990; 264:2406–2408.

5. DiPadova, Carlo, et al. "Effects of Ranitidine on Blood Alcohol Levels after Ethanol Ingestion." *JAMA* 1992; 267:83–86.

6. Caballeria J., et al. "Effects of Cimetidine on Gastric Alcohol Dehydrogenase Activity and Blood Ethanol Levels." *Gastroenterology* 1989; 96:388–392.

7. DiPadova, op. cit.

8. Levitt, M.D. "Review Article: Lack of Clinical Significance of the Interaction Between H_2-receptor Antagonists and Ethanol." *Aliment. Pharmacol. Ther.* 1993; 7:131–138.

9. F.D.C Reports: "The Pink Sheet." March 22, 1993, pp. 10–11.

10. Bauer, L.A., et al. "Verapamil Inhibits Ethanol Elimination and Prolongs the Perception of Intoxication." *Clin. Pharmacol. Ther.* 1992; 52:6–10.

11. Leo, M.A.: "Interaction of Ethanol with B-Carotene: Delayed Blood Clearance and Enhanced Hepatotoxicity." *Hepatology* 1992; 15:883–891.

References for the Drug/Alcohol Interactions Table

DiPadova, C., et al. "Effects of Ranitidine on Blood Alcohol Levels after Ethanol Ingestion." *JAMA* 1992; 267:83–86.

Graedon, J. *The People's Pharmacy-2.* New York: Avon, 1980.

Graedon, J., and T. Graedon. *The People's Pharmacy (Totally New & Revised).* New York: St. Martin's Press, 1985.

Hansten, P. D., and J.R. Horn, eds. *Drug Interactions and Updates.* Vancouver, Wash.: Applied Therapeutics, 1993.

Holford, N. "Clinical Pharmacokinetics of Ethanol." *Clin. Pharmacokinet.* 1987; 13:273–292.

Leo, M.A., et al. "Interaction of Ethanol with ß-Carotene: Delayed Blood Clearance and Enhanced Hepatotoxicity." *Hepatology* 1992; 15:883–891.

Palmer, R.H., et al. "Effects of Various Concomitant Medications on Gastric Alcohol Dehydrogenase and the First-Pass Metabolism of Ethanol." *Am J. Gastroenterology* 1991; 86:1749–1755.

Roine, R., et al. "Aspirin Increases Blood Alcohol Concentrations in Humans after Ingestion of Ethanol." *JAMA* 1990; 264:2406–2408.

Tatro, D., ed. *Drug Interaction Facts.* St. Louis: Facts & Comparisons (A Wolters Kluwer Company), 1993.

Yamanaka-Yuen, N. "Ethanol and Drug Interactions." *Drug Interactions Newsletter* 1985; 5:45–58.

Guides to Dangerous
Drug Interactions

Attention

These guides are not intended as a substitute for the medical advice of physicians. Due to space limitations, the charts do not include every serious or potentially deadly drug interaction that has been reported in the medical literature.

This is a constantly changing field. After we completed the book, controversial interactions continued to come to our attention. For example, **Luvox** (fluvoxamine), a **Prozac**-like drug that is prescribed for obsessive-compulsive disorder, has the potential for very dangerous interactions with **Anafranil** (clomipramine), **Elavil** (amitriptyline), **Eldepryl** (selegiline), **Hismanal** (astemizole), **Nardil** (phenelzine), **Parnate** (tranylcypromine), **Surmontil** (trimipramine), and **Tofranil** (imipramine). Doubtless other serious interactions will come to light.

Please remember that certain drugs with potentially lethal interactions can be successfully used together if appropriate monitoring and other precautions are undertaken. To better use these guides, take a moment to review the explanation on pages 15 to 19. Anyone who discovers an interaction in this book that is of concern must consult a physician before making any changes in drug therapy. **Every reader must consult with his or her physician before starting or stopping any medication.** Any side effects should be reported promptly to a physician.

Anti-Anxiety Drugs (BENZODIAZEPINES)

Ativan	Dalmane	Doral	Halcion	Klonopin
Librium	Paxipam	ProSom	Restoril	Serax
Tranxene	Valium	Versed	Xanax	

DANGEROUS

Alcohol beer liquor wine
Antibiotics (macrolides) E.E.S. E-Mycin ERYC EryPed
Ery-Tab Erythrocin Ilosone PCE Pediazole Tao
Drugs for Schizophrenia Clozaril Loxitane
Heart Drug (digoxin) Lanoxin

TROUBLESOME

Anticonvulsants (hydantoins) Dilantin Mesantoin
Peganone
Antidepressant (serotonin type) Prozac
Heart/Blood Pressure Drugs (beta-blockers) Inderal
Lopressor Toprol XL
Ulcer Drugs Prilosec Tagamet

Not every benzodiazepine drug interacts with each drug listed on this tree. See individual descriptions for details. Be sure to check with your physician and pharmacist if you must take any other drugs in combination with a benzodiazepine.

Never take or stop medication without your doctor's advice.

| **Anti-Anxiety Drugs** | **Alcohol** |

(BENZODIAZEPINES)

DANGEROUS

BRAND NAME	GENERIC NAME	NAME
Ativan	lorazepam	beer
Dalmane	flurazepam	liquor
Doral	quazepam	wine
Halcion	triazolam	medicines that contain alcohol
Klonopin	clonazepam	
Librium	chlordiazepoxide	
Paxipam	halazepam	
ProSom	estazolam	
Restoril	temazepam	
Serax	oxazepam	
Tranxene	clorazepate	
Valium	diazepam	
Versed	midazolam	
Xanax	alprazolam	

INSTRUCTIONS

The absorption and effects of alcohol are magnified if you drink on an empty stomach. Fatty food can delay alcohol absorption. If you drink, do so in moderation, and never drive.

INSTRUCTIONS

These drugs may be taken with food, especially if they upset the digestive tract.

INTERACTIONS

Benzodiazepines such as Valium, Librium, and Xanax can make people more relaxed, uncoordinated, confused, sedated, and unsteady. Reflexes and judgment may also be affected. Alcohol can cause many of the same effects. Combine alcohol with an anti-anxiety agent and driving becomes extremely hazardous, as does any task that requires alertness, good reflexes, and judgment. Older people may be more likely to fall. That could lead to a hip fracture, which can be devastating or lethal. Be safe; don't mix alcohol with sedating drugs.

Symptoms of Alcohol or Benzodiazepine Overdose

This interaction could lead to symptoms of overdose such as disorientation, unsteadiness, confusion, slurred speech, drowsiness, dizziness, or loss of motor coordination. Driving or operating machinery would be a mistake. Contact your physician if such symptoms occur.

Never take or stop medication without your doctor's advice.

Anti-Anxiety Drugs	Antibiotics
(BENZODIAZEPINES)	(MACROLIDES)

DANGEROUS

BRAND NAME	GENERIC NAME
Halcion	triazolam
Versed	midazolam
(other benzodiazepines may also be affected)	

INSTRUCTIONS

Halcion may be taken with food, especially if it upsets the digestive tract. It should be taken just before bedtime.

BRAND NAME	GENERIC NAME
E.E.S.	erythromycin
E-Mycin	erythromycin
ERYC	erythromycin
EryPed	erythromycin
Ery-Tab	erythromycin
Erythrocin	erythromycin
Ilosone	erythromycin
PCE	erythromycin
Pediazole	erythromycin
Tao	troleandomycin

INSTRUCTIONS

Some forms of erythromycin must be taken on an empty stomach; others may be taken with food See the table of Food and Drug Compatibility on pages 73–91 for specifics.

INTERACTION

Erythromycin and Tao appear to have a profound effect on the metabolism of certain benzodiazepines. Blood levels of Halcion could be doubled by erythromycin. Tao has increased blood levels of Halcion by over 100 percent and has prolonged the action of the drug in the body. Elevated levels of Halcion can lead to cognitive impairment and amnesia.

Erythromycin may also have an important impact on Versed, and can cause blood levels of this preanesthetic to climb. This could create increased sedation during or after surgery. Anyone taking such antibiotics must alert the surgeon and anesthesiologist before surgery so that they can anticipate any potential problems due to this interaction.

Symptoms of Benzodiazepine Overdose

This interaction could lead to symptoms of overdose such as disorientation, unsteadiness, confusion, slurred speech, drowsiness, dizziness, amnesia, and loss of motor coordination. Some other benzodiazepines may also be affected by these antibiotics. Contact your physician if such symptoms occur.

Never take or stop medication without your doctor's advice.

Anti-Anxiety Drugs
(BENZODIAZEPINES)

Drugs for Schizophrenia

DANGEROUS

BRAND NAME	GENERIC NAME
Ativan	lorazepam
Valium	diazepam

BRAND NAME	GENERIC NAME
Clozaril	clozapine
Loxitane	loxapine

INSTRUCTIONS

Ativan and Valium may be taken with food, especially if they upset the digestive tract.

INSTRUCTIONS

The dose should be individualized. Driving is dangerous. Those on Loxitane should avoid sunlight (unless adequately protected) because it may cause a bad sunburn. Clozaril patients require weekly blood tests. They should notify the doctor promptly of fever above 100.4°F.

INTERACTION

A number of cases in the medical literature point to an interaction between loxapine and lorazepam, as well as between Clozaril and Valium or Ativan. These patients, treated with both drugs, developed difficulty breathing and very low blood pressure. In some instances respiration slowed to between four and eight breaths a minute. One patient died, although it is unclear whether the interaction was responsible. Many patients fell deeply asleep and could not be roused. The stupor lasted a number of hours.

Research on this interaction is incomplete and many patients do well with a benzodiazepine and one of these schizophrenia medicines. Because there is potential for a dangerous interaction, though, it would seem prudent to try to avoid such a combination if possible. If these drugs are prescribed simultaneously, patients should have vital signs monitored closely!

Symptoms of an Adverse Lorazepam/Loxapine or Diazepam/ Clozapine Reaction

Dizziness, drowsiness, and fatigue may occur quickly and lead to delirium or stupor, low blood pressure, and very slow breathing. Blue fingernails and lips are a danger sign. Careful monitoring of respiration and blood pressure are essential. Notify the physician immediately of any such symptoms of an adverse interaction.

Never take or stop medication without your doctor's advice.

Anti-Anxiety Drugs
(BENZODIAZEPINES)

Heart Drug
(DIGOXIN)

DANGEROUS

BRAND NAME	GENERIC NAME
Ativan	lorazepam
Dalmane	flurazepam
Doral	quazepam
Halcion	triazolam
Klonopin	clonazepam
Librium	chlordiazepoxide
Paxipam	halazepam
ProSom	estazolam
Restoril	temazepam
Serax	oxazepam
Tranxene	clorazepate
Valium	diazepam
Versed	midazolam
Xanax	alprazolam

INSTRUCTIONS
These drugs may be taken with food, especially if they upset the digestive tract.

BRAND NAME	GENERIC NAME
Lanoxin	digoxin

INSTRUCTIONS
Digoxin should be taken in a consistent fashion, preferably with food but not with a meal high in fiber. Bran may limit the absorption of this drug.

Do not stop this medicine unless your doctor so directs.

INTERACTION
Valium (diazepam) has been shown to raise the blood levels of digoxin. One woman had a dramatic jump in digoxin after she started taking Xanax at bedtime for insomnia. She experienced symptoms of digoxin toxicity, including digestive tract upset, fatigue, and "head pressure." This Xanax and digoxin interaction remains unconfirmed in a more scientific study, however. Other benzodiazepines have not be adequately tested. Until such research is completed, people should have their digoxin levels monitored frequently if they need to take a benzodiazepine-type drug simultaneously.

Symptoms of Digoxin Toxicity
Nausea, vomiting, loss of appetite, diarrhea, stomach pain, visual disturbances (green or yellow tint and a halo around lights), weakness, drowsiness, depression, confusion, palpitations, rash, headaches, and hallucinations. Notify the doctor immediately if you experience any of these symptoms.

Never take or stop medication without your doctor's advice.

Anti-Anxiety Drugs (BENZODIAZEPINES)	**Anticonvulsants** (HYDANTOINS)

TROUBLESOME

BRAND NAME	GENERIC NAME	BRAND NAME	GENERIC NAME
Ativan	lorazepam	**Dilantin**	phenytoin
Dalmane	flurazepam	**Mesantoin**	mephenytoin
Doral	quazepam	**Peganone**	ethotoin
Halcion	triazolam		
Librium	chlordiazepoxide		
Paxipam	halazepam		
ProSom	estazolam		
Restoril	temazepam		
Serax	oxazepam		
Tranxene	clorazepate		
Valium	diazepam		
Xanax	alprazolam		

INSTRUCTIONS (Anticonvulsants)
Any of these medicines could upset the stomach. This is less likely if they are taken with food. All of them can cause drowsiness or blurred vision and could make driving dangerous.

INSTRUCTIONS (Anti-Anxiety)
These drugs may be taken with food, especially if they upset the digestive tract.

INTERACTION

This is a confusing interaction. The data are contradictory and no firm conclusions can be drawn. Nevertheless, there is some concern that Dilantin (phenytoin) levels may be increased by Valium or Librium. Some patients have apparently experienced symptoms of phenytoin toxicity as a result of this combination. Experts suggest that if patients need a benzodiazepine in addition to Dilantin, their blood phenytoin levels be monitored carefully, especially when starting or stopping the benzodiazepine. Although there is no information about anti-anxiety drugs other than Valium and Librium, the possibility exists that other benzodiazepines might interact as well.

Symptoms of Phenytoin Toxicity

Uncontrollable eye movements (nystagmus), unsteadiness, difficulty speaking clearly, dizziness, and stupor. Notify your physician immediately of any of these symptoms.

Never take or stop medication without your doctor's advice.

Anti-Anxiety Drugs (BENZODIAZEPINES)	**Antidepressant** (SEROTONIN-BASED)

TROUBLESOME

BRAND NAME	GENERIC NAME
Valium	diazepam
Xanax	alprazolam

INSTRUCTIONS
These drugs may be taken with food, especially if they upset the digestive tract.

BRAND NAME	GENERIC NAME
Prozac	fluoxetine

INSTRUCTIONS
Prozac is taken in the morning, or, if a higher dose has been prescribed, in the morning and at noon. It may be taken without regard to meals. Taking it with food may reduce stomach upset. A few patients experience serious weight loss on this medication. If this occurs, the doctor should be notified.

INTERACTION

This is not a particularly worrisome interaction. In fact, physicians may often prescribe drugs such as Valium or Xanax to counteract the jittery feelings and insomnia that are sometime associated with Prozac. If this combination is contemplated, however, there should be some consideration for the potential of these drugs to interact. Reports have surfaced linking Prozac to slightly higher blood levels of diazepam. Diazepam lasted longer in the body when people were also taking Prozac. The clinical significance of this interaction is unclear. Data on Xanax and Prozac are contradictory. One study demonstrated a slight effect while another showed no impact. There may be no cause for concern, but until further research is done people should be alert for increased effects from Valium or Xanax. Tasks that require coordination and attentiveness, like driving, could be affected.

Symptoms of Benzodiazepine Overdose
Disorientation, unsteadiness, confusion, slurred speech, drowsiness, dizziness, amnesia, and loss of motor coordination are tipoffs to overdose. Driving is hazardous! Contact the physician immediately if any such signs of overdose appear.

Never take or stop medication without your doctor's advice.

Anti-Anxiety Drugs
(BENZODIAZEPINES)

Heart/Blood Pressure Drugs
(BETA-BLOCKERS)

TROUBLESOME

BRAND NAME	GENERIC NAME
Dalmane	flurazepam
Halcion	triazolam
Librium	chlordiazepoxide
Tranxene	clorazepate
Valium	diazepam
Xanax	alprazolam

INSTRUCTIONS
These drugs may be taken with food, especially if they upset the digestive tract.

BRAND NAME	GENERIC NAME
Inderal	propranolol
Lopressor	metoprolol
Toprol XL	metoprolol

INSTRUCTIONS
Propranolol and metoprolol are best absorbed with meals, but consistency is the most important factor. These drugs should be taken at about the same time every day. Do not stop any of these medicines suddenly except on doctor's orders. Serious side effects could result.

INTERACTION

Blood levels of diazepam may be slightly increased by beta-blockers such as metoprolol or propranolol. The anti-anxiety agent also appears to persist longer in the body. People may find they are less alert when on such a combination and their visual acuity and reaction time might be affected. Serax does not seem to be impacted by propranolol. Be sensitive for any change in consciousness.

Symptoms of Benzodiazepine Overdose
This interaction could lead to symptoms of overdose such as disorientation, unsteadiness, confusion, slurred speech, drowsiness, dizziness, amnesia, or loss of motor coordination. Some other benzodiazepines may also be affected by these beta-blockers. Contact your physician if such symptoms occur.

Never take or stop medication without your doctor's advice.

Anti-Anxiety Drugs
(BENZODIAZEPINES)

Ulcer Drugs

TROUBLESOME

BRAND NAME	GENERIC NAME
Ativan	lorazepam
Dalmane	flurazepam
Doral	quazepam
Halcion	triazolam
Klonopin	clonazepam
Librium	chlordiazepoxide
Paxipam	halazepam
ProSom	estazolam
Restoril	temazepam
Serax	oxazepam
Tranxene	clorazepate
Valium	diazepam
Versed	midazolam
Xanax	alprazolam

INSTRUCTIONS
These drugs may be taken with food, especially if they upset the digestive tract.

BRAND NAME	GENERIC NAME
Prilosec	omeprazole
Tagamet	cimetidine

INSTRUCTIONS
Tagamet is usually taken with meals and/or at bedtime. Antacids may reduce absorption of Tagamet; do not take one for at least two hours after taking Tagamet. Prilosec should be taken just before eating, preferably in the morning.

INTERACTION
Tagamet can increase blood levels of benzodiazepines and prolong their stay in the body. Sedation and impairment could result, especially for older people. This interaction remains controversial since the data are contradictory. Be vigilant for any drowsiness or incoordination. Prilosec may have even more potential to increase blood levels of drugs such as diazepam and prolong their action. Sleeping pills such as Dalmane and Halcion may be affected by Prilosec. Unsteadiness is a possible complication.

Symptoms of Benzodiazepine Overdose
This interaction could lead to symptoms of overdose such as disorientation, unsteadiness, confusion, slurred speech, drowsiness, dizziness, amnesia, and loss of motor coordination. Some other benzodiazepines may also be affected by these ulcer drugs. Contact your physician if such symptoms occur.

Never take or stop medication without your doctor's advice.

Antibiotics (CO-TRIMOXAZOLE)

| Bactrim | Cotrim | Septra |
| SMZ-TMP | Sulfatrim | Uroplus |

LIFE-THREATENING

Anticoagulant Coumadin
Methotrexate Folex Mexate Rheumatrex
Transplant Drug Sandimmune

DANGEROUS

Diabetes Drugs DiaBeta Diabinese Dymelor
Glucotrol Glynase Micronase Orinase Tolinase

TROUBLESOME

Amantadine Symadine Symmetrel
Tuberculosis Drug (rifampin) Rifadin Rifamate
Rimactane

Interactions listed on this list are the most important but not the only medicines with which co-trimoxazole interacts. See individual descriptions for details. Be sure to check with your physician and pharmacist if you must take any other drugs in combination with this antibiotic.

Antibiotics (C0-TRIMOXAZOLE)	**Anticoagulant** (WARFARIN)

LIFE-THREATENING

BRAND NAME

Bactrim

Cotrim

Septra

SMZ-TMP

Sulfatrim

Uroplus

(All co-trimoxazole, formerly known as trimethoprim-sulfa-methoxazole)

INSTRUCTIONS

This drug is best absorbed when taken on an empty stomach, at least one hour before or two hours after a meal. It may be taken with food if it upsets the stomach. Drink at least eight cups of water a day to help keep the drug from crystallizing in the kidneys, and avoid large doses of vitamin C.

BRAND NAME   GENERIC NAME

Coumadin   warfarin

INSTRUCTIONS

Warfarin tablets can be swallowed with food or on an empty stomach. Try to avoid large variations in the quantity of vitamin-K-containing vegetables—such as broccoli, cabbage, or spinach—that you eat each day. Consuming much more or less than usual could change the action of the drug.

INTERACTION

Sulfa antibiotics such as Bactrim can substantially increase the effects of warfarin. *This interaction could trigger life-threatening bleeding.*

Apparently, co-trimoxazole interferes with the metabolism of warfarin in the liver, leading to higher blood levels of the anticoagulant. When this combination of medications is required, the doctor will order frequent blood tests to check prothrombin (clotting) time.

Symptoms of Warfarin Overdose

There may be no early warning signs of danger. Blood tests are essential. Symptoms include any unusual bleeding, including rectal or urinary tract bleeding, excessive menstrual bleeding, nosebleeds, bleeding around gums, bruising, red or tar-black stools, vomiting blood, red or dark-brown urine. Notify your doctor immediately if you suspect a problem.

Never take or stop medication without your doctor's advice.

Antibiotics (CO-TRIMOXAZOLE)	**Methotrexate**

LIFE-THREATENING

BRAND NAME

Bactrim

Cotrim

Septra

SMZ-TMP

Sulfatrim

Uroplus

(All co-trimoxazole, formerly known as trimethoprim-sulfa-methoxazole)

INSTRUCTIONS

This drug is best absorbed when taken on an empty stomach, at least one hour before or two hours after a meal. It may be taken with food if it upsets the stomach. Drink at least eight cups of water a day to help keep the drug from crystallizing in the kidneys, and avoid large doses of vitamin C.

BRAND NAME

Folex

Mexate

Rheumatrex

INSTRUCTIONS

Follow your doctor's instructions on dose and timing for methotrexate, which is taken **once a week** for psoriasis or rheumatoid arthritis. Do not drink alcohol or take salicylates such as aspirin or Pepto-Bismol while on this drug. Methotrexate can increase sensitivity to ultra-violet light, so protect your skin from exposure to sun or tanning lamps.

INTERACTION

People taking methotrexate for leukemia or other cancers may be more susceptible to infection than healthy people. Bactrim, Septra, and other brands of co-trimoxazole are useful for ear infections, urinary tract infections, and so forth. Reports indicate, however, that Bactrim or other sulfa antibiotics (including Gantanol and Gantrisin) can increase the toxicity of methotrexate to the blood system, resulting in bone marrow suppression, anemia, or changes in blood tests. *This interaction can be life threatening.* **Deaths have been reported.**

If both medications are prescribed, ask if another antibiotic would work as well. If both medicines are needed, the doctor should follow closely with frequent blood tests.

Symptoms of Methotrexate Toxicity

Nausea, vomiting, diarrhea, mouth sores, rash, itching, black sticky stools, stomach pain, sore throat, fever, chills, unusual bleeding or bruising, yellow skin or eyes, shortness of breath, cough, dark or bloody urine, and swelling of the legs or feet. Notify the physician immediately.

Never take or stop medication without your doctor's advice.

Antibiotics	Transplant Drug
(CO-TRIMOXAZOLE)	

LIFE-THREATENING

BRAND NAME

Bactrim

Cotrim

Septra

SMZ-TMP

Sulfatrim

Uroplus

(All co-trimoxazole, formerly known as trimethoprim-sulfamethoxazole)

INSTRUCTIONS

This drug is best absorbed when taken on an empty stomach, at least one hour before or two hours after a meal. It may be taken with food if it upsets the stomach. Drink at least eight cups of water a day to help keep the drug from crystallizing in the kidneys, and avoid large doses of vitamin C.

BRAND NAME   GENERIC NAME

Sandimmune   cyclosporine

INSTRUCTIONS

Sandimmune comes as an oral solution with a taste reminiscent of castor oil. It should be mixed in a glass with milk, chocolate milk, or orange juice at room temperature and drunk at once. Then the glass (no plastic) should be rinsed and the rinsing fluid drunk to get the full dose. Do not take Sandimmune with grapefruit juice unless the physician is monitoring blood levels of the drug closely. (See page 53.)

Due to a possible interaction between cyclosporine and oral contraceptives, barrier methods of contraception should be used while taking this drug.

Regular monitoring is important. Do not stop this medicine unless your doctor so directs.

INTERACTION

A transplant patient who comes down with an infection needs an antibiotic, and co-trimoxazole may be appropriate. This should be undertaken only with very careful follow-up and monitoring. Co-trimoxazole and other sulfa antibiotics may reduce the blood level of Sandimmune to a point so low that the drug becomes ineffective. Patients on this combination have experienced rejection episodes. *Although we are aware of no deaths, this interaction could be life threatening.*

In addition, kidney damage appears to occur more often with this combination of medications than with either drug alone. Frequent blood and urine tests may be required to detect a serious reaction.

Never take or stop medication without your doctor's advice.

Antibiotics
(CO-TRIMOXAZOLE)

Diabetes Drugs

DANGEROUS

BRAND NAME
Bactrim
Cotrim
Septra
SMZ-TMP
Sulfatrim
Uroplus
(All co-trimoxazole, formerly known as trimethoprim-sulfa-methoxazole)

INSTRUCTIONS
This drug is best absorbed when taken on an empty stomach, at least one hour before or two hours after a meal. It may be taken with food if it upsets the stomach. Drink at least eight cups of water a day to help keep the drug from crystallizing in the kidneys, and avoid large doses of vitamin C.

BRAND NAME	GENERIC NAME
DiaBeta, Glynase,	
Micronase	glyburide
Diabinese	chlorpropamide
Dymelor	acetohexamide
Glucotrol	glipizide
Orinase	tolbutamide
Tolinase	tolazamide

INSTRUCTIONS
DiaBeta, Glucotrol, and Micronase should be taken 15 minutes to half an hour before meals. The others may be taken with food if they upset the stomach. Blood glucose monitoring is important. Notify the doctor immediately if you experience rash, fever, sore throat, or unusual bleeding or bruising.

INTERACTION
These oral diabetes drugs last longer in the body when a person also takes a sulfa antibiotic such as Bactrim or Septra. Some patients have experienced hypoglycemia as a consequence. Orinase and Diabinese have been implicated most frequently, but there is one case report of this interaction causing hypoglycemia in a patient on Glucotrol. *This interaction could be dangerous.* DiaBeta, Glynase, and Micronase do not appear to interact with co-trimoxazole to cause hypoglycemia. Still, if you are on any oral diabetes drug and need to take this antibiotic, monitor your blood sugar carefully and be alert for hypoglycemia.
Symptoms of Hypoglycemia (Low Blood Sugar)
Shaking, sweating, tiredness, low temperature, faintness, palpitations, hunger, headache, confusion, irritability, visual disturbances, coma. Close observation (preferably in the hospital) is recommended for two or three days after such a reaction.

Never take or stop medication without your doctor's advice.

Antibiotics
(CO-TRIMOXAZOLE)

Amantadine

TROUBLESOME

BRAND NAME

Bactrim

Cotrim

Septra

SMZ-TMP

Sulfatrim

Uroplus

(All co-trimoxazole, formerly known as trimethoprim-sulfamethoxazole)

INSTRUCTIONS

This drug is best absorbed when taken on an empty stomach, at least one hour before or two hours after a meal. It may be taken with food if it upsets the stomach. Drink at least eight cups of water a day to help keep the drug from crystallizing in the kidneys, and avoid large doses of vitamin C.

BRAND NAME

Symadine

Symmetrel

INSTRUCTIONS

There is no information on whether amantadine should be taken with meals or on an empty stomach. It should not be discontinued suddenly, as that has triggered symptoms of Parkinson's disease in some patients.

INTERACTION

There is one case of an elderly man becoming very confused while taking this combination. When co-trimoxazole is taken in combination with amantadine, blood levels of both medications may be increased. *This interaction could be troublesome; stay alert for symptoms of confusion.*

Never take or stop medication without your doctor's advice.

Antibiotics (CO-TRIMOXAZOLE)	**Tuberculosis Drug** (RIFAMPIN)

TROUBLESOME

BRAND NAME
Bactrim
Cotrim
Septra
SMZ-TMP
Sulfatrim
Uroplus
(All co-trimoxazole, formerly known as trimethoprim-sulfamethoxazole)

INSTRUCTIONS
This drug is best absorbed when taken on an empty stomach, at least one hour before or two hours after a meal. It may be taken with food if it upsets the stomach. Drink at least eight cups of water a day to help keep the drug from crystallizing in the kidneys, and avoid large doses of vitamin C.

BRAND NAME	GENERIC NAME
Rifadin	rifampin
Rifamate	isoniazid/ rifampin
Rimactane	rifampin

INSTRUCTIONS
Rifampin should be taken on an empty stomach, at least one hour before or two hours after meals. If you develop fever, chills, unusual tiredness, unusual bleeding or bruising, sore throat, muscle and bone pain, or yellow skin and eyes, contact your physician immediately.

INTERACTION
A urinary tract or other infection in a tuberculosis patient might require that these drugs be taken at the same time. Co-trimoxazole can raise blood levels of rifampin when these two medicines are taken together. *This interaction could be troublesome; notify your doctor of unusual symptoms.*
Symptoms of Rifampin Overdose
Nausea, lethargy, or even, rarely, abnormal liver function tests, liver tenderness, or yellow skin and eyes. Notify the physician promptly of any such symptoms.

Never take or stop medication without your doctor's advice.

Anticoagulant (WARFARIN)

Coumadin

LIFE-THREATENING

Antibiotic (co-trimoxazole) Bactrim Cotrim Septra SMZ-TMP Sulfatrim Uroplus
Antibiotic (metronidazole) Flagyl Protostat
Aspirin
Arthritis Drugs (NSAIDs)
Barbiturates Amytal Butisol Mebaral Nembutal phenobarbital Seconal Tuinal
Breast Cancer Drug Nolvadex
Endometriosis Drug Danocrine
Heart Drug Cordarone
Ulcer Drug Tagamet

DANGEROUS

Anabolic Steroids Anadrol-50 Halotestin Metandren etc.
Antibiotics (macrolides) Biaxin E.E.S E-Mycin ERYC EryPed Ery-Tab Erythrocin Ilosone PCE Pediazole etc.
Antibiotics (tetracyclines) Achromycin V doxycycline Minocin Vibramycin etc.
Antidepressants (serotonin-based) Paxil Prozac Zoloft
Antifungal Drugs Diflucan Monistat
Cholesterol Drug Mevacor
Heart Drug (quinidine) Cardioquin Quinaglute Quinidex Quinora

TROUBLESOME

Anticonvulsant Tegretol
Cholesterol Drugs Colestid Questran
Thyroid Hormone Armour Thyroid Cytomel Levothroid Synthroid Thyroid Strong etc.
Tuberculosis Drug (rifampin) Rifadin Rifamate Rimactane
Vitamin E
Vitamin K

Interactions listed are the most important but not the only medicines with which warfarin interacts. See individual descriptions for details. Be sure to check with your physician and pharmacist if you must take any other drugs in combination with this anticoagulant.

Anticoagulant
(WARFARIN)

Antibiotic
(CO-TRIMOXAZOLE)

LIFE-THREATENING

BRAND NAME   GENERIC NAME
Coumadin   warfarin

INSTRUCTIONS
Warfarin tablets can be swallowed with food or on an empty stomach. Try to avoid large variations in the quantity of vitamin-K–containing vegetables—such as broccoli, cabbage, or spinach—that you eat each day. Consuming much more or less than usual could change the action of the drug.

BRAND NAME
Bactrim
Cotrim
Septra
SMZ-TMP
Sulfatrim
Uroplus
(All co-trimoxazole, formerly known as trimethoprim-sulfamethoxazole)

INSTRUCTIONS
This drug is best absorbed when taken on an empty stomach, at least one hour before or two hours after a meal. It may be taken with food if it upsets the stomach. Drink at least eight cups of water a day to help keep the drug from crystallizing in the kidneys, and avoid large doses of vitamin C.

INTERACTION
Sulfa antibiotics such as Bactrim can substantially increase the effects of warfarin. *This interaction could trigger life-threatening bleeding.*

Apparently, co-trimoxazole interferes with the metabolism of warfarin in the liver, leading to higher blood levels of the anticoagulant. When this combination of medications is required, the doctor will order frequent blood tests to check prothrombin (clotting) time.

Symptoms of Warfarin Overdose
There may be no early warning signs of danger. Blood tests are essential. Symptoms include any unusual bleeding, including rectal or urinary tract bleeding, excessive menstrual bleeding, nosebleeds, bleeding around gums, bruising, red or tar-black stools, vomiting blood, and red or dark-brown urine. Notify your doctor immediately if you suspect a problem.

Never take or stop medication without your doctor's advice.

Anticoagulant (WARFARIN)	**Antibiotic** (METRONIDAZOLE)
LIFE-THREATENING	

BRAND NAME	GENERIC NAME	BRAND NAME	GENERIC NAME
Coumadin	warfarin	**Flagyl**	metronidazole
		Protostat	metronidazole

INSTRUCTIONS

Warfarin tablets can be swallowed with food or on an empty stomach. Try to avoid large variations in the quantity of vitamin-K–containing vegetables—such as broccoli, cabbage, or spinach—that you eat each day. Consuming much more or less than usual could change the action of the drug.

INSTRUCTIONS

Metronidazole may be taken with meals to reduce stomach upset. Avoid alcohol while on this drug and for a day after stopping it, because the combination could trigger flushing, headache, nausea, and vomiting.

INTERACTION

Metronidazole can interfere with the body's elimination of warfarin, leading to higher blood levels of the anticoagulant. *This interaction could trigger life-threatening bleeding.*

This interaction is expected in many or most patients taking both warfarin and metronidazole. The doctor will probably order frequent blood tests to see if the dose of warfarin should be adjusted. Contact your physician without delay if there are any signs of unusual bleeding. *Symptoms of Warfarin Overdose*

There may be no early warning signs of danger. Blood tests are essential. Symptoms include any unusual bleeding, including rectal or urinary tract bleeding, excessive menstrual bleeding, nosebleeds, bleeding around gums, bruising, red or tar-black stools, vomiting blood, and red or dark-brown urine. Notify your doctor immediately if you suspect a problem.

Never take or stop medication without your doctor's advice.

Anticoagulant	**Aspirin and**
(WARFARIN)	**Arthritis Drugs**
	(NSAIDS)

LIFE-THREATENING

BRAND NAME   GENERIC NAME

Coumadin   warfarin

INSTRUCTIONS

Warfarin tablets can be swallowed with food or on an empty stomach. Try to avoid large variations in the quantity of vitamin-K–containing vegetables—such as broccoli, cabbage, or spinach—that you eat each day. Consuming much more or less than usual could change the action of the drug.

BRAND NAME   GENERIC NAME

Alka-Seltzer acetylsalicylic acid

Anacin   acetylsalicylic acid

Ascriptin   acetylsalicylic acid

Bayer   acetylsalicylic acid

Ecotrin, etc. acetylsalicylic acid

INSTRUCTIONS

Aspirin may be taken with food or milk to reduce stomach upset, always with a full eight ounces of liquid. Pregnant women should take aspirin only under the doctor's supervision. Children with flu or chickenpox must avoid aspirin because it increases the risk of Reye's syndrome.

INTERACTION

Both aspirin and warfarin are effective anticlotting agents, although they work through different pathways. Large doses of aspirin can significantly increase bleeding in people taking warfarin. *This interaction could prove life threatening.*

Low doses of aspirin together with warfarin may only slightly increase the risk of bleeding. A study (CARS) currently underway will test this combination. Until the results are in, aspirin and warfarin should be combined only under close monitoring. Prothrombin time should be tested, but serious bleeding may occur even without major changes in this test.

Symptoms of Warfarin Overdose

There may be no early warning signs of danger. Blood tests are essential. Symptoms include any unusual bleeding, including rectal or urinary tract bleeding, excessive menstrual bleeding, nosebleeds, bleeding around gums, bruising, red or tar-black stools, vomiting blood, and red or dark-brown urine. Notify your doctor immediately if you suspect a problem.

Never take or stop medication without your doctor's advice.

Anticoagulant	Barbiturates
(WARFARIN)	-

LIFE-THREATENING

BRAND NAME	GENERIC NAME
Coumadin	warfarin

INSTRUCTIONS
Warfarin tablets can be swallowed with food or on an empty stomach. Try to avoid large variations in the quantity of vitamin-K–containing vegetables—such as broccoli, cabbage, or spinach—that you eat each day. Consuming much more or less than usual could change the action of the drug.

BRAND NAME	GENERIC NAME
Alurate	aprobarbital
Amytal	amobarbital
Butisol	butabarbital
Lotusate	talbutal
Mebaral	mephobarbital
Nembutal	pentobarbital
Seconal	secobarbital
Solfoton	phenobarbital
Tuinal	amobarbital/
	secobarbital

INSTRUCTIONS
Any of these medications can cause drowsiness and limit attention. Take them at a time when you will not need to drive or do other complicated tasks.

INTERACTION
Barbiturates can rev up the liver enzymes that process warfarin, thus lowering both the blood levels and the effectiveness of this anticoagulant. *In such a situation, there is a risk of dangerous blood clots. Even more serious is the risk of life-threatening bleeding when a person on warfarin stops taking a barbiturate.* People vary a great deal in their response to this interaction. It is essential, however, that prothrombin time be tested frequently during the two weeks a barbiturate is started and the two weeks after it is stopped. Dosage adjustments may be necessary.

Symptoms of Warfarin Overdose
There may be no early warning signs of danger. Blood tests are essential. Symptoms include any unusual bleeding, including rectal or urinary tract bleeding, excessive menstrual bleeding, nosebleeds, bleeding around gums, bruising, red or tar-black stools, vomiting blood, and red or dark-brown urine. Notify your doctor immediately if you suspect a problem.

Never take or stop medication without your doctor's advice.

Anticoagulant	**Breast Cancer Drug**
(WARFARIN)	(TAMOXIFEN)

LIFE-THREATENING

BRAND NAME   GENERIC NAME
Coumadin   warfarin

INSTRUCTIONS
Warfarin tablets can be swallowed with food or on an empty stomach. Try to avoid large variations in the quantity of vitamin-K–containing vegetables—such as broccoli, cabbage, or spinach—that you eat each day. Consuming much more or less than usual could change the action of the drug.

BRAND NAME   GENERIC NAME
Nolvadex   tamoxifen

INSTRUCTIONS
Nolvadex may be taken with or without food. If you experience exceptional weakness, sleepiness, confusion, shortness of breath, or swollen, painful areas in the legs, contact the doctor immediately.

INTERACTION
In one case, a 65-year-old woman nearly died of hemorrhage several weeks after she was put on tamoxifen to battle breast cancer. She had been on the same dose of warfarin for many years prior to starting tamoxifen. Apparently, tamoxifen increased her blood level of warfarin to a dangerous degree. The doctors were able to save her life in the hospital and she was sent home on both drugs, but with the warfarin dose much reduced. *This interaction may be rare, but it could be life threatening.*

Prudence suggests frequent blood tests to check on warfarin's effectiveness during the weeks after Nolvadex is started or stopped. Notify the doctor immediately of any signs of bleeding.

Symptoms of Warfarin Overdose
There may be no early warning signs of danger. Blood tests are essential. Symptoms include any unusual bleeding, including rectal or urinary tract bleeding, excessive menstrual bleeding, nosebleeds, bleeding around gums, bruising, red or tar-black stools, vomiting blood, and red or dark-brown urine. Notify your doctor immediately if you suspect a problem.

Never take or stop medication without your doctor's advice.

Anticoagulant (WARFARIN)	**Endometriosis Drug** (DANAZOL)
LIFE-THREATENING	

BRAND NAME GENERIC NAME	BRAND NAME GENERIC NAME
Coumadin warfarin	**Danocrine** danazol

INSTRUCTIONS

Warfarin tablets can be swallowed with food or on an empty stomach. Try to avoid large variations in the quantity of vitamin-K–containing vegetables—such as broccoli, cabbage, or spinach—that you eat each day. Consuming much more or less than usual could change the action of the drug.

INSTRUCTIONS

Danocrine may be taken either with food or on an empty stomach. During Danocrine therapy, sexually active women should use barrier contraceptives (such as a diaphragm or condoms).

INTERACTION

Danocrine seems to increase the body's sensitivity to warfarin and may increase bleeding dramatically. *This interaction could be life threatening.*

The physician will probably order frequent blood tests for a period of time if danazol is stopped or started in a patient taking warfarin, to see if the dose of warfarin should be adjusted. If you experience unusual bleeding, let the physician know at once.

Symptoms of Warfarin Overdose

There may be no early warning signs of danger. Blood tests are essential. Symptoms include any unusual bleeding, including rectal or urinary tract bleeding, excessive menstrual bleeding, nosebleeds, bleeding around gums, bruising, red or tar-black stools, vomiting blood, and red or dark-brown urine. Notify your doctor immediately if you suspect a problem.

Never take or stop medication without your doctor's advice.

Anticoagulant (WARFARIN)	**Heart Drug** (AMIODARONE)

LIFE-THREATENING

BRAND NAME	GENERIC NAME	BRAND NAME	GENERIC NAME
Coumadin	warfarin	**Cordarone**	amiodarone

INSTRUCTIONS

Warfarin tablets can be swallowed with food or on an empty stomach. Try to avoid large variations in the quantity of vitamin-K–containing vegetables—such as broccoli, cabbage, or spinach—that you eat each day. Consuming much more or less than usual could change the action of the drug.

INSTRUCTIONS

Follow the physician's directions carefully. Tell your doctor if you notice shortness of breath, or changes in vision, or if your skin turns blue.

INTERACTION

Complicated cardiovascular problems may call for both an anticoagulant and a powerful heart drug. Cordarone increases the effect of warfarin so much that severe bleeding may occur. The dose of warfarin may need to be cut 30 to 50 percent if Cordarone is added. *This interaction could be life threatening.* Frequent blood tests are needed during the first month of combined therapy to check the warfarin dose. Cordarone lingers in the body a long time. If it is discontinued, blood tests will be needed for several months so that the dose of warfarin can be adjusted to avoid the risk of serious clotting.

Symptoms of Warfarin Overdose

There may be no early warning signs of danger. Blood tests are essential. Symptoms include any unusual bleeding, including rectal or urinary tract bleeding, excessive menstrual bleeding, nosebleeds, bleeding around gums, bruising, red or tar-black stools, vomiting blood, and red or dark-brown urine. Notify your doctor immediately if a problem.

Never take or stop medication without your doctor's a

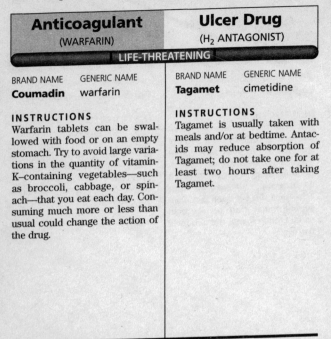

Anticoagulant (WARFARIN)	**Ulcer Drug** (H$_2$ ANTAGONIST)

LIFE-THREATENING

BRAND NAME	GENERIC NAME	BRAND NAME	GENERIC NAME
Coumadin	warfarin	**Tagamet**	cimetidine

INSTRUCTIONS

Warfarin tablets can be swallowed with food or on an empty stomach. Try to avoid large variations in the quantity of vitamin-K–containing vegetables—such as broccoli, cabbage, or spinach—that you eat each day. Consuming much more or less than usual could change the action of the drug.

INSTRUCTIONS

Tagamet is usually taken with meals and/or at bedtime. Antacids may reduce absorption of Tagamet; do not take one for at least two hours after taking Tagamet.

INTERACTION

Although warfarin may cause nausea, loss of appetite, stomach cramping, or diarrhea, taking Tagamet to treat these symptoms might trigger serious problems. Tagamet affects metabolism and increases Coumadin's blood-thinning potential. This prolongs prothrombin time (a measure of clotting) and could lead to serious hemorrhaging. *The interaction is potentially lethal.* Experts warn against this combination of drugs. If an ulcer medicine is needed with warfarin, the drugs Axid, Pepcid, or Zantac may be a safer alternative than Tagamet. Prothrombin time should be monitored when taking warfarin with an ulcer drug.

Symptoms of Warfarin Overdose

There may be no early warning signs of danger. Blood tests are essential. Symptoms include any unusual bleeding, including rectal or urinary tract bleeding, excessive menstrual bleeding, nosebleeds, bleeding around gums, bruising, red or tar-black stools, vomiting blood, and red or dark-brown urine. Notify your doctor immediately if you suspect a problem.

Never take or stop medication without your doctor's advice.

Anticoagulant (WARFARIN)	Anabolic Steroids

DANGEROUS

BRAND NAME	GENERIC NAME
Coumadin	warfarin

INSTRUCTIONS
Warfarin tablets can be swallowed with food or on an empty stomach. Try to avoid large variations in the quantity of vitamin-K–containing vegetables—such as broccoli, cabbage, or spinach—that you eat each day. Consuming much more or less than usual could change the action of the drug.

BRAND NAME	GENERIC NAME
Anadrol-50	oxymetholone
Halotestin	fluoxymesterone
Metandren	methyl-testosterone
Winstrol	stanozolol

INSTRUCTIONS
These drugs may cause nausea and vomiting. Tell the doctor if this becomes a problem, or if you develop swollen ankles or yellow skin. These medications may affect blood sugar control, so diabetics require close monitoring.

INTERACTION

Anabolic steroids increase the effects of warfarin against clotting. If one of these drugs is needed, prothrombin time should monitored closely to guide a possible adjustment in warfarin dose. Blood tests may also be required for several days after one of these medicines is discontinued. *This interaction could be dangerous.*

Symptoms of Warfarin Overdose
There may be no early warning signs of danger. Blood tests are essential. Symptoms include any unusual bleeding, including rectal or urinary tract bleeding, excessive menstrual bleeding, nosebleeds, bleeding around gums, bruising, red or tar-black stools, vomiting blood, and red or dark-brown urine. Notify your doctor immediately if you suspect a problem.

Never take or stop medication without your doctor's advice

Anticoagulant
(WARFARIN)

Antibiotics
(MACROLIDES)

DANGEROUS

BRAND NAME	GENERIC NAME
Coumadin	warfarin

INSTRUCTIONS

Warfarin tablets can be swallowed with food or on an empty stomach. Try to avoid large variations in the quantity of vitamin-K–containing vegetables—such as broccoli, cabbage, or spinach—that you eat each day. Consuming much more or less than usual could change the action of the drug.

BRAND NAME	GENERIC NAME
Biaxin	clarithromycin
E.E.S.	erythromycin
E-Mycin	erythromycin
ERYC	erythromycin
EryPed	erythromycin
Ery-Tab	erythromycin
Erythrocin	erythromycin
Ilosone	erythromycin
PCE	erythromycin
Pediazole	erythromycin
Tao	troleandomycin
Zithromax	azithromycin

INSTRUCTIONS

Some forms of erythromycin must be taken on an empty stomach; others may be taken with food. See the table of Food and Drug Compatibility on pages 73–91 for specifics. Biaxin can be taken without regard to meals. Zithromax is best taken on an empty stomach.

INTERACTION

Erythromycin increases the body's response to warfarin. In several cases, this has resulted in serious bleeding. Tests of prothrombin (clotting) time should be done frequently when erythromycin must be added to warfarin. Blood tests may also be required for several days after one of these medicines is discontinued. *This interaction could be dangerous.*

Biaxin and Zithromax may not interact with warfarin in the same way as the other macrolides. It would be wise, however, to consider the possibility of an interaction and to monitor prothrombin time closely if one of these antibiotics must be taken together with warfarin.

Symptoms of Warfarin Overdose

There may be no early warning signs of danger. Blood tests are essential. Symptoms include any unusual bleeding, including rectal or urinary tract bleeding, excessive menstrual bleeding, nosebleeds, bleeding around gums, bruising, red or tar-black stools, vomiting blood, and red or dark-brown urine. Notify your doctor immediately if you suspect a problem.

Never take or stop medication without your doctor's advice.

Anticoagulant	Antibiotics
(WARFARIN)	(TETRACYCLINES)

BRAND NAME	GENERIC NAME
Coumadin	warfarin

INSTRUCTIONS

Warfarin tablets can be swallowed with food or on an empty stomach. Try to avoid large variations in the quantity of vitamin-K–containing vegetables—such as broccoli, cabbage, or spinach—that you eat each day. Consuming much more or less than usual could change the action of the drug.

BRAND NAME	GENERIC NAME
Achromycin V	tetracycline
Declomycin	demeclocycline
Doryx	doxycycline
Minocin	minocycline
Panmycin	tetracycline
Robitet	tetracycline
Rondomycin	methacycline
Sumycin	tetracycline
Terramycin	oxytetracycline
Uri-Tet	oxytetracycline
Vibramycin	doxycycline

INSTRUCTIONS

Take most forms of tetracycline on an empty stomach. See the table of Food and Drug Compatibility on pages 73–91 for specifics. Do not take these drugs with antacids, calcium or iron supplements, or dairy products because they could interfere with absorption. Never take outdated tetracycline, which may be toxic to the kidneys.

INTERACTION

Tetracycline antibiotics appear capable of increasing warfarin's effects in some people. Prothrombin (clotting) time should be tested frequently when a tetracycline is started or stopped, and the dosage of warfarin adjusted accordingly; *otherwise, this interaction could lead to dangerous bleeding.*

Symptoms of Warfarin Overdose

There may be no early warning signs of danger. Blood tests are essential. Symptoms include any unusual bleeding, including rectal or urinary tract bleeding, excessive menstrual bleeding, nosebleeds, bleeding around gums, bruising, red or tar-black stools, vomiting blood, and red or dark-brown urine. Notify your doctor immediately if you suspect a problem.

Never take or stop medication without your doctor's advice.

Anticoagulant	**Antidepressants**
(WARFARIN)	(SEROTONIN-BASED)

DANGEROUS

BRAND NAME	GENERIC NAME	BRAND NAME	GENERIC NAME
Coumadin	warfarin	**Paxil**	paroxetine
		Prozac	fluoxetine
		Zoloft	sertraline

INSTRUCTIONS

Warfarin tablets can be swallowed with food or on an empty stomach. Try to avoid large variations in the quantity of vitamin-K–containing vegetables—such as broccoli, cabbage, or spinach—that you eat each day. Consuming much more or less than usual could change the action of the drug.

INSTRUCTIONS

Paxil and Zoloft are taken once a day, usually in the morning. Prozac is taken in the morning, or, if a higher dose has been prescribed, in the morning and at noon. It may be taken without regard to meals. Taking it with food may reduce stomach upset. A few patients experience serious weight loss on these medications. If this occurs, the doctor should be notified.

INTERACTION

Although there are only a few reports of interaction between any of these antidepressants and warfarin, it appears that in some cases these serotonin-based medications can increase the risk of bleeding associated with warfarin. *This interaction could be dangerous.*

It is possible that many patients will have no trouble with this combination, but the physician should monitor carefully for a potential interaction. Prothrombin time or international normalized ratio (INR) may be increased. Notify your physician immediately if you experience any symptoms of bleeding.

Symptoms of Warfarin Overdose

There may be no early warning signs of danger. Blood tests are essential. Symptoms include any unusual bleeding, including rectal or urinary tract bleeding, excessive menstrual bleeding, nosebleeds, bleeding around gums, bruising, red or tar-black stools, vomiting blood, and red or dark-brown urine. Notify your doctor immediately if you suspect a problem.

Never take or stop medication without your doctor's advice.

Anticoagulant
(WARFARIN)

Antifungal Drugs

DANGEROUS

BRAND NAME   GENERIC NAME
Coumadin   warfarin

INSTRUCTIONS
Warfarin tablets can be swallowed with food or on an empty stomach. Try to avoid large variations in the quantity of vitamin-K–containing vegetables—such as broccoli, cabbage, or spinach—that you eat each day. Consuming much more or less than usual could change the action of the drug.

BRAND NAME   GENERIC NAME
Diflucan   fluconazole
Monistat   miconazole

INSTRUCTIONS
Ask your doctor for precise instructions on how to take Diflucan. Doses are individualized, depending on the infection treated, and the first dose is often higher than the rest. Unprotected sexual intercourse should be avoided during Monistat treatment.

INTERACTION
Monistat is principally a vaginal preparation, but when given systemically (intravenously), it inhibits an important liver enzyme that processes warfarin. As a result, levels of the anticoagulant build up and prothrombin time may increase as much as four or five times. *This interaction could be dangerous, resulting in serious bleeding.* Even when Monistat is used as a vaginal cream, some is absorbed into the body. Precautions are appropriate. When either Diflucan or Monistat is taken together with warfarin, prothrombin time should be monitored frequently (at least every two days) and the dose of warfarin adjusted as necessary.

Symptoms of Warfarin Overdose
There may be no early warning signs of danger. Blood tests are essential. Symptoms include any unusual bleeding, including rectal or urinary tract bleeding, excessive menstrual bleeding, nosebleeds, bleeding around gums, bruising, red or tar-black stools, vomiting blood, and red or dark-brown urine. Notify your doctor immediately if you suspect a problem.

Never take or stop medication without your doctor's advice.

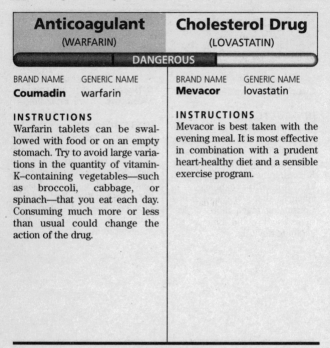

Anticoagulant
(WARFARIN)

Cholesterol Drug
(LOVASTATIN)

DANGEROUS

BRAND NAME | GENERIC NAME
Coumadin warfarin

BRAND NAME | GENERIC NAME
Mevacor lovastatin

INSTRUCTIONS
Warfarin tablets can be swallowed with food or on an empty stomach. Try to avoid large variations in the quantity of vitamin-K–containing vegetables—such as broccoli, cabbage, or spinach—that you eat each day. Consuming much more or less than usual could change the action of the drug.

INSTRUCTIONS
Mevacor is best taken with the evening meal. It is most effective in combination with a prudent heart-healthy diet and a sensible exercise program.

INTERACTION

Mevacor appears to increase the effects of warfarin in some patients. Two middle-aged men requiring warfarin were later put on Mevacor for elevated cholesterol. Each of them developed unexpected bleeding and prolonged prothrombin times. *This interaction could be dangerous.* If Mevacor and warfarin are both needed, frequent blood tests will guide warfarin dose adjustment. There is no evidence that the other cholesterol-lowering drugs, Pravachol (generic: pravastatin) or Zocor (generic: simvastatin), interact with warfarin in the same fashion. Because they are similar to Mevacor, however, caution is probably advisable.

Symptoms of Warfarin Overdose
There may be no early warning signs of danger. Blood tests are essential. Symptoms include any unusual bleeding, including rectal or urinary tract bleeding, excessive menstrual bleeding, nosebleeds, bleeding around gums, bruising, red or tar-black stools, vomiting blood, and red or dark-brown urine. Notify your doctor immediately if you suspect a problem.

Never take or stop medication without your doctor's advice.

Anticoagulant	**Heart Drug**
(WARFARIN)	(QUINIDINE)

DANGEROUS

BRAND NAME	GENERIC NAME
Coumadin	warfarin

INSTRUCTIONS
Warfarin tablets can be swallowed with food or on an empty stomach. Try to avoid large variations in the quantity of vitamin-K–containing vegetables—such as broccoli, cabbage, or spinach—that you eat each day. Consuming much more or less than usual could change the action of the drug.

BRAND NAME	GENERIC NAME
Cardioquin	quinidine
Quinaglute	quinidine
Quinidex	quinidine
Quinora	quinidine

INSTRUCTIONS
Quinidine may upset the stomach and should be taken with food. Sustained-release tablets should not be chewed or crushed.

It may provoke visual disturbances, ringing in the ears, headache, dizziness, nausea, skin rash, or breathing difficulties. Notify your doctor if you develop any of these symptoms.

INTERACTION
Quinine derivatives, including the heart drug quinidine, may increase the effectiveness of warfarin. *This interaction could be dangerous, resulting in serious bleeding.*

Prothrombin time should be tested when any of these medicines must be started or stopped, because the dose of warfarin might need adjustment. Notify the doctor of any problems.

Symptoms of Warfarin Overdose
There may be no early warning signs of danger. Blood tests are essential. Symptoms include any unusual bleeding, including rectal or urinary tract bleeding, excessive menstrual bleeding, nosebleeds, bleeding around gums, bruising, red or tar-black stools, vomiting blood, and red or dark-brown urine. Notify your doctor immediately if you suspect a problem.

Never take or stop medication without your doctor's advice.

Anticoagulant
(WARFARIN)

Anticonvulsant
(CARBAMAZÉPINE)

TROUBLESOME

BRAND NAME	GENERIC NAME
Coumadin	warfarin

INSTRUCTIONS
Warfarin tablets can be swallowed with food or on an empty stomach. Try to avoid large variations in the quantity of vitamin-K–containing vegetables—such as broccoli, cabbage, or spinach—that you eat each day. Consuming much more or less than usual could change the action of the drug.

BRAND NAME	GENERIC NAME
Tegretol	carbamazepine

INSTRUCTIONS
Carbamazepine may upset the stomach; if so, take it with food or milk. Do not stop taking this drug suddenly; seizures could result. To maintain its strength, it must be stored away from humidity and heat in a tightly closed container.

INTERACTION
Carbamazepine apparently reduces circulating levels of warfarin. The result could be a greater risk of blood clots. *This interaction could be troublesome.*

When a person on warfarin needs to start or stop taking this anticonvulsant, close monitoring of prothrombin time is appropriate. A few case reports feature patients whose prothrombin time was five or six times greater upon discontinuing carbamazepine, a situation that could lead to dangerous bleeding. The physician may need to adjust the dose of warfarin when Tegretol is discontinued.

Symptoms of Warfarin Overdose
There may be no early warning signs of danger. Blood tests are essential. Symptoms include any unusual bleeding, including rectal or urinary tract bleeding, excessive menstrual bleeding, nosebleeds, bleeding around gums, bruising, red or tar-black stools, vomiting blood, and red or dark-brown urine. Notify your doctor immediately if you suspect a problem.

Never take or stop medication without your doctor's advice.

Anticoagulant (WARFARIN)	**Cholesterol Drugs**

TROUBLESOME

BRAND NAME	GENERIC NAME
Coumadin	warfarin

INSTRUCTIONS
Warfarin tablets can be swallowed with food or on an empty stomach. Try to avoid large variations in the quantity of vitamin-K–containing vegetables—such as broccoli, cabbage, or spinach—that you eat each day. Consuming much more or less than usual could change the action of the drug.

BRAND NAME	GENERIC NAME
Colestid	colestipol
Questran	cholestyramine

INSTRUCTIONS
Questran and Colestid come in powder form and need to be mixed with a glassful of water. Questran should not be taken with carbonated beverages. These medications are usually taken before meals, but check with a physician or pharmacist for specific instructions.

INTERACTION
These cholesterol-lowering drugs appear to reduce the absorption of blood thinners such as Coumadin. This could lead to diminished effectiveness and increase the risk of blood clots. It would be better to avoid this interaction if at all possible. When that is not possible, at least six hours should separate the intake of Questran or Colestid and Coumadin. Maintain the same schedule each day to prevent variation in absorption. Blood should be monitored carefully to make sure proper anticoagulant action is obtained.

Symptoms of Warfarin Overdose
There may be no early warning signs of danger. Blood tests are essential. Symptoms include any unusual bleeding, including rectal or urinary tract bleeding, excessive menstrual bleeding, nosebleeds, bleeding around gums, bruising, red or tar-black stools, vomiting blood, and red or dark-brown urine. Notify your doctor immediately if you suspect a problem.

Never take or stop medication without your doctor's advice.

Anticoagulant (WARFARIN)	Thyroid Hormone

TROUBLESOME

BRAND NAME   GENERIC NAME
Coumadin   warfarin

INSTRUCTIONS
Warfarin tablets can be swallowed with food or on an empty stomach. Try to avoid large variations in the quantity of vitamin-K–containing vegetables—such as broccoli, cabbage, or spinach—that you eat each day. Consuming much more or less than usual could change the action of the drug.

BRAND NAME   GENERIC NAME
Armour Thyroid dessicated
                    thyroid
Cytomel   liothyronine
Levothroid   levothyroxine
Synthroid   levothyroxine
Thyroid Strong dessicated
                    thyroid

INSTRUCTIONS
Thyroid hormone is best taken on an empty stomach at the same time each day. It should not be taken together with iron supplements, which reduce absorption.

INTERACTION
Thyroid hormone can have a major impact on bleeding associated with Coumadin, greatly increasing prothrombin time. People with underactive thyroids may need higher doses of warfarin than usual. If they are then started on thyroid hormone replacement, the anticoagulant may become significantly more effective (50 to 400 percent). *This reaction could result in troublesome bleeding.*
Symptoms of Warfarin Overdose
There may be no early warning signs of danger. Blood tests are essential. Symptoms include any unusual bleeding, including rectal or urinary tract bleeding, excessive menstrual bleeding, nosebleeds, bleeding around gums, bruising, red or tar-black stools, vomiting blood, and red or dark-brown urine. Notify your doctor immediately if you suspect a problem.

Never take or stop medication without your doctor's advice.

Anticoagulant (WARFARIN)	**Tuberculosis Drug** (RIFAMPIN)

TROUBLESOME

BRAND NAME	GENERIC NAME
Coumadin	warfarin

INSTRUCTIONS
Warfarin tablets can be swallowed with food or on an empty stomach. Try to avoid large variations in the quantity of vitamin-K–containing vegetables—such as broccoli, cabbage, or spinach—that you eat each day. Consuming much more or less than usual could change the action of the drug.

BRAND NAME	GENERIC NAME
Rifadin	rifampin
Rifamate	isoniazid/ rifampin
Rimactane	rifampin

INSTRUCTIONS
Rifampin should be taken on an empty stomach, at least one hour before or two hours after meals. If you develop fever, chills, unusual tiredness, unusual bleeding or bruising, sore throat, muscle and bone pain, or yellow skin and eyes, contact your physician immediately.

INTERACTION
Rifampin may speed the body's elimination of warfarin and thus decrease circulating levels of the anticoagulant. The result could be a greater risk of blood clots. *This interaction could be troublesome.*

When a person on warfarin needs to start or stop this tuberculosis treatment, close monitoring of prothrombin time is appropriate. Because rifampin increases the requirement for warfarin by as much as 50 percent, the dose must be adjusted downward carefully when rifampin is discontinued to avoid excess bleeding.

Symptoms of Warfarin Overdose
There may be no early warning signs of danger. Blood tests are essential. Symptoms include any unusual bleeding, including rectal or urinary tract bleeding, excessive menstrual bleeding, nosebleeds, bleeding around gums, bruising, red or tar-black stools, vomiting blood, and red or dark-brown urine. Notify your doctor immediately if you suspect a problem.

Never take or stop medication without your doctor's advice.

Anticoagulant (WARFARIN)	**Vitamin E**

TROUBLESOME

BRAND NAME	GENERIC NAME
Coumadin	warfarin

INSTRUCTIONS

Warfarin tablets can be swallowed with food or on an empty stomach. Try to avoid large variations in the quantity of vitamin-K–containing vegetables—such as broccoli, cabbage, or spinach—that you eat each day. Consuming much more or less than usual could change the action of the drug.

BRAND NAME	GENERIC NAME
Aquasol E	tocopherol
E-Complex	tocopherol
Vitamin E	tocopherol
Vita-Plus E	tocopherol

INSTRUCTIONS

Vitamin E may be taken with meals or on an empty stomach. A doctor's supervision is prudent for doses of 800 IU daily or more.

INTERACTION

Vitamin E alone helps prevent blood clotting by keeping platelets from sticking together. In combination with warfarin, theoretically it could have an additive effect and lead to unexpected bleeding. *This interaction could be troublesome.*

One patient got into trouble by taking up to 1,200 IU of vitamin E a day on his own, in addition to his prescribed warfarin. After two months, he experienced unusual bleeding and his prothrombin time was increased. Doses of vitamin E over 400 IU daily may be required to trigger this interaction, but it makes sense to be careful even at lower doses. If you plan to take vitamin E supplements, consult your doctor. More frequent blood tests may be appropriate.

Symptoms of Warfarin Overdose

There may be no early warning signs of danger. Blood tests are essential. Symptoms include any unusual bleeding, including rectal or urinary tract bleeding, excessive menstrual bleeding, nosebleeds, bleeding around gums, bruising, red or tar-black stools, vomiting blood, and red or dark-brown urine. Notify your doctor immediately if you suspect a problem.

Never take or stop medication without your doctor's advice.

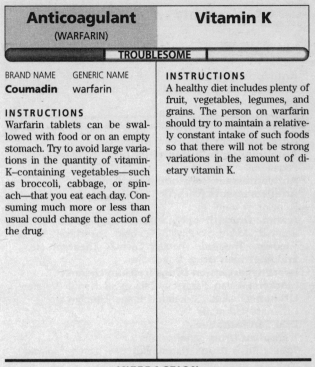

Anticoagulant (WARFARIN)

Vitamin K

TROUBLESOME

BRAND NAME   GENERIC NAME
Coumadin   warfarin

INSTRUCTIONS
Warfarin tablets can be swallowed with food or on an empty stomach. Try to avoid large variations in the quantity of vitamin-K–containing vegetables—such as broccoli, cabbage, or spinach—that you eat each day. Consuming much more or less than usual could change the action of the drug.

INSTRUCTIONS
A healthy diet includes plenty of fruit, vegetables, legumes, and grains. The person on warfarin should try to maintain a relatively constant intake of such foods so that there will not be strong variations in the amount of dietary vitamin K.

INTERACTION

Vitamin K is essential for proper clotting of blood. Warfarin works by suppressing certain vitamin-K–dependent factors needed for the formation of blood clots, but giving enough extra vitamin K can overwhelm the system and diminish the effects of warfarin. *While this action is useful in the hospital when bleeding threatens, it could be troublesome if vitamin K intake were inadvertent.*

It is important not to vary intake of vitamin K sources greatly. If fluctuations are likely, prothrombin time should probably be monitored.

Symptoms of Warfarin Overdose

There may be no early warning signs of danger. Blood tests are essential. Symptoms include any unusual bleeding, including rectal or urinary tract bleeding, excessive menstrual bleeding, nosebleeds, bleeding around gums, bruising, red or tar-black stools, vomiting blood, and red or dark-brown urine. Notify your doctor immediately if you suspect a problem.

Never take or stop medication without your doctor's advice.

Anticonvulsant (CARBAMAZEPINE)

Tegretol

LIFE-THREATENING

Antibiotics (macrolides) Biaxin E.E.S. E-Mycin PCE etc.
Pain Reliever (propoxyphene) Darvocet-N Darvon
Darvon-N Wygesic

DANGEROUS

Anticonvulsant Depakene Depakote
Anticonvulsants (hydantoins) Dilantin Mesantoin
Peganone
Antidepressant (serotonin-based) Prozac
Antidepressants (tricyclic) Elavil Norpramin
Pamelor Tofranil etc.
Asthma Drug (theophylline) Elixophyllin Quibron-T
Respbid Slo-bid Slo-Phyllin Theobid Theochron
Theoclear Theo-Dur Theolair Theo-24 Theovent etc.
Endometriosis Drug Danocrine
**Heart/Hypertension Drugs (calcium channel
blockers)** Calan Cardizem Dilacor XR Isoptin Verelan
Lithium Cibalith-S Eskalith Lithane Lithobid
Lithonate Lithotabs
Oral Contraceptives
Transplant Drug Sandimmune
Tuberculosis Drugs (isoniazid) INH Izonid Laniazid
Nydrazid Rifamate
Ulcer Drug Tagamet

TROUBLESOME

Antibiotic (doxycycline) Doryx Doxychel Hyclate
Monodox Vibramycin Vibra-Tabs
Anticoagulant Coumadin
Barbiturates Amytal Butisol Mebaral Nembutal
phenobarbital Seconal Tuinal
Drug for Schizophrenia Haldol
Influenza Vaccine

Carbamazepine interacts with many other medications. Some of
these interactions are potentially serious. We have included the
most common, but be sure to check with your physician and pharmacist if you must take any other drugs in conjunction with this
anticonvulsant.

Anticonvulsant
(CARBAMAZEPINE)

Antibiotics
(MACROLIDES)

LIFE-THREATENING

BRAND NAME	GENERIC NAME
Tegretol	carbamazepine

INSTRUCTIONS
Carbamazepine may upset the stomach; if so, take it with food or milk. Do not stop this drug suddenly; seizures could result. To maintain its strength, it must be stored away from humidity and heat in a tightly closed container.

BRAND NAME	GENERIC NAME
Biaxin	clarithromycin
E.E.S.	erythromycin
E-Mycin	erythromycin
ERYC	erythromycin
EryPed	erythromycin
Ery-Tab	erythromycin
Erythrocin	erythromycin
Ilosone	erythromycin
PCE	erythromycin
Pediazole	erythromycin
Tao	troleandomycin
Zithromax	azithromycin

INSTRUCTIONS
Some forms of erythromycin must be taken on an empty stomach; others may be taken with food. See pages 73–91 for specifics. Biaxin can be taken without regard to meals. Zithromax is best taken on an empty stomach.

INTERACTION

Erythromycin and other drugs in this category can interfere with the liver's processing of carbamazepine. The anticonvulsant can build up to toxic levels within a day or two. *This interaction can be life threatening, requiring hospitalization and resuscitation.*

If no other antibiotic is appropriate, carbamazepine levels must be monitored extremely closely. They may remain high for two or three days after the antibiotic is discontinued. The doctor may be able to adjust the dose of Tegretol to avoid a toxic reaction. Contact your physician without delay if there is any sign of problems.

Symptoms of Carbamazepine Toxicity
Nausea, vomiting, drowsiness, unsteadiness, incoordination, dizziness, muscle twitching or tremor, irregular breathing, rapid heartbeat, changes in blood pressure, changes in urination, and impaired consciousness. Notify your physician immediately of any such symptoms.

Never take or stop medication without your doctor's advice.

Anticonvulsant
(CARBAMAZEPINE)

Pain Reliever
(PROPOXYPHENE)

LIFE-THREATENING

BRAND NAME   GENERIC NAME
Tegretol   carbamazepine

INSTRUCTIONS
Carbamazepine may upset the stomach; if so, take it with food or milk. Do not stop this drug suddenly; seizures could result. To maintain its strength, it must be stored away from humidity and heat in a tightly closed container.

BRAND NAME   GENERIC NAME
Darvocet-N   propoxyphene/
   acetaminophen
Darvon   propoxyphene
Darvon-N   propoxyphene
Wygesic   propoxyphene/
   acetaminophen

INSTRUCTIONS
Propoxyphene should be taken with food to reduce the risk of nausea. If it causes constipation, a stool softener or fiber bulk agent (such as Metamucil) may be used. Do not drink alcohol while taking propoxyphene.

INTERACTION

Propoxyphene interferes with liver metabolism of Tegretol and leads to high blood levels of carbamazepine. This will probably occur in most people taking both medications, with blood levels of the anticonvulsant ranging from 66 to 300 percent higher than normal. *This interaction can result in life-threatening carbamazepine toxicity, with possible coma.*

Generally, the doctor will be able to prescribe an alternate pain medication. If this is not possible, frequent monitoring of carbamazepine blood levels is necessary to prevent a dangerous interaction.

Symptoms of Carbamazepine Toxicity
Nausea, vomiting, drowsiness, unsteadiness, incoordination, dizziness, muscle twitching or tremor, irregular breathing, rapid heartbeat, changes in blood pressure, changes in urination, and impaired consciousness. Notify your physician immediately of any such symptoms.

Never take or stop medication without your doctor's advice.

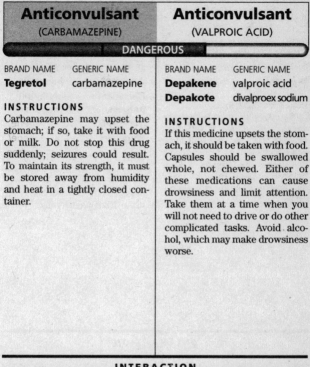

Anticonvulsant
(CARBAMAZEPINE)

Anticonvulsant
(VALPROIC ACID)

DANGEROUS

BRAND NAME   GENERIC NAME
Tegretol   carbamazepine

INSTRUCTIONS
Carbamazepine may upset the stomach; if so, take it with food or milk. Do not stop this drug suddenly; seizures could result. To maintain its strength, it must be stored away from humidity and heat in a tightly closed container.

BRAND NAME   GENERIC NAME
Depakene   valproic acid
Depakote   divalproex sodium

INSTRUCTIONS
If this medicine upsets the stomach, it should be taken with food. Capsules should be swallowed whole, not chewed. Either of these medications can cause drowsiness and limit attention. Take them at a time when you will not need to drive or do other complicated tasks. Avoid alcohol, which may make drowsiness worse.

INTERACTION
Carbamazepine and valproic acid may both be prescribed for a complex seizure disorder. This combination may be complicated, because Tegretol can speed the elimination of Depakene and other valproates from the body. This may result in lower blood levels, and possibly a loss of effectiveness. *Because of the risk of seizures, this interaction is dangerous.*

Valproic acid can also affect carbamazepine levels. The action may vary from one person to another. Regular blood tests to monitor levels of both drugs are desirable for at least one month after starting or stopping this combination. Dosage adjustments may be necessary.

Symptoms of Carbamazepine Toxicity
Nausea, vomiting, drowsiness, unsteadiness, incoordination, dizziness, muscle twitching or tremor, irregular breathing, rapid heartbeat, changes in blood pressure, changes in urination, and impaired consciousness. Notify your physician immediately of any such symptoms.

Never take or stop medication without your doctor's advice.

Anticonvulsant
(CARBAMAZEPINE)

Anticonvulsants
(HYDANTOINS)

DANGEROUS

BRAND NAME	GENERIC NAME
Tegretol	carbamazepine

INSTRUCTIONS
Carbamazepine may upset the stomach; if so, take it with food or milk. Do not stop this drug suddenly; seizures could result. To maintain its strength, it must be stored away from humidity and heat in a tightly closed container.

BRAND NAME	GENERIC NAME
Dilantin	phenytoin
Mesantoin	mephenytoin
Peganone	ethotoin

INSTRUCTIONS
Any of these medicines could upset the stomach. This is less likely if they are taken with food. All of them can cause drowsiness or blurred vision and could make driving dangerous.

INTERACTION

People who have had seizures often need more than one kind of medicine to prevent a recurrence. Carbamazepine and an anticonvulsant such as Dilantin may be prescribed together and can be helpful. They may interact in a complex and unpredictable way, however. Dilantin and similar drugs can lower blood levels of carbamazepine. No seizures have been reported as a result, but theoretically they are possible. In contrast, carbamazepine sometimes raises and sometimes lowers blood levels of Dilantin. Some cases of toxicity from excess phenytoin have been reported. *This interaction could well be dangerous.*

Frequent blood tests for both drugs are advised, especially when starting, stopping, or changing the dose of one of them. The dose of one or both may need to be adjusted.

Symptoms of Phenytoin Toxicity
Uncontrollable eye movements (nystagmus), unsteadiness, difficulty speaking clearly, dizziness, and stupor. Notify your physician immediately of any of these symptoms.

Never take or stop medication without your doctor's advice.

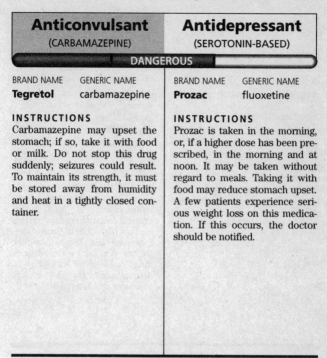

Anticonvulsant (CARBAMAZEPINE)	**Antidepressant** (SEROTONIN-BASED)

DANGEROUS

BRAND NAME   GENERIC NAME
Tegretol   carbamazepine

INSTRUCTIONS
Carbamazepine may upset the stomach; if so, take it with food or milk. Do not stop this drug suddenly; seizures could result. To maintain its strength, it must be stored away from humidity and heat in a tightly closed container.

BRAND NAME   GENERIC NAME
Prozac   fluoxetine

INSTRUCTIONS
Prozac is taken in the morning, or, if a higher dose has been prescribed, in the morning and at noon. It may be taken without regard to meals. Taking it with food may reduce stomach upset. A few patients experience serious weight loss on this medication. If this occurs, the doctor should be notified.

INTERACTION
A depressed person with epilepsy might need both Prozac and carbamazepine. This combination might also be prescribed to someone with bipolar depression who has not responded to the usual treatments. Prozac apparently interferes with carbamazepine metabolism and may increase blood levels of the anticonvulsant to the point of toxicity. *The interaction could be dangerous.*

Because Prozac can linger in the body, the problems may continue for some time even if the drug is discontinued. Notify your physician immediately if you experience symptoms. There are no documented problems with the related antidepressants Paxil and Zoloft, but be alert for such a possibility.

Symptoms of Carbamazepine Toxicity
Nausea, vomiting, drowsiness, unsteadiness, incoordination, dizziness, muscle twitching or tremor, irregular breathing, rapid heartbeat, changes in blood pressure, changes in urination, and impaired consciousness. Notify your physician immediately of any such symptoms.

Never take or stop medication without your doctor's advice.

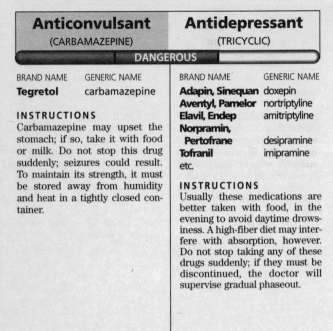

Anticonvulsant
(CARBAMAZEPINE)

Antidepressant
(TRICYCLIC)

DANGEROUS

BRAND NAME   GENERIC NAME

Tegretol   carbamazepine

INSTRUCTIONS
Carbamazepine may upset the stomach; if so, take it with food or milk. Do not stop this drug suddenly; seizures could result. To maintain its strength, it must be stored away from humidity and heat in a tightly closed container.

BRAND NAME   GENERIC NAME

Adapin, Sinequan doxepin
Aventyl, Pamelor nortriptyline
Elavil, Endep amitriptyline
**Norpramin,
  Pertofrane**   desipramine
Tofranil   imipramine
etc.

INSTRUCTIONS
Usually these medications are better taken with food, in the evening to avoid daytime drowsiness. A high-fiber diet may interfere with absorption, however. Do not stop taking any of these drugs suddenly; if they must be discontinued, the doctor will supervise gradual phaseout.

INTERACTION
There are many reasons (including bipolar disorder) a patient might require both carbamazepine and a tricyclic antidepressant. There are indications from the medical literature that people taking both types of drug may have lower blood levels of the tricyclic antidepressant. It is not clear how often this has an impact on effectiveness. Conversely, at least one patient developed carbamazepine toxicity when she started taking desipramine. Blood levels of the anticonvulsant were dangerously high. *No one knows how often this interaction may occur, but it could be dangerous.*

Blood levels of both carbamazepine and tricyclic antidepressants should be checked when a person starts or stops this combination. Report any unusual symptoms to your doctor.

Symptoms of Carbamazepine Toxicity
Nausea, vomiting, drowsiness, unsteadiness, incoordination, dizziness, muscle twitching or tremor, irregular breathing, rapid heartbeat, changes in blood pressure, changes in urination, and impaired consciousness. Notify the physician immediately of any such symptoms.

Never take or stop medication without your doctor's advice.

Anticonvulsant	**Asthma Drug**
(CARBAMAZEPINE)	(THEOPHYLLINE)

DANGEROUS

BRAND NAME   GENERIC NAME

Tegretol   carbamazepine

INSTRUCTIONS

Carbamazepine may upset the stomach; if so, take it with food or milk. Do not stop this drug suddenly; seizures could result. To maintain its strength, it must be stored away from humidity and heat in a tightly closed container.

BRAND NAME

Aerolate	**Aquaphyllin**
Bronkodyl	**Elixomin**
Elixophyllin	**Quibron-T**
Slo-bid	**Slo-Phyllin**
Theobid	**Theochron**
Theoclear	**Theo-Dur**
Theolair	**Theo-24**
Theovent	**Uniphyl**

INSTRUCTIONS

Theophylline interacts with food in complex ways, so discuss this issue thoroughly with your doctor and pharmacist. Theophylline may upset the stomach. In some cases this problem can be alleviated by taking the drug with food. See pages 73–91 for more information.

INTERACTION

This interaction is complex and confusing, because carbamazepine may either increase or decrease blood levels of theophylline. Case reports confirm that both reactions occur.

Increased theophylline levels may lead to toxicity. Diminished levels may be associated with reduced efficacy. In addition, theophylline may reduce carbamazepine levels, leading to a seizure. *This interaction could be dangerous.*

It is important for your physician to check blood levels of both drugs. If you experience symptoms of toxicity, let your doctor know at once.
Symptoms of Theophylline Toxicity
Nausea, diarrhea, stomach pain, headache, insomnia, restlessness, and irritability. Severe toxicity (convulsions, heart rhythm changes, or death) may occur with no warning symptoms. Notify your doctor immediately if you suspect a problem.

Never take or stop medication without your doctor's advice.

Anticonvulsant | Endometriosis Drug
(CARBAMAZEPINE) | (DANAZOL)

DANGEROUS

BRAND NAME	GENERIC NAME	BRAND NAME	GENERIC NAME
Tegretol	carbamazepine	**Danocrine**	danazol

INSTRUCTIONS

Carbamazepine may upset the stomach; if so, take it with food or milk. Do not stop this drug suddenly; seizures could result. To maintain its strength, it must be stored away from humidity and heat in a tightly closed container.

INSTRUCTIONS

Danocrine may be taken either with food or on an empty stomach. During Danocrine therapy, sexually active women should use barrier contraceptives (such as a diaphragm or condoms).

INTERACTION

Danocrine may increase blood levels of carbamazepine to double the previous measurement. Several women on this combination of drugs experienced carbamazepine toxicity associated with high blood levels several days to a month after they added Danocrine to their regimen. *This interaction could be dangerous.*

A patient who requires both drugs should have carbamazepine blood levels monitored carefully when starting or stopping the Danocrine. She should also be aware that lethargy, dizziness, blurred vision, or unsteady gait may be signs of toxicity, and contact her doctor if she experiences any of them. The dose of carbamazepine may need adjustment.

Symptoms of Carbamazepine Toxicity

Nausea, vomiting, drowsiness, unsteadiness, incoordination, dizziness, muscle twitching or tremor, irregular breathing, rapid heartbeat, changes in blood pressure, changes in urination, and impaired consciousness. Notify your physician immediately of any such symptoms.

Never take or stop medication without your doctor's advice.

Anticonvulsant
(CARBAMAZEPINE)

Heart/Blood Pressure Drugs
(CALCIUM CHANNEL BLOCKERS)

DANGEROUS

BRAND NAME	GENERIC NAME
Tegretol	carbamazepine

INSTRUCTIONS
Carbamazepine may upset the stomach; if so, take it with food or milk. Do not stop this drug suddenly; seizures could result. To maintain its strength, it must be stored away from humidity and heat in a tightly closed container.

BRAND NAME	GENERIC NAME
Calan,	
Isoptin	verapamil
Cardizem,	
Dilacor XR	diltiazem
Plendil	felodipine
Verelan	verapamil

INSTRUCTIONS
Sustained-release forms, such as Calan SR or Dilacor XR, should not be chewed or crushed. Taking Plendil with grapefruit juice may lead to unexpectedly high blood levels. See pages 73–91 for specifics. If the drug must be discontinued, follow your doctor's instructions for gradual tapering.

INTERACTION
Both verapamil and diltiazem have been associated with elevated blood levels of carbamazepine, with the possibility of toxicity. *This interaction could be dangerous.*

Carbamazepine concentrations should be monitored closely if this drug is taken with a calcium channel blocker. Nifedipine may not interact, but the dose of carbamazepine may need to be reduced by as much as 50 percent when combined with verapamil. Monitoring is crucial if a patient on Tegretol stops taking a calcium channel blocker.

If a patient on Plendil takes carbamazepine, blood pressure may not be controlled with the normal dose of Plendil. One study found that patients on Tegretol had only about 6 percent the amount of Plendil in their bloodstreams as people taking the Plendil alone. In such a case, your doctor may want to adjust the dose of Plendil.

Symptoms of Carbamazepine Toxicity
Nausea, vomiting, drowsiness, unsteadiness, incoordination, dizziness, muscle twitching or tremor, irregular breathing, rapid heartbeat, changes in blood pressure, changes in urination, and impaired consciousness. Notify the physician immediately of any such symptoms.

Never take or stop medication without your doctor's advice.

Anticonvulsant
(CARBAMAZEPINE)

Lithium

DANGEROUS

BRAND NAME | GENERIC NAME
Tegretol | carbamazepine

INSTRUCTIONS
Carbamazepine may upset the stomach; if so, take it with food or milk. Do not stop this drug suddenly; seizures could result. To maintain its strength, it must be stored away from humidity and heat in a tightly closed container.

BRAND NAME
Cibalith-S
Eskalith
Lithane
Lithobid
Lithonate
Lithotabs

INSTRUCTIONS
Lithium should be taken immediately after meals or with food or milk to reduce stomach upset. It is essential to drink 8 to 12 glasses of water or other fluid each day while on lithium. This medication can affect alertness, so activities such as driving or operating machinery can be dangerous for people on lithium.

INTERACTION
Carbamazepine appears to make lithium more effective, without necessarily boosting blood levels noticeably. In some patients, this interaction has been of benefit, helping to control the manic phase better. In others, however, it has resulted in symptoms of lithium toxicity. *This interaction could be dangerous.*

Lithium may interact with carbamazepine to improve white blood cell counts that may be depressed by the anticonvulsant. Both drugs can affect thyroid function, however, and together may impact more heavily on the thyroid (lower circulating thyroid hormone) than either separately. Monitoring of clinical status is important when someone on lithium starts or stops carbamazepine. Blood tests for lithium levels may not tell the whole story. Patients on this combination should have thyroid function checked regularly.

Symptoms of Lithium Toxicity
Nausea, diarrhea, incoordination, muscle weakness, and difficulty walking may be signs of toxicity. Ringing in the ears, visual problems, dizziness, slurred speech, confusion, agitation, and incontinence are more serious. Notify the physician promptly of any such symptoms.

Never take or stop medication without your doctor's advice.

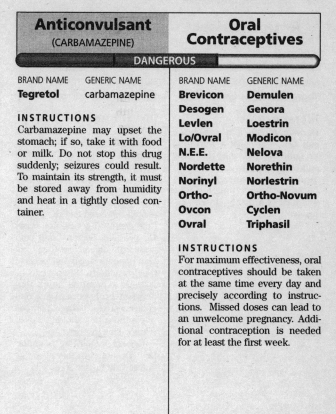

Anticonvulsant (CARBAMAZEPINE)	Oral Contraceptives

DANGEROUS

BRAND NAME	GENERIC NAME
Tegretol	carbamazepine

INSTRUCTIONS
Carbamazepine may upset the stomach; if so, take it with food or milk. Do not stop this drug suddenly; seizures could result. To maintain its strength, it must be stored away from humidity and heat in a tightly closed container.

BRAND NAME	GENERIC NAME
Brevicon	**Demulen**
Desogen	**Genora**
Levlen	**Loestrin**
Lo/Ovral	**Modicon**
N.E.E.	**Nelova**
Nordette	**Norethin**
Norinyl	**Norlestrin**
Ortho-	**Ortho-Novum**
Ovcon	**Cyclen**
Ovral	**Triphasil**

INSTRUCTIONS
For maximum effectiveness, oral contraceptives should be taken at the same time every day and precisely according to instructions. Missed doses can lead to an unwelcome pregnancy. Additional contraception is needed for at least the first week.

INTERACTION
A number of epileptic women (in one study, 3 out of 41) have become pregnant while taking oral contraceptives and carbamazepine. This seems to be the result of carbamazepine speeding clearance of both estrogen and progesterone from the body in less time than usual. *Because carbamazepine has also been associated with some birth defects, this interaction could be dangerous.*

A woman who must take carbamazepine should not rely on oral contraceptives alone.

Never take or stop medication without your doctor's advice.

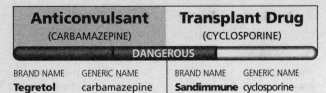

Anticonvulsant (CARBAMAZEPINE)	**Transplant Drug** (CYCLOSPORINE)

DANGEROUS

BRAND NAME	GENERIC NAME	BRAND NAME	GENERIC NAME
Tegretol	carbamazepine	**Sandimmune**	cyclosporine

INSTRUCTIONS

Carbamazepine may upset the stomach; if so, take it with food or milk. Do not stop this drug suddenly; seizures could result. To maintain its strength, it must be stored away from humidity and heat in a tightly closed container.

INSTRUCTIONS

Sandimmune comes as an oral solution with a taste reminiscent of castor oil. It should be mixed in a glass with milk, chocolate milk, or orange juice at room temperature and drunk at once. Then the glass (no plastic) should be rinsed and the rinsing fluid drunk to get the full dose. Do not take Sandimmune with grapefruit juice unless the physician is monitoring blood levels of the drug closely. (See page 53.) Due to a possible interaction between cyclosporine and oral contraceptives, barrier methods of contraception should be used while taking this drug.

Regular monitoring is important. Do not stop this medicine unless your doctor so directs

IINTERACTION

Carbamazepine can increase the speed with which the body disposes of Sandimmune. In some cases, blood levels of Sandimmune drop below detectable limits after carbamazepine is added. *This interaction could be dangerous, with the possibility of a rejection episode resulting.*

Anticonvulsants containing valproic acid (Depakene, etc.) do not appear to affect Sandimmune concentrations in the same way and may offer an alternative. If both Sandimmune and carbamazepine are needed, blood tests for Sandimmune levels are recommended.

Never take or stop medication without your doctor's advice.

Anticonvulsant	**Tuberculosis Drug**
(CARBAMAZEPINE)	(ISONIAZID)

DANGEROUS

BRAND NAME	GENERIC NAME
Tegretol	carbamazepine

INSTRUCTIONS
Carbamazepine may upset the stomach; if so, take it with food or milk. Do not stop this drug suddenly; seizures could result. To maintain its strength, it must be stored away from humidity and heat in a tightly closed container.

BRAND NAME	GENERIC NAME
INH	isoniazid
Izonid	isoniazid
Laniazid	isoniazid
Nydrazid	isoniazid
Rifamate	isoniazid/rifampin

INSTRUCTIONS
Isoniazid is best taken on an empty stomach, at least one hour before meals or two hours after. It may be taken with food if it upsets the stomach. Alcohol increases the risk of a potentially fatal liver reaction. Foods high in tyramine interact with isoniazid to raise blood pressure dangerously; see the list on page 59. Symptoms of B_6 deficiency may develop; supplements may be required.

INTERACTION
Isoniazid can interfere with carbamazepine metabolism, leading to a buildup of the anticonvulsant in the body. Most patients on this combination will have higher blood levels of the anticonvulsant than they did before starting the tuberculosis drug. *This interaction can be dangerous, with carbamazepine toxicity developing rather quickly.*

There is some evidence that carbamazepine, in turn, can make isoniazid more toxic to the liver. If both drugs are required, blood levels of both carbamazepine and liver enzymes should be monitored closely. Contact your doctor at the first sign of trouble.

Symptoms of Carbamazepine Toxicity
Nausea, vomiting, drowsiness, unsteadiness, incoordination, dizziness, muscle twitching or tremor, irregular breathing, rapid heartbeat, changes in blood pressure, changes in urination, and impaired consciousness. Notify the physician immediately of any such symptoms.

Never take or stop medication without your doctor's advice.

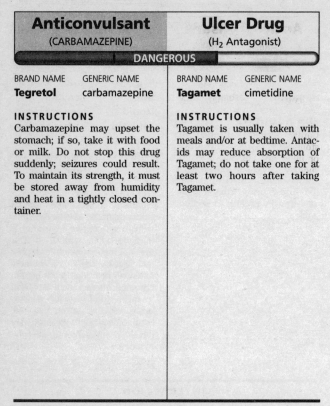

Anticonvulsant (CARBAMAZEPINE)	**Ulcer Drug** (H$_2$ Antagonist)

DANGEROUS

BRAND NAME	GENERIC NAME	BRAND NAME	GENERIC NAME
Tegretol	carbamazepine	**Tagamet**	cimetidine

INSTRUCTIONS
Carbamazepine may upset the stomach; if so, take it with food or milk. Do not stop this drug suddenly; seizures could result. To maintain its strength, it must be stored away from humidity and heat in a tightly closed container.

INSTRUCTIONS
Tagamet is usually taken with meals and/or at bedtime. Antacids may reduce absorption of Tagamet; do not take one for at least two hours after taking Tagamet.

INTERACTION

Tagamet appears to modify the metabolism of carbamazepine. The problem is that Tagamet affects liver enzymes and may make them less capable of processing these anticonvulsants. As a result, blood levels can rise. *This could lead to dangerous toxicity.*

While Tagamet and Tegretol seem less likely to interact if Tegretol has been taken for longer than four weeks, physicians should be cautious when considering such a combination.

Symptoms of Carbamazepine Toxicity
Nausea, vomiting, drowsiness, unsteadiness, incoordination, dizziness, muscle twitching or tremor, irregular breathing, rapid heartbeat, changes in blood pressure, changes in urination, and impaired consciousness. Notify the physician immediately of any such symptoms.

Never take or stop medication without your doctor's advice.

Anticonvulsant	**Antibiotic**
(CARBAMAZEPINE)	(DOXYCYCLINE)

TROUBLESOME

BRAND NAME	GENERIC NAME
Tegretol	carbamazepine

INSTRUCTIONS

Carbamazepine may upset the stomach; if so, take it with food or milk. Do not stop this drug suddenly; seizures could result. To maintain its strength, it must be stored away from humidity and heat in a tightly closed container.

BRAND NAME	GENERIC NAME
Doryx	doxycycline
Doxi Film	doxycycline
Doxy-Caps	doxycycline
Doxychel Hyclate	
	doxycycline
Doxy-D	doxycycline
Monodox	doxycycline
Vibramycin	doxycycline
Vibra-Tabs	doxycycline

INSTRUCTIONS

Doxycycline may be taken with food or milk to reduce stomach upset, always with a full eight ounces of liquid. Do not take this medicine with antacids, calcium supplements, or iron pills, as they could interfere with absorption of the drug. Never take outdated doxycycline, which may be toxic to the kidneys.

INTERACTION

Tegretol can speed the liver's processing of this antibiotic, potentially lowering blood levels and making it less effective. *This interaction could be troublesome, as the infection might not be eradicated.*

Other tetracyclines do not appear to interact with carbamazepine in this manner. If doxycycline is best, the doctor will want to keep a careful watch on the patient's progress, as a higher dose of doxycycline may be needed.

Never take or stop medication without your doctor's advice.

Anticonvulsant
(CARBAMAZEPINE)

Anticoagulant
(WARFARIN)

TROUBLESOME

BRAND NAME   GENERIC NAME
Tegretol   carbamazepine

BRAND NAME   GENERIC NAME
Coumadin   warfarin

INSTRUCTIONS
Carbamazepine may upset the stomach; if so, take it with food or milk. Do not stop this drug suddenly; seizures could result. To maintain its strength, it must be stored away from humidity and heat in a tightly closed container.

INSTRUCTIONS
Warfarin tablets can be swallowed with food or on an empty stomach. Try to avoid large variations in the quantity of vitamin-K–containing vegetables—such as broccoli, cabbage, or spinach—that you eat each day. Consuming much more or less than usual could change the action of the drug.

INTERACTION
Carbamazepine apparently reduces circulating levels of warfarin. The result could be a greater risk of blood clots. *This interaction could be troublesome.*

When a person on warfarin needs to start or stop taking this anticonvulsant, close monitoring of prothrombin time is appropriate. A few case reports feature patients whose prothrombin time was five or six times greater upon discontinuing carbamazepine, a situation that could lead to dangerous bleeding. The physician may need to adjust the dose of warfarin when Tegretol is discontinued.

Symptoms of Warfarin Overdose
There may be no early warning signs of danger. Blood tests are essential. Symptoms include any unusual bleeding, including rectal or urinary tract bleeding, excessive menstrual bleeding, nosebleeds, bleeding around gums, bruising, red or tar-black stools, vomiting blood, and red or dark-brown urine. Notify your doctor immediately if you suspect a problem.

Never take or stop medication without your doctor's advice.

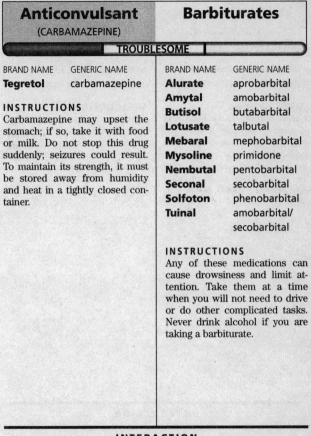

Anticonvulsant
(CARBAMAZEPINE)

Barbiturates

TROUBLESOME

BRAND NAME	GENERIC NAME
Tegretol	carbamazepine

INSTRUCTIONS
Carbamazepine may upset the stomach; if so, take it with food or milk. Do not stop this drug suddenly; seizures could result. To maintain its strength, it must be stored away from humidity and heat in a tightly closed container.

BRAND NAME	GENERIC NAME
Alurate	aprobarbital
Amytal	amobarbital
Butisol	butabarbital
Lotusate	talbutal
Mebaral	mephobarbital
Mysoline	primidone
Nembutal	pentobarbital
Seconal	secobarbital
Solfoton	phenobarbital
Tuinal	amobarbital/ secobarbital

INSTRUCTIONS
Any of these medications can cause drowsiness and limit attention. Take them at a time when you will not need to drive or do other complicated tasks. Never drink alcohol if you are taking a barbiturate.

INTERACTION

In complex seizure situations, a combination of carbamazepine and barbiturates may be appropriate for the control of epilepsy. Caution is required with this combination, however. Barbiturates can rev up the liver enzymes that process carbamazepine, speeding its elimination from the body. This generally leads to lower blood levels of the anticonvulsant than when it is taken alone. *This interaction might be troublesome if the anticonvulsant becomes less effective.*

Seizures are possible. They occurred in one case in which the barbiturate Mysoline evidently interfered with carbamazepine.

Never take or stop medication without your doctor's advice.

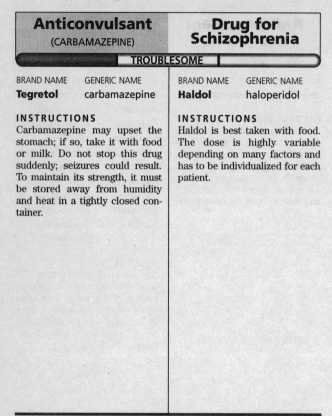

Anticonvulsant
(CARBAMAZEPINE)

Drug for Schizophrenia

TROUBLESOME

BRAND NAME	GENERIC NAME
Tegretol	carbamazepine

INSTRUCTIONS
Carbamazepine may upset the stomach; if so, take it with food or milk. Do not stop this drug suddenly; seizures could result. To maintain its strength, it must be stored away from humidity and heat in a tightly closed container.

BRAND NAME	GENERIC NAME
Haldol	haloperidol

INSTRUCTIONS
Haldol is best taken with food. The dose is highly variable depending on many factors and has to be individualized for each patient.

INTERACTION

This interaction is exceptionally confusing, because studies and clinical reports do not agree on its direction and impact. In some situations, patients do well on this combination of medications. Other reports show significantly (up to 60 percent) lower blood levels of Haldol when carbamazepine is added to the regimen. In some cases, this has resulted in lower efficacy, with a recurrence of hallucinations, delusions, and schizophrenic behavior. *This interaction could be troublesome.*

If a patient needs both medications, the doctor will need to monitor the clinical status carefully. The dosage of Haldol may require adjustment.

Never take or stop medication without your doctor's advice.

Anticonvulsant
(CARBAMAZEPINE)

Influenza Vaccine

TROUBLESOME

BRAND NAME	GENERIC NAME
Tegretol	carbamazepine

INSTRUCTIONS
Carbamazepine may upset the stomach; if so, take it with food or milk. Do not stop this drug suddenly; seizures could result. To maintain its strength, it must be stored away from humidity and heat in a tightly closed container.

BRAND NAME	GENERIC NAME
Fluogen	
FluShield	
Fluvirin	
Fluzone	
influenza virus vaccine trivalent	

INSTRUCTIONS
Vaccination is recommended for people over age 65, for those with chronic conditions, especially of the heart or lungs, and for the caregivers or household contacts of those at high risk. People who are allergic to chicken egg may also be allergic to the vaccine. Appropriate precautions are advised.

INTERACTION
Flu vaccine may interfere with the normal metabolism of carbamazepine, allowing blood levels of the anticonvulsant to rise. There is a possibility of carbamazepine toxicity for a few days following vaccination. Carbamazepine levels should be monitored. Notify your physician if you feel drowsy, lethargic, dizzy, or unsteady on your feet. *This interaction may be troublesome.*

Symptoms of Carbamazepine Toxicity
Nausea, vomiting, drowsiness, unsteadiness, incoordination, dizziness, muscle twitching or tremor, irregular breathing, rapid heartbeat, changes in blood pressure, changes in urination, and impaired consciousness. Notify your physician immediately of any such symptoms.

Never take or stop medication without your doctor's advice.

Anticonvulsants (HYDANTOINS)

Dilantin   Mesantoin   Peganone

LIFE-THREATENING

Transplant Drug Sandimmune

DANGEROUS

Anticonvulsant Tegretol
Anticonvulsant (valproic acid) Depakene Depakote
Anticonvulsant Mysoline
Antidepressant (serotonin-based) Prozac
Antifungal Drugs Diflucan Monistat
Heart Drug Cordarone
Oral Contraceptives
Tuberculosis Drugs (isoniazid) INH Izonid Laniazid
Nydrazid Rifamate
Ulcer Drugs Prilosec Tagamet

TROUBLESOME

Anti-Anxiety Drugs (benzodiazepines) Librium
Valium
Antibiotic (doxycycline) Doryx Monodox
Vibramycin Vibra-Tabs
Asthma Drug (theophylline) Elixophyllin Quibron-T
Slo-bid Theobid Theo-Dur Theo-24 Theovent etc.
Folic Acid
Heart Drug Mexitil
Heart Drug (quinidine) Cardioquin Quinaglute
Quinalan Quinidex Quinora
Pain Reliever (acetaminophen) Anacin-3 Darvocet-N
Panadol Tylenol etc.
Tuberculosis Drugs (rifampin) Rifadin Rifamate
Rimactane

Dilantin and other hydantoin anticonvulsants interact with many other medications. Some of these interactions are potentially serious. We have included the most common, but be sure to check with your physician and pharmacist if you must take any other drugs in conjunction with the anticonvulsants listed above.

Anticonvulsants (HYDANTOINS)	**Transplant Drug** (CYCLOSPORINE)

LIFE-THREATENING

BRAND NAME	GENERIC NAME
Dilantin	phenytoin
Mesantoin	mephenytoin
Peganone	ethotoin

INSTRUCTIONS

Any of these medicines could upset the stomach. This is less likely if they are taken with food. All of them can cause drowsiness or blurred vision and could make driving dangerous.

BRAND NAME	GENERIC NAME
Sandimmune	cyclosporine

INSTRUCTIONS

Sandimmune comes as an oral solution with a taste reminiscent of castor oil. It should be mixed in a glass with milk, chocolate milk, or orange juice at room temperature and drunk at once. Then the glass (no plastic) should be rinsed and the rinsing fluid drunk to get the full dose. Do not take Sandimmune with grapefruit juice unless the physician is monitoring blood levels of the drug closely. (See page 53.)

Due to a possible interaction between cyclosporine and oral contraceptives, barrier methods of contraception should be used while taking this drug.

Regular monitoring is important. Do not stop this medicine unless your doctor so directs.

INTERACTION

Dilantin, and presumably the other drugs in its class, seems to interfere significantly with the absorption of Sandimmune. Patients on this combination have only half as much of the transplant drug circulating in their bodies as they had before starting Dilantin. The interaction sets in within two days of starting on Dilantin, and disappears within a week of stopping the anticonvulsant. Taking the medicines at different times does not seem to help. *Although we are aware of no deaths as a consequence of this interaction, such low levels of Sandimmune could lead to a life-threatening rejection episode.*

A person who needs both drugs should have Sandimmune levels monitored closely. The dose may need adjustment to maintain adequate blood levels. Contact your physician without delay if there is any sign of trouble.

Never take or stop medication without your doctor's advice.

Anticonvulsants
(HYDANTOINS)

Anticonvulsant
(CARBAMAZEPINE)

DANGEROUS

BRAND NAME	GENERIC NAME
Dilantin	phenytoin
Mesantoin	mephenytoin
Peganone	ethotoin

INSTRUCTIONS
Any of these medicines could upset the stomach. This is less likely if they are taken with food. All of them can cause drowsiness or blurred vision and could make driving dangerous.

BRAND NAME	GENERIC NAME
Tegretol	carbamazepine

INSTRUCTIONS
Carbamazepine may upset the stomach; if so, take it with food or milk. Do not stop this drug suddenly; seizures could result. To maintain its strength, it must be stored away from humidity and heat in a tightly closed container.

∎INTERACTION

People who have had seizures often need more than one kind of medicine to prevent a recurrence. Carbamazepine and an anticonvulsant such as Dilantin may be prescribed together and can be helpful. They may interact in a complex and unpredictable way, however. Dilantin and similar drugs can lower blood levels of carbamazepine. No seizures have been reported as a result, but theoretically they are possible. In contrast, carbamazepine sometimes raises and sometimes lowers blood levels of Dilantin. Some cases of toxicity from excess phenytoin have been reported. *This interaction could well be dangerous.*

Frequent blood tests for both drugs are advised, especially when starting, stopping, or changing the dose of one of them. The dose of one or both may need to be adjusted.

Symptoms of Phenytoin Toxicity
Uncontrollable eye movements (nystagmus), unsteadiness, difficulty speaking clearly, dizziness, and stupor. Notify your physician immediately of any of these symptoms.

Never take or stop medication without your doctor's advice.

Anticonvulsants (HYDANTOINS)	**Anticonvulsants** (VALPROIC ACID)

DANGEROUS

BRAND NAME	GENERIC NAME	BRAND NAME	GENERIC NAME
Dilantin	phenytoin	**Depakene**	valproic acid
Mesantoin	mephenytoin	**Depakote**	divalproex
Peganone	ethotoin		sodium

INSTRUCTIONS

Any of these medicines could upset the stomach. This is less likely if they are taken with food. All of them can cause drowsiness or blurred vision and could make driving dangerous.

INSTRUCTIONS

If this medicine upsets the stomach, it should be taken with food. Capsules should be swallowed whole, not chewed. Any of these medications can cause drowsiness and limit attention. Take them at a time when you will not need to drive or do other complicated tasks. Avoid alcohol, which may make drowsiness worse.

INTERACTION

Doctors may prescribe Dilantin and valproic acid together for a complex seizure disorder. Getting the dosage of the combination correct, however, may be complicated. Valproic acid competes with phenytoin for metabolic enzymes and carriers in the blood. The usual result is greater activity of Dilantin. Toxicity may occur even when blood levels are within the normal range.

Phenytoin may also reduce valproic acid levels, which might result in a loss of seizure control. Interpreting blood tests for these drugs is difficult because the interaction is extremely complex. Levels of both drugs should be monitored, however, so that doses can be adjusted if necessary. *The risk of toxicity or seizures makes this interaction dangerous.*

Symptoms of Phenytoin Toxicity

Uncontrollable eye movements (nystagmus), unsteadiness, difficulty speaking clearly, dizziness, and stupor. Notify your physician immediately of any of these symptoms.

Never take or stop medication without your doctor's advice.

Anticonvulsants
(HYDANTOINS)

Anticonvulsant
(PRIMIDONE)

DANGEROUS

BRAND NAME	GENERIC NAME
Dilantin	phenytoin
Mesantoin	mephenytoin
Peganone	ethotoin

INSTRUCTIONS
Any of these medicines could upset the stomach. This is less likely if they are taken with food. All of them can cause drowsiness or blurred vision and could make driving dangerous.

BRAND NAME	GENERIC NAME
Mysoline	primidone

INSTRUCTIONS
This drug may upset the stomach. If so, it should be taken with food. It can cause drowsiness or blurred vision and could make driving or other complex tasks more dangerous.

INTERACTION
People who have had seizures may need more than one kind of medicine to prevent a recurrence. Dilantin and Mysoline may be prescribed together to good effect. Blood levels must be monitored when starting or stopping Dilantin, however, because this and similar drugs can alter the metabolism of primidone. Mysoline is broken down in the body into phenobarbital, among other chemicals, and blood levels of phenobarbital increase by up to 50 percent when primidone and Dilantin are taken together. There is a potential for primidone to reach toxic levels. *This interaction could be dangerous.*

Symptoms of Primidone Toxicity
Unsteadiness, nausea, vomiting, uncontrollable eye movements (nystagmus), dizziness, drowsiness, and impaired consciousness. Notify your physician immediately about any of these symptoms.

Never take or stop medication without your doctor's advice.

Anticonvulsants (HYDANTOINS)	**Antidepressants** (SEROTONIN-BASED)

DANGEROUS

BRAND NAME	GENERIC NAME
Dilantin	phenytoin
Mesantoin	mephenytoin
Peganone	ethotoin

INSTRUCTIONS

Any of these medicines could upset the stomach. This is less likely if they are taken with food. All of them can cause drowsiness or blurred vision and could make driving dangerous.

BRAND NAME	GENERIC NAME
Prozac	fluoxetine

INSTRUCTIONS

Prozac is taken in the morning, or, if a higher dose has been prescribed, in the morning and at noon. It may be taken without regard to meals. Taking it with food may reduce stomach upset. A few patients experience serious weight loss on this medication. If this occurs, the doctor should be notified.

INTERACTION

A depressed person with epilepsy might need both Prozac and an anticonvulsant medicine. Prozac apparently interferes with the metabolism of these compounds and may increase blood levels of Dilantin or similar anticonvulsants to the point of toxicity. *The interaction could be dangerous.*

Because Prozac can linger in the body, interaction problems may continue for some time even if Prozac is discontinued. Notify your physician immediately if you experience symptoms such as unsteadiness, slurred speech, blurred vision, incoordination, dizziness, drowsiness, or confusion. Blood tests for a few weeks after starting or a few weeks after stopping Prozac are advisable.

Symptoms of Phenytoin Toxicity

Uncontrollable eye movements (nystagmus), unsteadiness, difficulty speaking clearly, dizziness, and stupor. Notify the physician immediately of any of these symptoms.

Never take or stop medication without your doctor's advice.

Anticonvulsants
(HYDANTOINS)

Antifungal Drugs

DANGEROUS

BRAND NAME	GENERIC NAME
Dilantin	phenytoin
Mesantoin	mephenytoin
Peganone	ethotoin

INSTRUCTIONS

Any of these medicines could upset the stomach. This is less likely if they are taken with food. All of them can cause drowsiness or blurred vision and could make driving dangerous.

BRAND NAME	GENERIC NAME
Diflucan	fluconazole
Monistat	miconazole

INSTRUCTIONS

Ask your doctor for precise instructions on how to take Diflucan. Doses are individualized, depending on the infection treated, and the first dose is often higher than the rest. Unprotected sexual intercourse should be avoided during Monistat treatment.

INTERACTION

Monistat is commonly used as a vaginal cream, which could result in blood levels too low to trigger this reaction. Clinical studies and case reports indicate that Diflucan can raise blood levels of Dilantin substantially and make it last longer. Toxicity is definitely a possibility. Toxicity associated with elevated phenytoin levels has also occurred when Monistat was given intravenously in conjunction with Dilantin. *This interaction could be dangerous.*

Blood levels of the anticonvulsant should be checked more frequently when someone must start or stop treatment with one of these antifungal drugs. Report any symptoms of toxicity to the doctor.

Symptoms of Phenytoin Toxicity

Uncontrollable eye movements (nystagmus), unsteadiness, difficulty speaking clearly, dizziness, and stupor. Notify the physician immediately of any of these symptoms.

Never take or stop medication without your doctor's advice.

Anticonvulsants	**Heart Drug**
(HYDANTOINS)	(AMIODARONE)

DANGEROUS

BRAND NAME	GENERIC NAME
Dilantin	phenytoin
Mesantoin	mephenytoin
Peganone	ethotoin

INSTRUCTIONS
Any of these medicines could upset the stomach. This is less likely if they are taken with food. All of them can cause drowsiness or blurred vision and could make driving dangerous.

BRAND NAME	GENERIC NAME
Cordarone	amiodarone

INSTRUCTIONS
Follow the physician's directions carefully. Tell your doctor if you notice shortness of breath or changes in vision, or if your skin turns blue.

INTERACTION

Cordarone may interfere with the metabolism of Dilantin and similar drugs, leading to blood levels of the anticonvulsants that are twice as high as normal. In this case, a patient might experience symptoms of phenytoin toxicity. Cordarone is metabolized more rapidly in the presence of Dilantin. In theory, levels as much as 49 percent lower than normal could reduce its effectiveness against arrhythmias. *We are not aware of any cases, but the interaction could be quite dangerous.*

This interaction may show up slowly, so blood levels of phenytoin should be monitored. Be alert for signs of toxicity. Because Cordarone lasts a long time in the body, it may take weeks for blood levels to return to normal unless the doctor is able to adjust the dose.

Symptoms of Phenytoin Toxicity
Uncontrollable eye movements (nystagmus), unsteadiness, difficulty speaking clearly, dizziness, and stupor. Notify the physician immediately of any of these symptoms.

Never take or stop medication without your doctor's advice.

Anticonvulsants
(HYDANTOINS)

Oral Contraceptives

DANGEROUS

BRAND NAME	GENERIC NAME
Dilantin	phenytoin
Mesantoin	mephenytoin
Peganone	ethotoin

INSTRUCTIONS
Any of these medicines could upset the stomach. This is less likely if they are taken with food. All of them can cause drowsiness or blurred vision and could make driving dangerous.

BRAND NAME

Brevicon	**Demulen**
Desogen	**Genora**
Levlen	**Loestrin**
Lo/Ovral	**Modicon**
N.E.E.	**Nelova**
Nordette	**Norethin**
Norinyl	**Norlestrin**
Ortho-Cyclen	**Ortho-Novum**
Ovcon	**Ovral**
Triphasil	

INSTRUCTIONS
Oral contraceptives should be taken at the same time every day and precisely according to instructions. Missed doses can lead to an unwelcome pregnancy. Additional contraception is needed for at least the first week.

INTERACTION

Epileptic women have become pregnant while taking oral contraceptives in conjunction with anticonvulsants. The risk is approximately 25 times higher than the normally very low risk of pregnancy using birth control pills. Hydantoins may speed clearance of both estrogen and progesterone from the body in less time than usual. *Because these anticonvulsants have been associated with some birth defects, this interaction could be dangerous.*

Oral contraceptives may also increase the blood levels of anticonvulsants such as Mesantoin, resulting in toxicity. Other contraceptive methods are advisable, if possible.

Symptoms of Phenytoin Toxicity
Uncontrollable eye movements (nystagmus), unsteadiness, difficulty speaking clearly, dizziness, and stupor. Notify the physician immediately of any of these symptoms.

Never take or stop medication without your doctor's advice.

Anticonvulsants (HYDANTOINS)	**Tuberculosis Drug** (ISONIAZID)

DANGEROUS

BRAND NAME	GENERIC NAME	BRAND NAME	GENERIC NAME
Dilantin	phenytoin	**INH**	isoniazid
Mesantoin	mephenytoin	**Izonid**	isoniazid
Peganone	ethotoin	**Laniazid**	isoniazid
		Nydrazid	isoniazid
		Rifamate	isoniazid/ rifampin

INSTRUCTIONS

Any of these medicines could upset the stomach. This is less likely if they are taken with food. All of them can cause drowsiness or blurred vision and could make driving dangerous.

INSTRUCTIONS

Isoniazid is best taken on an empty stomach, at least one hour before meals or two hours after. It may be taken with food if it upsets the stomach. Alcohol increases the risk of a potentially fatal liver reaction, so don't drink. Foods high in tyramine interact with isoniazid to raise blood pressure dangerously; see the list on page 59. Fish such as skipjack and tuna may trigger an unpleasant histamine reaction. Symptoms of B_6 deficiency may develop; supplements may be required.

INTERACTION

One-tenth to almost a third of the people who must take both the tuberculosis medicine and one of these anticonvulsants will experience phenytoin toxicity. This is a far higher proportion than those who may have toxicity reactions while taking one of the hydantoins alone. *This interaction could be dangerous.*

   It is important for your physician to check blood levels of Dilantin or a similar medication if you start or stop taking isoniazid. If you experience symptoms of toxicity, notify the doctor at once.

Symptoms of Phenytoin Toxicity

Uncontrollable eye movements (nystagmus), unsteadiness, difficulty speaking clearly, dizziness, and stupor. Notify your physician immediately of any of these symptoms.

Never take or stop medication without your doctor's advice.

Anticonvulsants
(HYDANTOINS)

Ulcer Drugs

DANGEROUS

BRAND NAME	GENERIC NAME
Dilantin	phenytoin
Mesantoin	mephenytoin
Peganone	ethotoin

INSTRUCTIONS
Any of these medicines could upset the stomach. This is less likely if they are taken with food. All of them can cause drowsiness or blurred vision and could make driving dangerous.

BRAND NAME	GENERIC NAME
Prilosec	omeprazole
Tagamet	cimetidine

INSTRUCTIONS
Tagamet is usually taken with meals and/or at bedtime. Antacids may reduce absorption of Tagamet; do not take one for at least two hours after taking Tagamet. Prilosec should be taken just before eating, preferably in the morning.

INTERACTION

Tagamet appears to modify the metabolism of Dilantin. Tagamet also seems likely to affect the metabolism of Mesantoin and Peganone, although this interaction has not yet been documented in the medical literature. The problem is that Tagamet affects liver enzymes so that they are less capable of processing these particular anticonvulsants. As a result, blood levels of the anticonvulsants can rise, leading to toxicity. A similar, but weaker, interaction has been noted in studies of Prilosec and Dilantin. *This interaction could be dangerous.*

Symptoms of Phenytoin Toxicity
Uncontrollable eye movements (nystagmus), unsteadiness, difficulty speaking clearly, dizziness, and stupor. Notify your physician immediately of any of these symptoms.

Never take or stop medication without your doctor's advice.

Anticonvulsants
(HYDANTOINS)

Anti-Anxiety Drugs
(BENZODIAZEPINES)

TROUBLESOME

BRAND NAME	GENERIC NAME
Dilantin	phenytoin
Mesantoin	mephenytoin
Peganone	ethotoin

INSTRUCTIONS
Any of these medicines could upset the stomach. This is less likely if they are taken with food. All of them can cause drowsiness or blurred vision and could make driving dangerous.

BRAND NAME	GENERIC NAME
Ativan	lorazepam
Dalmane	flurazepam
Doral	quazepam
Halcion	triazolam
Librium	chlordiazepoxide
Paxipam	halazepam
ProSom	estazolam
Restoril	temazepam
Serax	oxazepam
Tranxene	clorazepate
Valium	diazepam
Xanax	alprazolam

INSTRUCTIONS
These drugs may be taken with food, especially if they upset the digestive tract.

INTERACTION

This is a confusing interaction. The data are contradictory and no firm conclusions can be drawn. Nevertheless, there is some concern that Dilantin (phenytoin) levels may be increased by Valium or Librium. Some patients have apparently experienced symptoms of phenytoin toxicity as a result of this combination. Experts suggest that if patients need a benzodiazepine in addition to Dilantin, their blood phenytoin levels be monitored carefully, especially when starting or stopping the benzodiazepine. Although there is no information about anti-anxiety drugs other than Valium and Librium, the possibility exists that other benzodiazepines might interact with phenytoin as well.

Symptoms of Phenytoin Toxicity
Uncontrollable eye movements (nystagmus), unsteadiness, difficulty speaking clearly, dizziness, and stupor. Notify the physician immediately of any of these symptoms.

Never take or stop medication without your doctor's advice.

Anticonvulsants
(HYDANTOINS)

Antibiotic
(DOXYCYCLINE)

TROUBLESOME

BRAND NAME	GENERIC NAME
Dilantin	phenytoin
Mesantoin	mephenytoin
Peganone	ethotoin

INSTRUCTIONS

Any of these medicines could upset the stomach. This is less likely if they are taken with food. All of them can cause drowsiness or blurred vision and could make driving dangerous.

BRAND NAME	GENERIC NAME
Doryx	doxycycline
Doxi Film	doxycycline
Doxy-Caps	doxycycline
Doxychel Hyclate	doxycycline
Doxy-D	doxycycline
Monodox	doxycycline
Vibramycin	doxycycline
Vibra-Tabs	doxycycline

INSTRUCTIONS

Doxycycline may be taken with food or milk to reduce stomach upset, always with a full eight ounces of liquid. Do not take this medicine with antacids, calcium supplements, or iron pills, as they could interfere with absorption of the drug. Never take outdated doxycycline, which may be toxic to the kidneys.

INTERACTION

Dilantin, like Tegretol, can significantly reduce the amount of time it takes for the liver to process and eliminate doxycycline. As a consequence, blood levels of this antibiotic may be lower than expected when it is taken in conjunction with one of the hydantoins, and infections might not heal as quickly or as well as anticipated. *This interaction could certainly be troublesome.*

The doctor may decide to double the dose of doxycycline to ensure therapeutic success. In any event, progress on the antibiotic should be monitored closely in patients on hydantoin anticonvulsants.

Never take or stop medication without your doctor's advice.

Anticonvulsants
(HYDANTOINS)

Asthma Drug
(THEOPHYLLINE)

TROUBLESOME

BRAND NAME	GENERIC NAME
Dilantin	phenytoin
Mesantoin	mephenytoin
Peganone	ethotoin

INSTRUCTIONS
Any of these medicines could upset the stomach. This is less likely if they are taken with food. All of them can cause drowsiness or blurred vision and could make driving dangerous.

BRAND NAME

Aerolate	**Aquaphyllin**
Asmalix	**Bronkodyl**
Elixomin	**Elixophyllin**
Quibron-T	**Respbid**
Slo-bid	**Slo-Phyllin**
Theobid	**Theochron**
Theoclear	**Theo-Dur**
Theolair	**Theo-24**
Theovent	**Theo-X**
T-Phyl	**Uniphyl**

INSTRUCTIONS
Theophylline interacts with food in complex ways, so discuss this issue thoroughly with your doctor and pharmacist. Theophylline may upset the stomach. In some cases this problem can be alleviated by taking the drug with food. See the table of Food and Drug Interactions on pages 73–91 for more information.

INTERACTION
This is a double interaction, because both theophylline and the anticonvulsants can lead to lower blood levels of the other drug. The effect of the anticonvulsants, especially Dilantin, is to speed up removal of theophylline from the system by as much as 65 percent. *This interaction could be troublesome, leading to asthma symptoms.*

The interaction may become noticeable within about five days of taking the two drugs together. If both are needed, blood levels of each should be monitored so that doses can be adjusted appropriately by your doctor.

Never take or stop medication without your doctor's advice.

| **Anticonvulsants** (HYDANTOINS) | **Folic Acid** |

TROUBLESOME

BRAND NAME	GENERIC NAME	BRAND NAME	GENERIC NAME
Dilantin	phenytoin	**Folvite**	folic acid
Mesantoin	mephenytoin		
Peganone	ethotoin		

INSTRUCTIONS

Any of these medicines could upset the stomach. This is less likely if they are taken with food. All of them can cause drowsiness or blurred vision and could make driving dangerous.

INSTRUCTIONS

Fruits and vegetables, whole grains, and legumes are rich sources of this vitamin. Supplements of up to 800 micrograms (0.8 mg) are available without prescription, although most people maintain adequate stores of this vitamin on an intake of 100 to 200 micrograms daily.

INTERACTION

Dilantin can deplete folic acid levels, especially with long-term therapy. Relatively few patients develop frank megaloblastic anemia, but the clinician should be on the lookout for deficiency. Unfortunately, this interaction works both ways. Folic acid can reduce blood levels of phenytoin, so treatment should be supervised by an experienced physician. Occasionally folic acid supplementation (at levels greater than 2 mg/day) has reduced the efficacy of the anticonvulsant, with seizures occurring as a result. *This interaction could be troublesome.*

Dilantin has other potential nutritional impacts, and may lower levels of vitamin B_6, vitamin D, and vitamin K as well as folic acid. A person who expects to take this anticonvulsant for a long time might benefit from consultation with a knowledgeable dietitian.

Never take or stop medication without your doctor's advice.

Anticonvulsants (HYDANTOINS)	**Heart Drug** (MEXILETINE)

TROUBLESOME

BRAND NAME	GENERIC NAME
Dilantin	phenytoin
Mesantoin	mephenytoin
Peganone	ethotoin

INSTRUCTIONS
Any of these medicines could upset the stomach. This is less likely if they are taken with food. All of them can cause drowsiness or blurred vision and could make driving dangerous.

BRAND NAME	GENERIC NAME
Mexitil	mexiletine

INSTRUCTIONS
Mexitil may irritate the digestive tract, so it should be taken with food or an antacid. Dramatic changes in diet should be avoided. Notify the doctor immediately if fever, yellow skin and eyes, sore throat, or unusual tiredness develop.

INTERACTION

Dilantin and the other anticonvulsants in this class can affect the metabolism of Mexitil so that blood levels of this heart drug are reduced. This interaction was confirmed through a clinical study of healthy volunteers. There have been no reports to date, however, of lowered effectiveness resulting from the lower blood levels. *This interaction is potentially troublesome.*

Armed with knowledge of this interaction, the physician will wish to monitor blood levels of mexiletine when a patient starts or stops one of the hydantoin anticonvulsants. The doctor may need to adjust the dose of the heart medication.

Never take or stop medication without your doctor's advice.

Anticonvulsants
(HYDANTOINS)

Heart Drug
(QUINIDINE)

TROUBLESOME

BRAND NAME	GENERIC NAME
Dilantin	phenytoin
Mesantoin	mephenytoin
Peganone	ethotoin

INSTRUCTIONS
Any of these medicines could upset the stomach. This is less likely if they are taken with food. All of them can cause drowsiness or blurred vision and could make driving dangerous.

BRAND NAME	GENERIC NAME
Cardioquin	quinidine
Quinaglute	quinidine
Quinalan	quinidine
Quinidex	quinidine
Quinora	quinidine

INSTRUCTIONS
Quinidine may upset the stomach. Taking it with food may help alleviate this problem. Sustained-release tablets (Quinaglute Dura-Tabs, Quinalan, Quinidex Extentabs) should not be chewed or crushed.

Quinidine may provoke visual disturbances, ringing in the ears, headache, dizziness, nausea, skin rash, or breathing difficulties. Notify your doctor if you develop any of these symptoms. Do not stop this medicine unless your doctor so directs.

INTERACTION
Several case reports have demonstrated that Dilantin can speed elimination of quinidine from the system. It appears to do this through an effect on the liver enzymes responsible for metabolism. In some patients, quinidine levels are reduced by half, and the effectiveness of the medication is compromised. *This interaction could be troublesome.*

If phenytoin is to be added or deleted from a person's treatment regimen, blood levels of quinidine should be monitored carefully. The physician may need to adjust the dose.

Never take or stop medication without your doctor's advice.

Anticonvulsants	**Pain Reliever**
(HYDANTOINS)	(ACETAMINOPHEN)

TROUBLESOME

BRAND NAME	GENERIC NAME
Dilantin	phenytoin
Mesantoin	mephenytoin
Peganone	ethotoin

INSTRUCTIONS

Any of these medicines could upset the stomach. This is less likely if they are taken with food. All of them can cause drowsiness or blurred vision and could make driving dangerous.

BRAND NAME	GENERIC NAME
Anacin-3	acetaminophen
Darvocet-N	acetaminophen/ propoxyphene
Panadol	acetaminophen
Tylenol	acetaminophen
Vicodin	acetaminophen/ hydrocodone

INSTRUCTIONS

Acetaminophen may be taken with meals or on an empty stomach; pain relief is more rapid if it is taken without food. Fasting may make acetaminophen more dangerous to the liver. Never take large doses of acetaminophen if you are not able to eat regularly.

INTERACTION

Regular use of Dilantin or a similar anticonvulsant may make a person more susceptible to liver damage due to acetaminophen taken at high doses or for a long time. The more rapid metabolism of acetaminophen in the presence of hydantoins means it could be somewhat less effective. *This interaction could be troublesome.*

If acetaminophen does not appear to be offering the expected pain relief at normal doses, it would be more prudent to consider an alternate pain medication than to increase the dose of this drug. High doses could contribute to liver problems.

Never take or stop medication without your doctor's advice.

Anticonvulsants
(HYDANTOINS)

Tuberculosis Drug
(RIFAMPIN)

TROUBLESOME

BRAND NAME	GENERIC NAME
Dilantin	phenytoin
Mesantoin	mephenytoin
Peganone	ethotoin

INSTRUCTIONS

Any of these medicines could upset the stomach. This is less likely if they are taken with food. All of them can cause drowsiness or blurred vision and could make driving dangerous.

BRAND NAME	GENERIC NAME
Rifadin	rifampin
Rifamate	isoniazid/ rifampin
Rimactane	rifampin

INSTRUCTIONS

Rifampin should be taken on an empty stomach, at least one hour before or two hours after meals. If you develop fever, chills, unusual tiredness, unusual bleeding or bruising, sore throat, muscle and bone pain, or yellow skin and eyes, contact your physician immediately.

INTERACTION

A person who needs one of these tuberculosis medicines as well as Dilantin or a similar anticonvulsant may process the anticonvulsant more quickly. This could result in lower blood levels of the anticonvulsant than when it is taken alone. *This interaction might be troublesome, as the anticonvulsant could be less effective.*

Seizures are theoretically possible. Blood levels of Dilantin should be monitored when a person starts or stops rifampin therapy.

Never take or stop medication without your doctor's advice.

Antidepressants (SEROTONIN-BASED)

Paxil   Prozac   Zoloft

LIFE-THREATENING

Antidepressants (MAO inhibitors) Eldepryl Marplan
Nardil Parnate

DANGEROUS

Anticoagulant Coumadin
Anticonvulsants Depakene Dilantin Tegretol
Antidepressant Desyrel
Antidepressants (tricyclic) Adapin Aventyl Elavil
Endep Norpramin Pamelor Pertofrane Sinequan
Tofranil etc.
Drug for Obsessive-Compulsive Disorder Anafranil
Heart/Blood Pressure Drugs (beta-blockers)
Inderal Lopressor Toprol XL

TROUBLESOME

Anti-Anxiety Drugs (benzodiazepines) Valium
Xanax
Antihistamine Periactin
**Heart/Blood Pressure Drugs (calcium channel
blockers)** Adalat Calan Isoptin Procardia Verelan
Lithium Cibalith-S Eskalith Lithane Lithobid
Lithotabs

Not every serotonin-based antidepressant listed above interacts with
each medication listed on this list. See individual descriptions for
details. Be sure to check with your physician and pharmacist if you
must take any other drugs in combination with one of these
antidepressants.

Antidepressants
(SEROTONIN-BASED)

Antidepressants
(MAO INHIBITORS)

LIFE-THREATENING

BRAND NAME	GENERIC NAME
Paxil	paroxetine
Prozac	fluoxetine
Zoloft	sertraline

INSTRUCTIONS
Prozac, Paxil, and Zoloft are usually taken once a day, often in the morning. Prozac may be taken without regard to meals. Taking it with food may reduce stomach upset. A few patients experience serious weight loss on these medications. If this occurs, the doctor should be notified.

BRAND NAME	GENERIC NAME
Eldepryl	selegiline
Marplan	isocarboxazid
Nardil	phenelzine
Parnate	tranycypromine

INSTRUCTIONS
MAO inhibitors can interact in dangerous ways with tyramine-containing foods and beverages. See page 59. Consult your doctor before taking other prescription or over-the-counter drugs. Notify him or her if you notice a skin rash, severe headache, yellow eyes or skin, or dark urine. Do not stop this medicine unless your doctor so advises.

INTERACTION
When a patient does not get adequate relief of depression from one medication, the doctor may add a different antidepressant. The literature accompanying serotonin-based antidepressants warns against this combination. *Fatalities have resulted from this interaction.* Some people who have received this combination experience "serotonin syndrome," a very serious, potentially lethal reaction. Because these drugs last in the body for quite some time, at least two weeks should pass after discontinuing an MAO inhibitor before starting on Prozac, Zoloft, or Paxil. The manufacturer of Prozac recommends waiting five weeks after stopping Prozac before beginning an MAO inhibitor antidepressant. For Zoloft and Paxil, at least two weeks should elapse after stopping the serotonin-based antidepressant before beginning Marplan, Nardil, or Parnate. Eldepryl may also interact with the serotonin-based antidepressants.

Symptoms of Serotonin Syndrome
Severe shivering, agitation, confusion, restlessness, muscle twitches or rigidity, diarrhea, elevated temperature, sweating, changes in blood pressure, and coma. Notify your doctor at once if you experience any of these symptoms.

Never take or stop medication without your doctor's advice.

Antidepressants (SEROTONIN-BASED)	**Anticoagulant** (WARFARIN)

DANGEROUS

BRAND NAME	GENERIC NAME
Paxil	paroxetine
Prozac	fluoxetine
Zoloft	sertraline

INSTRUCTIONS

Prozac, Paxil, and Zoloft are usually taken once a day, often in the morning. Prozac may be taken without regard to meals. Taking it with food may reduce stomach upset. A few patients experience serious weight loss on these medications. If this occurs, the doctor should be notified.

BRAND NAME	GENERIC NAME
Coumadin	warfarin

INSTRUCTIONS

Warfarin tablets can be swallowed with food or on an empty stomach. Try to avoid large variations in the quantity of vitamin-K–containing vegetables—such as broccoli, cabbage, or spinach—that you eat each day. Consuming much more or less than usual could change the action of the drug.

INTERACTION

Although there are only a few reports of interaction between any of these antidepressants and warfarin, it appears that in some cases these serotonin-based medications can increase the risk of bleeding associated with warfarin. *This interaction could be dangerous.*

It is possible that many patients will have no trouble with this combination, but the physician should monitor carefully for a potential interaction. Prothrombin time or international normalized ratio (INR) may be increased. Notify your physician immediately if you experience any symptoms of bleeding.

Symptoms of Warfarin Overdose

There may be no early warning signs of danger. Blood tests are essential. Symptoms include any unusual bleeding, including rectal or urinary tract bleeding, excessive menstrual bleeding, nosebleeds, bleeding around gums, bruising, red or tar-black stools, vomiting blood, and red or dark-brown urine. Notify your doctor immediately if you suspect a problem.

Never take or stop medication without your doctor's advice.

Antidepressants
(SEROTONIN-BASED)

Anticonvulsants

DANGEROUS

BRAND NAME	GENERIC NAME
Prozac	fluoxetine

INSTRUCTIONS

Prozac is taken in the morning, or, if a higher dose has been prescribed, in the morning and at noon. It may be taken without regard to meals. Taking it with food may reduce stomach upset. A few patients experience serious weight loss on this medication. If this occurs, the doctor should be notified.

BRAND NAME	GENERIC NAME
Depakene	valproic acid
Dilantin	phenytoin
Tegretol	carbamazepine

INSTRUCTIONS

Do not discontinue any of these medicines unless your doctor supervises the process carefully. Suddenly stopping these drugs could trigger seizures. These pills should be taken with food to reduce the possibility of stomach upset. Notify the physician immediately of any unusual bruising, bleeding, or yellowing of the skin and eyes.

INTERACTION

A depressed person with epilepsy might need both Prozac and an anticonvulsant medicine. The combination might also be prescribed to someone with bipolar depression who has not responded to the usual treatments. Prozac apparently interferes with metabolism of these compounds and may increase blood levels of Tegretol, Dilantin, or Depakene to the point of toxicity. *The interaction could be dangerous.*

Because Prozac can linger in the body, interaction problems may continue for some time even if Prozac is discontinued. Contact your physician immediately if you experience symptoms such as unsteadiness, drowsiness, or confusion. Blood tests for a few weeks after starting or a few weeks after stopping Prozac are advisable.

Symptoms of Anticonvulsant Toxicity

Nausea, vomiting, digestive upset, slurred speech, blurred vision, incoordination, dizziness, confusion, yellow skin or eyes, unusual bleeding or bruising, headache, and fever. Notify your physician immediately of any of these symptoms.

Never take or stop medication without your doctor's advice.

Antidepressants
(SEROTONIN-BASED)

Antidepressant
(TRAZODONE)

DANGEROUS

BRAND NAME	GENERIC NAME
Paxil	paroxetine
Prozac	fluoxetine

INSTRUCTIONS
Paxil is taken once a day, usually in the morning. Prozac is taken in the morning, or, if a higher dose has been prescribed, in the morning and at noon. Prozac may be taken without regard to meals. Taking it with food may reduce stomach upset. A few patients experience serious weight loss on these medications. If this occurs, the doctor should be notified.

BRAND NAME	GENERIC NAME
Desyrel	trazodone

INSTRUCTIONS
Usually Desyrel is better taken with food, in the evening, to avoid daytime drowsiness. Activities that require mental attention such as driving or operating machinery can be dangerous for people on Desyrel. Never stop taking this drug suddenly. If Desyrel needs to be discontinued, this process should be monitored carefully by a physician.

INTERACTION
If a patient does not respond well to one antidepressant, the physician sometimes adds a different medication to try to reverse the depression. However, Prozac and Paxil slow down the liver enzyme that is essential to the metabolism of some older antidepressants such as Desyrel, and can cause blood levels of Desyrel to rise, potentially to toxic levels. *Although we are aware of no fatalities, this interaction could be quite serious.*

Because Prozac lasts a long time in the body, the problems may continue for a few weeks after it is discontinued. Generally, if both drugs are needed, the doctor should adjust the dose of each and monitor the effects closely.

Signs of Desyrel Overdose
Drowsiness, vomiting, dizziness, disorientation, difficulty speaking, difficulty walking, palpitations, prolonged penile erections, breathing difficulties, and seizures. Contact your physician immediately if any such signs of overdose appear.

Never take or stop medication without your doctor's advice.

Antidepressants
(SEROTONIN-BASED)

Antidepressants
(TRICYCLIC)

DANGEROUS

BRAND NAME	GENERIC NAME
Paxil	paroxetine
Prozac	fluoxetine

INSTRUCTIONS

Paxil is taken once a day, usually in the morning. Prozac is taken in the morning, or, if a higher dose has been prescribed, in the morning and at noon. Prozac may be taken without regard to meals. Taking it with food may reduce stomach upset. A few patients experience serious weight loss on these medications. If this occurs, your doctor should be notified.

BRAND NAME	GENERIC NAME
Adapin, Sinequan	doxepin
Aventyl, Pamelor	nortriptyline
Elavil, Endep	amitriptyline
Norpramin, Pertofrane	desipramine
Tofranil	imipramine
etc.	

INSTRUCTIONS

Usually these medications are better taken with food, in the evening to avoid daytime drowsiness. A high-fiber diet may interfere with absorption, however. Sinequan Concentrate should be mixed with four ounces of milk, water, or juice just before taking, not ahead of time. Do not stop taking any of these drugs suddenly; if they must be discontinued, your doctor will supervise gradual phaseout.

INTERACTION

If a patient does not respond well to one antidepressant, the physician sometimes adds a different medication to try to reverse the depression. However, Prozac and Paxil slow down the liver enzyme that is essential to the metabolism of the older antidepressants listed above, and can cause blood levels of these medications to rise markedly, often 100 to 400 percent. This may result in toxic levels. *Although we are aware of no fatalities, this interaction is quite serious.*

Adverse effects may include, in extreme cases, delirium and seizures. Because Prozac lasts a long time in the body, the problems may continue for a few weeks after it is discontinued. Generally, if both drugs are needed, your doctor should adjust the dose of each and monitor the effects closely.

Symptoms of Tricyclic Antidepressant Overdose

Nausea, constipation, confusion, sleepiness, palpitations, dizziness, dry mouth, blurred vision, and fever. Contact the physician immediately if any such signs of overdose appear.

Never take or stop medication without your doctor's advice.

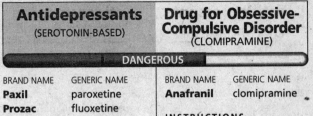

Antidepressants
(SEROTONIN-BASED)

Drug for Obsessive-Compulsive Disorder
(CLOMIPRAMINE)

DANGEROUS

BRAND NAME	GENERIC NAME
Paxil	paroxetine
Prozac	fluoxetine

INSTRUCTIONS
Paxil is taken once a day, usually in the morning. Prozac is taken in the morning, or, if a higher dose has been prescribed, in the morning and at noon. Prozac may be taken without regard to meals. Taking it with food may reduce stomach upset. A few patients experience serious weight loss on these medications. If this occurs, your doctor should be notified.

BRAND NAME	GENERIC NAME
Anafranil	clomipramine

INSTRUCTIONS
Anafranil is best taken with food, preferably in the evening to avoid daytime drowsiness. Do not stop taking Anafranil suddenly, because that could result in unpleasant withdrawal symptoms. If it must be discontinued, your doctor will supervise gradual phaseout.

INTERACTION

A doctor might prescribe both these medications for a patient with obsessive-compulsive disorder complicated by depression. In addition, Prozac may be prescribed for obsessions or compulsions and is often effective. If a patient does not respond well to one of these agents, however, the physician might try for a greater effect by adding the other. Both Prozac and Paxil slow down the liver enzyme critical for metabolizing Anafranil, and may cause blood levels of Anafranil to soar. *This interaction could be dangerous.*

Adverse effects may include, in extreme cases, delirium and seizures. Because Prozac lasts a long time in the body, the problems may continue for a few weeks after it is discontinued. Generally, if both drugs are needed, your doctor should adjust the dose of both and monitor the effects closely.

Symptoms of Anafranil Overdose
Nausea, constipation, confusion, sleepiness, palpitations, dizziness, dry mouth, blurred vision, and fever. Contact your physician immediately if any such signs of overdose appear.

Never take or stop medication without your doctor's advice.

Antidepressants (SEROTONIN-BASED)	Heart/Blood Pressure Drugs (BETA-BLOCKERS)

DANGEROUS

BRAND NAME	GENERIC NAME
Prozac	fluoxetine

INSTRUCTIONS
Prozac is taken in the morning, or, if a higher dose has been prescribed, in the morning and at noon. It may be taken without regard to meals. Taking it with food may reduce stomach upset. A few patients experience serious weight loss on this medication. If this occurs, your doctor should be notified.

BRAND NAME	GENERIC NAME
Inderal	propranolol
Lopressor	metoprolol
Toprol XL	metoprolol

INSTRUCTIONS
Propranolol and metoprolol are best absorbed with meals, but consistency is the most important factor. These drugs should be taken at about the same time every day. Do not stop any of these medicines suddenly except on doctor's orders. Serious side effects could result.

INTERACTION

Because metoprolol and propranolol are both widely prescribed, it is likely that some people may take one of these drugs together with Prozac. There are a few case reports of increased toxicity of the beta-blocker attributed to this combination. One man developed a potentially life-threatening rhythm disturbance called heart block after adding Prozac to propranolol. A patient with angina experienced a dangerously slow pulse two days after Prozac was added to his heart medicine, metoprolol.

Anyone on a beta-blocker such as propranolol or metoprolol should be monitored very carefully if Prozac is added to the regimen. Dosage adjustments may be necessary. Because the effects of Prozac may persist in the body for up to two weeks after the drug is discontinued, caution must also be exercised if a beta-blocker is prescribed to someone who has recently stopped Prozac.

Symptoms of Beta-Blocker Toxicity
Slow heart rate, abnormal electrocardiogram, very low blood pressure, disorientation, lightheadedness, lethargy, or heart failure. Notify your physician immediately of any such symptoms.

Never take or stop medication without your doctor's advice.

Antidepressants
(SEROTONIN-BASED)

Anti-Anxiety Drugs
(BENZODIAZEPINES)

TROUBLESOME

BRAND NAME	GENERIC NAME
Prozac	fluoxetine

INSTRUCTIONS
Prozac is taken in the morning, or, if a higher dose has been prescribed, in the morning and at noon. It may be taken without regard to meals. Taking it with food may reduce stomach upset. A few patients experience serious weight loss on this medication. If this occurs, your doctor should be notified.

BRAND NAME	GENERIC NAME
Valium	diazepam
Xanax	alprazolam

INSTRUCTIONS
These drugs may be taken with food, especially if they upset the digestive tract.

INTERACTION
This is not a particularly worrisome interaction. In fact, physicians may often prescribe drugs such as Valium or Xanax to counteract the jittery feelings and insomnia that are sometimes associated with Prozac. If this combination is contemplated, however, there should be some consideration for the potential of these drugs to interact. Reports have surfaced linking Prozac to slightly higher blood levels of diazepam. Diazepam also lasted longer in the body when people were also taking Prozac. The clinical significance of this interaction is unclear. Data on Xanax and Prozac are contradictory. One study demonstrated a slight effect while another showed no impact. There may be no cause for concern, but until further research is done patients should be alert for increased effects from Valium or Xanax. Tasks that require coordination and attentiveness, like driving, could be affected.

Symptoms of Benzodiazepine Overdose
Disorientation, unsteadiness, confusion, slurred speech, drowsiness, dizziness, amnesia, or loss of motor coordination are tipoffs to overdose. Driving is hazardous! Contact your physician immediately if any such signs of overdose appear.

Never take or stop medication without your doctor's advice.

Antidepressants	**Antihistamine**
(SEROTONIN-BASED)	

TROUBLESOME

BRAND NAME	GENERIC NAME	BRAND NAME	GENERIC NAME
Prozac	fluoxetine	**Periactin**	cyproheptadine

INSTRUCTIONS

Prozac is taken in the morning, or, if a higher dose has been prescribed, in the morning and at noon. It may be taken without regard to meals. Taking it with food may reduce stomach upset. A few patients experience serious weight loss on this medication. If this occurs, your doctor should be notified.

INSTRUCTIONS

Periactin is best taken with food to reduce the risk of stomach upset or nausea. Because of the possibility of experiencing drowsiness, dizziness, confusion, and blurred vision people, should rarely, if ever, drive or operate machinery while taking Periactin.

INTERACTION

People who take Prozac may experience sexual side effects including lowered libido, difficulty ejaculating, and lack of orgasm. Because sexual dysfunction is thought to be caused by the serotonin-enhancing effect of Prozac, physicians have tried to reverse this unpleasant consequence by administering an antiserotonin drug such as Periactin. They were successful in restoring sexuality, but symptoms of depression also returned.

Two female patients taking Prozac for bulimia (binge eating and purging) also experienced a reemergence of their symptoms when Periactin was prescribed. It appears that the serotonin-blocking action of Periactin can reverse the benefits of Prozac. Although no reports have yet appeared regarding the interaction between Periactin and Paxil or Zoloft, there is every reason to believe it could be a problem. If depression returns, suicidal thoughts might occur. *This interaction could be troublesome.*

Never take or stop medication without your doctor's advice.

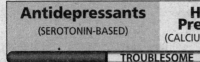

| Antidepressants (SEROTONIN-BASED) | Heart/Blood Pressure Drugs (CALCIUM CHANNEL BLOCKERS) |

TROUBLESOME

BRAND NAME	GENERIC NAME
Prozac	fluoxetine

INSTRUCTIONS

Prozac is taken in the morning, or, if a higher dose has been prescribed, in the morning and at noon. It may be taken without regard to meals. Taking it with food may reduce stomach upset. A few patients experience serious weight loss on this medication. If this occurs, your doctor should be notified.

BRAND NAME	GENERIC NAME
Adalat, Procardia	nifedipine
Calan, Isoptin, Verelan	verapamil

INSTRUCTIONS

These drugs come in a variety of doses; follow the doctor's directions carefully to get the right dose. Sustained-release forms, such as Calan SR or Dilacor XR, should not be chewed or crushed and are best taken with food. Avoid taking Adalat or Procardia with grapefruit juice, as this could boost blood levels unexpectedly. See the table on pages 73–91 for specific instructions. Withdrawal symptoms, especially chest pain, may occur if these drugs are stopped suddenly. Follow the doctor's instructions for tapering slowly if the medicine must be discontinued.

INTERACTION

There are a few case reports of increased toxicity of calcium channel blockers such as Calan and Procardia due to this combination. *This interaction could be troublesome.*

Side Effects of Calcium Channel Blockers

Nausea, constipation, skin rash, dizziness, headache, drowsiness, insomnia, shortness of breath, fluid retention, and changes in heart rate or rhythm. Contact your physician promptly if any such adverse effects appear while you are on Prozac and one of the calcium channel blockers.

Never take or stop medication without your doctor's advice.

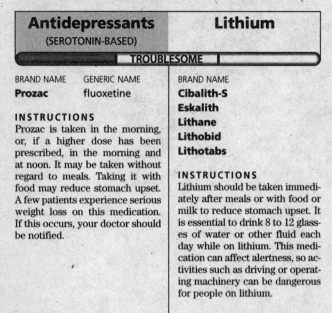

Antidepressants
(SEROTONIN-BASED)

Lithium

TROUBLESOME

BRAND NAME   GENERIC NAME
Prozac   fluoxetine

INSTRUCTIONS
Prozac is taken in the morning, or, if a higher dose has been prescribed, in the morning and at noon. It may be taken without regard to meals. Taking it with food may reduce stomach upset. A few patients experience serious weight loss on this medication. If this occurs, your doctor should be notified.

BRAND NAME
Cibalith-S
Eskalith
Lithane
Lithobid
Lithotabs

INSTRUCTIONS
Lithium should be taken immediately after meals or with food or milk to reduce stomach upset. It is essential to drink 8 to 12 glasses of water or other fluid each day while on lithium. This medication can affect alertness, so activities such as driving or operating machinery can be dangerous for people on lithium.

INTERACTION
For someone with bipolar depression, the psychiatrist may prescribe both lithium, to prevent or treat the manic phase, and Prozac, to relieve the depressive stage. Paxil did not interact with lithium in a five-week study, and Zoloft resulted in an insignificant reduction in lithium levels. There is at least one report of a clinical interaction between lithium and Prozac, however. A 44-year-old woman who had been on lithium for 20 years with no problems developed dizziness, unsteadiness and difficulty walking, stiff arms and legs, and other signs of lithium toxicity shortly after starting Prozac. Her blood lithium levels were high and Prozac was stopped. She recovered fully. It is unclear how many others might also be susceptible to a similar reaction. *This interaction could be troublesome.*

Symptoms of Lithium Toxicity
Drowsiness, incoordination, dizziness, blurred vision, ringing in the ears, slurred speech, confusion, seizures, and coma. Notify your physician immediately of any of these symptoms.

Never take or stop medication without your doctor's advice.

Antihistamines (NONSEDATING)

Hismanal

LIFE-THREATENING

Antibiotics (macrolides) Biaxin E.E.S. E-Mycin ERYC EryPed Ery-Tab Erythrocin Ilosone PCE Pediazole Tao Zithromax

Antifungal Drugs Diflucan Nizoral Sporanox

DANGEROUS

Grapefruit Juice

TROUBLESOME

Cholesterol Drug Lorelco

Drugs for Schizophrenia Haldol Mellaril

Heart Drugs Betapace Cardioquin disopyramide Norpace procainamide Procan SR Pronestyl Quinaglute Quinidex quinidine Quinora

The most serious known interactions with this antihistamine are listed here. See the individual summaries for details. Be sure to check with your pharmacist and physician before taking other drugs in combination with any nonsedating antihistamine.

Antihistamines	Antibiotics
(NONSEDATING)	(MACROLIDES)

LIFE-THREATENING

BRAND NAME	GENERIC NAME
Hismanal	astemizole

INSTRUCTIONS

Hismanal works best when taken on an empty stomach (either one hour before meals or two hours after eating).

BRAND NAME	GENERIC NAME
Biaxin	clarithromycin
E.E.S.	erythromycin
E-Mycin	erythromycin
ERYC	erythromycin
EryPed	erythromycin
Ery-Tab	erythromycin
Erythrocin	erythromycin
Ilosone	erythromycin
PCE	erythromycin
Pediazole	erythromycin
Zithromax	azithromycin

INSTRUCTIONS

Some forms of erythromycin must be taken on an empty stomach; others may be taken with food. See pages 73–91 for specifics. Biaxin can be taken without regard to meals. Zithromax is best taken on an empty stomach.

INTERACTION

People with allergies may be prone to ear, nose, throat, and respiratory tract infections that might call for one of the listed antibiotics. These antibiotics affect the liver to slow metabolism of the antihistamines. Blood levels of Hismanal may rise to dangerous levels. *The interaction is potentially lethal.* **Deaths have been reported.**

Abnormal electrocardiograms (prolongation of the QT interval), irregular heartbeats, and cardiac arrest are associated with elevated blood levels of Hismanal. Erythromycin, Biaxin, and Tao have been reported to produce this effect. Although no case reports implicate Zithromax, it should be combined with these antihistamines only under careful medical supervision.

Symptoms of Hismanal Toxicity

Except for subtle changes on an electrocardiogram, there may be no warning signs of danger. Heart palpitations, dizziness, fainting, chest discomfort, or shortness of breath require emergency treatment.

Never take or stop medication without your doctor's advice.

Antihistamines (NONSEDATING)	**Antifungal Drugs**

BRAND NAME	GENERIC NAME
Hismanal	astemizole

INSTRUCTIONS

Hismanal works best when taken on an empty stomach (either one hour before meals or two hours after eating).

BRAND NAME	GENERIC NAME
Diflucan	fluconazole
Nizoral	ketoconazole
Sporanox	itraconazole

INSTRUCTIONS

Nizoral and Sporanox are best taken with food to reduce stomach upset. The dose of Diflucan must be individualized depending upon the type of infection being treated.

INTERACTION

Nizoral and Sporanox can affect the metabolism of the antihistamine Hismanal. They do this by knocking out a crucial enzyme in the liver called cytochrome P-450-3A4. Without adequate amounts of this enzyme, blood levels of Hismanal can rise, in some cases to dangerous levels. *The interaction is potentially lethal.* **Deaths have been reported.**

Abnormal electrocardiograms, irregular heartbeats, and cardiac arrest are associated with elevated blood levels of Hismanal. At the time of this writing only Nizoral and Sporanox have been reported to interact with Hismanal to produce this effect. It is not clear if Diflucan will also interact with nonsedating antihistamines. Caution is appropriate until more is known.

Symptoms of Hismanal Toxicity

Except for subtle changes on an electrocardiogram, there may be no warning signs of danger. Heart palpitations, dizziness, fainting, chest discomfort, or shortness of breath require emergency treatment.

Never take or stop medication without your doctor's advice.

Antihistamines
(NONSEDATING)

Grapefruit Juice

DANGEROUS

BRAND NAME   GENERIC NAME
Hismanal   astemizole

INSTRUCTIONS
Hismanal works best when taken on an empty stomach (either one hour before meals or two hours after eating).

INSTRUCTIONS
Research on the effects of grapefruit juice on drug metabolism is still in its infancy. No one knows how many medications may be affected. To be on the safe side, do not take your medicines with grapefruit or grapefruit juice unless advised to do so by a physician. Preliminary data suggest that grapefruit is far less likely to affect blood levels if ingested four or more hours after taking medicine (Dr. David Flockhart, personal communication).

INTERACTION

The first warning that grapefruit juice could interact with drugs came during a study of the blood pressure medicine Plendil (felodipine). Blood levels of the drug jumped way beyond predicted levels when the medicine was swallowed with grapefruit juice. Other studies have confirmed that grapefruit juice magnifies the drug's effects and side effects.

A 1993 article in *The Journal of the American Medical Association* (Vol. 269, p. 1535-1536) suggested that grapefruit juice might also affect Seldane. This was later confirmed, and Hismanal too was found to be affected. When blood levels of these antihistamines rise there is a risk of dangerous, if not deadly, heart rhythm abnormalities. The concern is great enough to discourage taking grapefruit juice with such pills.

Symptoms of Hismanal Toxicity
Except for subtle changes on an electrocardiogram, there may be no warning signs of danger. Heart palpitations, dizziness, fainting, chest discomfort, or shortness of breath require emergency treatment.

Never take or stop medication without your doctor's advice.

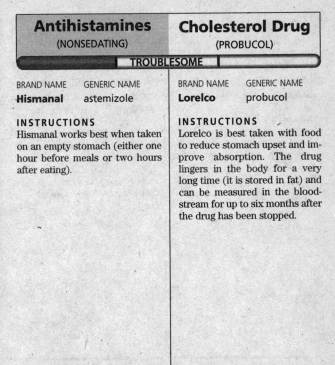

Antihistamines
(NONSEDATING)

Cholesterol Drug
(PROBUCOL)

TROUBLESOME

BRAND NAME   GENERIC NAME
Hismanal   astemizole

INSTRUCTIONS
Hismanal works best when taken on an empty stomach (either one hour before meals or two hours after eating).

BRAND NAME   GENERIC NAME
Lorelco   probucol

INSTRUCTIONS
Lorelco is best taken with food to reduce stomach upset and improve absorption. The drug lingers in the body for a very long time (it is stored in fat) and can be measured in the bloodstream for up to six months after the drug has been stopped.

INTERACTION
This interaction is, at the time of this writing, purely theoretical. There have been, to our knowledge, no published reports of deaths or serious adverse reactions resulting from the combination of Lorelco and Hismanal. Nevertheless, an article in *The Journal of the American Medical Association* (1993; Vol. 269, p. 1536) cautions physicians about "combining terfenadine [Seldane] therapy with other drugs that . . . prolong the QT interval."

Since both Lorelco and Hismanal may prolong the QT interval, the risk of a serious irregular heart rhythm must be weighed carefully by a physician before prescribing Lorelco together with this nonsedating antihistamine. *Such arrhythmias could be life threatening.*

Symptoms of Hismanal Toxicity
Except for subtle changes on an electrocardiogram, there may be no warning signs of danger. Heart palpitations, dizziness, fainting, chest discomfort, or shortness of breath require emergency treatment.

Never take or stop medication without your doctor's advice.

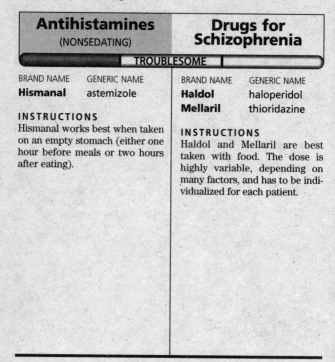

Antihistamines
(NONSEDATING)

Drugs for Schizophrenia

TROUBLESOME

BRAND NAME   GENERIC NAME
Hismanal   astemizole

INSTRUCTIONS
Hismanal works best when taken on an empty stomach (either one hour before meals or two hours after eating).

BRAND NAME   GENERIC NAME
Haldol   haloperidol
Mellaril   thioridazine

INSTRUCTIONS
Haldol and Mellaril are best taken with food. The dose is highly variable, depending on many factors, and has to be individualized for each patient.

INTERACTION

This interaction is, at the time of this writing, purely theoretical. There have been, to our knowledge, no published reports of deaths or serious adverse reactions resulting from the combination of Haldol or Mellaril with Hismanal. Nevertheless, an article in *The Journal of the American Medical Association* (1993; Vol. 269, p. 1536) cautions physicians about "combining terfenadine [Seldane] therapy with other drugs that . . . prolong the QT interval."

Hismanal may prolong the QT interval, as can Haldol and Mellaril. The risk of a serious irregular heart rhythm must be weighed carefully by a physician before prescribing either Haldol or Mellaril with this nonsedating antihistamine. *Such arrhythmias could be life threatening.*

Symptoms of Hismanal Toxicity
Except for subtle changes on an electrocardiogram, there may be no warning signs of danger. Heart palpitations, dizziness, fainting, chest discomfort, or shortness of breath require emergency treatment.

Never take or stop medication without your doctor's advice.

Antihistamines (NONSEDATING)	**Heart Drugs**

TROUBLESOME

BRAND NAME	GENERIC NAME
Hismanal	astemizole

INSTRUCTIONS

Hismanal works best when taken on an empty stomach (either one hour before meals or two hours after eating).

BRAND NAME	GENERIC NAME
Betapace	sotalol
Cardioquin	quinidine
Norpace	disopyramide
Procan SR	procainamide
Pronestyl	procainamide
Quinaglute	quinidine
Quinidex	quinidine
Quinora	quinidine

INSTRUCTIONS

Quinidine is best taken with food to reduce stomach upset. Procainamide is absorbed better on an empty stomach but it causes GI problems and may be taken at mealtime. Check with a physician and pharmacist on proper dosing for all of these drugs because the dose must be individualized and timed carefully.

INTERACTION

This interaction is, at the time of this writing, purely theoretical. We know of no published reports of deaths or serious reactions resulting from the combination of antiarrhythmics and Hismanal. Nevertheless, an article in *The Journal of the American Medical Association* (1993; Vol. 269, p. 1536) cautions physicians about combining Seldane with other drugs that prolong the QT interval or increase the risk of heart irregularities. Hismanal is similar.

Mixing drugs that have the potential to cause heart rhythm disturbances could be dangerous. The risk of a serious arrhythmia must be weighed carefully by a physician before prescribing such heavy-duty heart pills with this nonsedating antihistamine. *Such arrhythmias could be life threatening.*

Symptoms of Hismanal Toxicity

Except for subtle changes on an electrocardiogram, there may be no warning signs of danger. Heart palpitations, dizziness, fainting, chest discomfort, or shortness of breath require emergency treatment.

Never take or stop medication without your doctor's advice.

Arthritis Drugs (NSAIDS)

Advil   Aleve   Anaprox Ansaid   aspirin   Clinoril
Feldene ibuprofen Lodine Motrin   Naprosyn Nuprin
Relafen Tolectin Toradol Voltaren etc.

LIFE-THREATENING

Anticoagulant Coumadin
Methotrexate Folex Mexate Rheumatrex

DANGEROUS

Diuretics (potassium-sparing) Aldactazide
Aldactone Dyazide Dyrenium Maxzide Midamor
Moduretic
Diuretics (potassium-wasting) Bumex Diucardin
Diuril Edecrin Enduron Esidrix HydroDIURIL Hygroton
Lasix Lozol etc.
Heart/Blood Pressure Drugs (ACE inhibitors)
Accupril Capoten Lotensin Prinivil Vasotec Zestril etc.
Heart/Blood Pressure Drugs (beta-blockers)
Blocadren Corgard Inderal Lopressor Tenormin
Toprol XL Visken
Lithium Cibalith-S Eskalith Lithane Lithobid
Lithotabs

TROUBLESOME

Alcohol beer liquor wine medicines that contain
alcohol

Not every nonsteroidal anti-inflammatory drug (NSAID) listed above
interacts with each medicine on this list. See individual summaries for
details. These NSAIDs interact with many other medications. Be sure
to check with your physician and pharmacist if you must take any
other drugs in combination with one of them.

| **Arthritis Drugs** (NSAIDS) | **Anticoagulant** (WARFARIN) |

LIFE-THREATENING

BRAND NAME GENERIC NAME

Advil, Motrin,
Nuprin ibuprofen
Aleve,
Naprosyn naproxen
Ansaid flurbiprofen
Aspirin aspirin
Indocin indomethacin
Lodine etodolac
Relafen nabumetone
Toradol ketorolac
etc.

INSTRUCTIONS

Take with food to reduce the risk of stomach irritation. (See table on pages 73–91.) Aspirin and OTC ibuprofen or naproxen should not be mixed with prescription NSAIDs or each other.

BRAND NAME GENERIC NAME

Coumadin warfarin

INSTRUCTIONS

Warfarin tablets can be swallowed with food or on an empty stomach. Try to avoid large variations in the quantity of vitamin-K–containing vegetables—such as broccoli, cabbage, or spinach—that you eat each day. Consuming much more or less than usual could change the action of the drug.

INTERACTION

Large doses of aspirin can significantly increase bleeding in people taking warfarin. *This interaction could prove life threatening.* See page 18 for recommendations on low-dose aspirin and Coumadin.

People who take NSAIDs for pain and inflammation and also warfarin may dramatically increase their risk of a bleeding ulcer. One study (*Arch. Intern. Med.*, Jul 26, 1993;153:1665-1670) reported that such combinations were associated with a 13-fold rise in GI hemorrhage. *Bleeding ulcers can be fatal.* If an arthritis medicine such as the ones listed here is prescribed with Coumadin, extreme caution must be exercised!

Symptoms of NSAID/Warfarin Adverse Interaction

Notify your doctor immediately if you detect any unusual bleeding, including rectal or urinary tract bleeding, excessive menstrual bleeding, bruising, red or tar-black stools, and red or dark brown urine. A silent or bleeding ulcer can occur with no symptoms. Indigestion, heartburn, anemia, fatigue, and weight loss may be early symptoms of trouble.

Never take or stop medication without your doctor's advice.

| **Arthritis Drugs** (NSAIDS) | **Methotrexate** |

LIFE-THREATENING

BRAND NAME	GENERIC NAME
Advil, Motrin, Nuprin	ibuprofen
Aleve, Naprosyn	naproxen
Ansaid	flurbiprofen
Aspirin	aspirin
Indocin	indomethacin
Lodine	etodolac
Relafen	nabumetone
Toradol	ketorolac
etc.	

INSTRUCTIONS
Take with food to reduce the risk of stomach irritation. (See table on pages 73–91.) Aspirin and OTC ibuprofen or naproxen should not be mixed with prescription NSAIDs or each other

BRAND NAME
Folex
Mexate
Rheumatrex

INSTRUCTIONS
Follow your doctor's instructions on dose and timing for methotrexate, which is taken **once a week** for psoriasis or rheumatoid arthritis. Do not drink alcohol or take salicylates such as aspirin or Pepto-Bismol while on this drug. Methotrexate can increase sensitivity to ultraviolet light, so protect your skin from exposure to sun or tanning lamps.

INTERACTION

Arthritis drugs (NSAIDs and aspirin) can make methotrexate far more toxic than when it is taken alone. Since methotrexate, by itself, has the potential for serious side effects, such an interaction can be extremely dangerous. Blood levels of methotrexate can climb unpredictably in the presence of NSAIDs and should be monitored closely. Kidney damage, digestive tract difficulties, bone marrow suppression, and immune system impairment are potential complications. *This interaction could be life threatening.* Lower doses of methotrexate used to treat rheumatoid arthritis or psoriasis may interact less severely, but careful medical supervision is crucial.

Symptoms of Methotrexate Toxicity
Nausea, vomiting, diarrhea, mouth sores, rash, itching, black sticky stools, stomach pain, sore throat, fever, chills, unusual bleeding or bruising, yellow skin or eyes, shortness of breath, cough, dark or bloody urine, or swelling of the legs or feet. Notify your physician immediately.

Never take or stop medication without your doctor's advice.

Arthritis Drugs	Diuretics
(NSAIDS)	(POTASSIUM-SPARING)

DANGEROUS

BRAND NAME	GENERIC NAME
Advil, Motrin, Nuprin	ibuprofen
Aleve, Naprosyn	naproxen
Ansaid	flurbiprofen
Aspirin	aspirin
Indocin	indomethacin
Lodine	etodolac
Relafen	nabumetone
Voltaren	diclofenac
etc.	

INSTRUCTIONS

Take with food to reduce the risk of stomach irritation. (See table on pages 73–91.) Aspirin and OTC ibuprofen or naproxen should not be mixed with prescription NSAIDs or each other.

BRAND NAME	GENERIC NAME
Aldactazide	spironolactone, HCTZ
Aldactone	spironolactone
Dyazide	triamterene, HCTZ
Dyrenium	triamterene
Maxzide	triamterene, HCTZ
Midamor	amiloride
Moduretic	amiloride, HCTZ

INSTRUCTIONS

Midamor and Dyrenium may upset the stomach, so they are best taken right after meals. Maxzide can be taken without regard to meals. Midamor and Aldactone may interfere with the alertness and coordination necessary for driving. Periodic blood tests for magnesium and potassium are advisable.

INTERACTION

Some arthritis drugs may reduce the effectiveness of diuretics. Fluid may build up, posing a serious problem for patients with heart trouble. Thiazide diuretics such as hydrochlorothiazide (HCTZ) may be less effective in lowering blood pressure. If diuretics and arthritis drugs are taken simultaneously, blood pressure should be monitored carefully. Indocin may raise potassium levels to dangerous levels when combined with potassium-sparing diuretics like Moduretic. Measure potassium levels periodically. Potassium-sparing diuretics containing triamterene (Dyazide, Dyrenium, and Maxzide) may interact badly with ibuprofen, Indocin, or Voltaren (diclofenac). Kidney damage has been reported. Other arthritis drugs may also interact.

Symptoms of Heart and Kidney Problems

Notify your doctor of sudden weight gain, swollen legs and feet, change in the color of the urine, unusual back pain, fatigue, cough, or breathlessness. Elevated serum creatinine may mean kidney trouble. Monitor blood pressure frequently.

Never take or stop medication without your doctor's advice.

Arthritis Drugs (NSAIDS)	Diuretics (POTASSIUM-WASTING)

DANGEROUS

BRAND NAME	GENERIC NAME	BRAND NAME	GENERIC NAME
Advil, Motrin,		**Bumex**	bumetanide
Nuprin	ibuprofen	**Diachlor,**	
Aleve,		**Diuril**	chlorothiazide
Naprosyn	naproxen	**Diucardin,**	
Clinoril	sulindac	**Saluron**	hydroflumethiazide
Aspirin	aspirin	**Edecrin**	ethacrynic acid
Indocin	indomethacin	**Enduron**	methyclothiazide
Lodine	etodolac	**Esidrix,**	
Relafen	nabumetone	**HydroDIURIL**	hydrochlorothiazide
Toradol	ketorolac	**Hygroton,**	
etc.		**Hylidone**	chlorthalidone
		Lasix	furosemide
		Lozol	indapamide
		etc.	

INSTRUCTIONS

Take with food to reduce the risk of stomach irritation. (See table on pages 73–91.) Aspirin and OTC ibuprofen or naproxen should not be mixed with prescription NSAIDs or each other.

INSTRUCTIONS

If a diuretic is taken early in the day it may reduce nighttime urination. If it causes stomach upset the drug may be taken with food or milk. See the Food and Drug Interaction Table on pages 73–91 for specifics.

INTERACTION

NSAIDs such as ibuprofen and Indocin appear to reduce the effectiveness of diuretics such as Bumex and Lasix. (Clinoril may also affect Bumex.) Fluid may build up and symptoms of heart failure could become worse. This is a very serious situation for people with heart trouble. Thiazide diuretics such as chlorthalidone, chlorothiazide, and hydrochlorothiazide may be less effective in lowering blood pressure, but this interaction does not seem so serious. Blood pressure should be monitored to make sure adequate control is maintained.

Symptoms of Heart Problems

Fluid retention, fatigue, cough, and breathlessness are possible signs of congestive heart failure. Monitor blood pressure frequently. Notify the physician immediately of symptoms.

Never take or stop medication without your doctor's advice.

Arthritis Drugs (NSAIDS)		**Heart/Blood Pressure Drugs** (ACE INHIBITORS)	
DANGEROUS			

BRAND NAME	GENERIC NAME	BRAND NAME	GENERIC NAME
Advil, Motrin,		**Accupril**	quinapril
Nuprin	ibuprofen	**Altace**	ramipril
Aleve,		**Capoten**	captopril
Naprosyn	naproxen	**Lotensin**	benazepril
Ansaid	flurbiprofen	**Monopril**	fosinopril
Aspirin	aspirin	**Prinivil,**	
Indocin	indomethacin	**Zestril**	lisinopril
Lodine	etodolac	**Vasotec**	enalapril
Relafen	nabumetone		
Toradol	ketorolac		
etc.			

INSTRUCTIONS

Take with food to reduce the risk of stomach irritation. (See table on pages 73–91.) Aspirin and OTC ibuprofen or naproxen should not be mixed with prescription NSAIDs or each other.

INSTRUCTIONS

Capoten should be taken one hour before meals. High-fat meals may reduce absorption of Accupril. Food does not affect the other drugs in this class.

INTERACTION

Some of the arthritis drugs on this list can drastically diminish the effectiveness of blood pressure medicines such as Capoten and Vasotec. Indocin can wipe out the blood-pressure-lowering power of these drugs; ibuprofen can interact similarly with Capoten. Even aspirin given with or before Vasotec can reduce that drug's benefit for treating congestive heart failure. Although some people do not react badly to this combination, it makes sense to assume that any arthritis medicine could interfere with any ACE medication, and keep careful tabs on blood pressure and cardiac function if both drugs are needed. *This interaction could be dangerous.*

Kidney problems are a rare but serious reaction to both these classes of drugs. Taking them in combination may increase the risk of this problem. *Notify your doctor immediately of sudden weight gain, swollen legs and feet, change in the color of the urine, or unusual back pain.* A kidney function test may be in order. **Monitor blood pressure regularly.**

Never take or stop medication without your doctor's advice.

Arthritis Drugs
(NSAIDS)

Heart/Blood Pressure Drugs
(BETA-BLOCKERS)

DANGEROUS

BRAND NAME	GENERIC NAME
Advil, Motrin,	
Nuprin	ibuprofen
Aleve,	
Naprosyn	naproxen
Ansaid	flurbiprofen
Aspirin	aspirin
Indocin	indomethacin
Lodine	etodolac
Relafen	nabumetone
Toradol	ketorolac

BRAND NAME	GENERIC NAME
Blocadren	timolol
Corgard	nadolol
Inderal	propranolol
Lopressor,	
Toprol XL	metoprolol
Tenormin	atenolol
Visken	pindolol
(Other beta-blockers may also interact.)	

INSTRUCTIONS

Take with food to reduce the risk of stomach irritation. (See table on pages 73–91.) Aspirin and OTC ibuprofen or naproxen should not be mixed with prescription NSAIDs or each other.

INSTRUCTIONS

Inderal and Lopressor are best absorbed with meals, but consistency is the most important factor. These drugs should be taken at about the same time every day. Do not stop any of these medicines suddenly except on doctor's orders. Serious side effects could result.

INTERACTION

This combination is of concern because so many people take beta-blockers for high blood pressure and heart problems. Millions rely on NSAIDs for pain relief. NSAIDs may reduce the effectiveness of blood-pressure-lowering beta-blockers. People may not realize a beta-blocker is not working as it should to control hypertension. Experts warn doctors to avoid this combination if possible. The arthritis drug Clinoril (sulindac) may be less likely to interact with beta-blockers, but no matter which arthritis drug is used, people taking an arthritis drug in combination with a beta-blocker will need to have blood pressure monitored frequently. If hypertension becomes a problem, the physician should adjust the dose of beta-blocker or reconsider treatment options.

Symptoms of Beta-Blocker Undertreatment

Blood pressure may climb and heart symptoms might appear. Be alert for chest pain or palpitations and notify your doctor immediately. Monitor blood pressure carefully.

Never take or stop medication without your doctor's advice.

Arthritis Drugs (NSAIDS)	Lithium

DANGEROUS

BRAND NAME	GENERIC NAME
Advil, Motrin, Nuprin	ibuprofen
Aleve, Naprosyn	naproxen
Ansaid	flurbiprofen
Aspirin	aspirin
Indocin	indomethacin
Lodine	etodolac
Relafen	nabumetone
Toradol	ketorolac
etc.	

INSTRUCTIONS
Take with food to reduce the risk of stomach irritation. (See table on pages 73–91.) Aspirin and OTC ibuprofen or naproxen should not be mixed with prescription NSAIDs or each other.

BRAND NAME	GENERIC NAME
Cibalith-S	
Eskalith	
Lithane	
Lithobid	
Lithotabs	

INSTRUCTIONS
Lithium should be taken immediately after meals or with food or milk to reduce stomach upset. It is essential to drink 8 to 12 glasses of water or other fluid each day while on lithium. This medication can affect alertness, so activities such as driving or operating machinery can be dangerous for people on lithium.

INTERACTION

Arthritis drugs can alter the way the body eliminates lithium, possibly through their effects on the kidney. The result is that lithium levels may climb, sometimes to toxic levels. It may take a week or two for this reaction to occur, so serum lithium levels should be measured several times during the first few weeks after starting or stopping one of these nonsteroidal anti-inflammatory drugs. People who are taking over-the-counter ibuprofen or Aleve (naproxen) should be sure to notify their doctors so that proper monitoring can be conducted.

Symptoms of Lithium Toxicity
Nausea, diarrhea, stomach pain, vomiting, incoordination, muscle weakness, and difficulty walking may be signs of early toxicity. Ringing in the ears, visual problems, dizziness, muscle twitching, difficulty speaking clearly, confusion, agitation, and incontinence are more serious signs of trouble. These symptoms require immediate medical attention.

Never take or stop medication without your doctor's advice.

Arthritis Drugs (NSAIDS)	**Alcohol**

TROUBLESOME

BRAND NAME	GENERIC NAME
Advil, Motrin,	
Nuprin	ibuprofen
Aleve,	
Naprosyn	naproxen
Aspirin	aspirin
Indocin	indomethacin
Lodine	etodolac
Relafen	nabumetone
Toradol	ketorolac
etc.	

INSTRUCTIONS
Take with food to reduce the risk of stomach irritation. (See table on pages 73–91.) Aspirin and OTC ibuprofen or naproxen should not be mixed with prescription NSAIDs or each other.

BRAND NAME	GENERIC NAME
NAME	
beer	
liquor	
wine	
medicines that contain alcohol	

INSTRUCTIONS
The absorption and effects of alcohol are magnified if you drink on an empty stomach. Fatty food can delay alcohol absorption. If you drink, do so in moderation, and never drive.

INTERACTION

Arthritis medicine (NSAIDs and aspirin) can be hard on the stomach. People often walk a tightrope between adequate pain relief and stomach upset or ulcers. Alcohol makes that balancing act far more difficult. Alcohol itself can be irritating to the digestive tract, and it also alters the natural protective lining of the stomach. Studies have shown that aspirin causes greater bleeding from the GI tract if people have been drinking. *This interaction could be troublesome.*

One study showed that normal doses of aspirin increase blood alcohol levels. The clinical significance of this research is controversial, but some people might have higher blood alcohol levels than expected if they take aspirin before a social drink. Don't combine aspirin or other NSAIDs and alcohol.

Symptoms of NSAID or Alcohol Toxicity

Nausea, stomach pain, indigestion, and heartburn are tipoffs to trouble. Bleeding from the stomach may occur with no symptoms. Ulcers and more serious digestive tract inflammation may not always be detectable without medical testing.

Never take or stop medication without your doctor's advice.

Asthma Drug (THEOPHYLLINE)

Elixophyllin Quibron-T Respbid Slo-bid Slo-Phyllin
Theo-24 Theobid Theochron Theoclear Theo-Dur
Theolair Theovent etc.

LIFE-THREATENING

Antibiotics (quinolones) Cipro Noroxin Penetrex
Ulcer Drug (H$_2$ antagonist) Tagamet

DANGEROUS

Antibiotics (macrolides) Biaxin E.E.S. E-Mycin ERYC
EryPed Ery-Tab Erythrocin Ilosone PCE Pediazole Tao
Anticonvulsant Tegretol
Heart/Blood Pressure Drugs (beta-blockers)
Blocadren Cartrol Inderal Levatol Timoptic Visken
Heart/Blood Pressure (calcium channel blockers)
Adalat Calan Cardizem Dilacor XR Isoptin Procardia
Verelan
Heart Drug Mexitil
Oral Contraceptives

TROUBLESOME

Alzheimer's Disease Drug Cognex
Anticonvulsants (hydantoins) Dilantin Mesantoin
Peganone
Barbiturates Alturate Amytal Butisol Lotusate
Mebaral Nembutal phenobarbital Seconal Solfoton
Tuinal
Tuberculosis Drug (rifampin) Rifadin Rifamate
Rimactane

Theophylline interacts with many other medications. Be sure to check with your physician and pharmacist if you must take any other drugs in combination with theophylline.

Asthma Drug
(THEOPHYLLINE)

Antibiotics
(QUINOLONES)

LIFE-THREATENING

BRAND NAME

Aerolate	**Aquaphyllin**
Bronkodyl	**Elixomin**
Elixophyllin	**Quibron-T**
Slo-bid	**Slo-Phyllin**
Theobid	**Theochron**
Theoclear	**Theo-Dur**
Theolair	**Theo-24**
Theovent	**Uniphyl**

BRAND NAME	GENERIC NAME
Cipro	ciprofloxacin
Noroxin	norfloxacin
Penetrex	enoxacin

INSTRUCTIONS
Theophylline interacts with food in complex ways, so discuss this issue thoroughly with your doctor and pharmacist. Theophylline may upset the stomach. In some cases this problem can be alleviated by taking the drug with food. See table of Food and Drug Compatibility on pages 73–91 for more information.

INSTRUCTIONS
These drugs come in a variety of doses; it is important to follow the doctor's directions to get the proper dose. See the table of Food and Drug Compatibility on pages 73–91 for details on how to take each one. Antacids or other products containing aluminum, magnesium, iron, zinc, or bismuth should not be taken within two hours of the medicine. These medicines boost caffeine levels; it's best to drink less coffee, tea, or cola than usual.

INTERACTION
People with asthma are often susceptible to respiratory infections, for which these antibiotics are often prescribed. If both medications are needed, theophylline levels should be monitored carefully. Cipro, Noroxin, and Penetrex can raise blood levels of theophylline significantly, resulting in toxicity. *This interaction could be lethal.* **Deaths have been reported.**

Maxaquin and Floxin may not interact with theophylline in the same way. Still, the prudent doctor will monitor theophylline levels and the wise patient will report any symptoms of theophylline toxicity to the doctor.

Symptoms of Theophylline Toxicity
Nausea, diarrhea, stomach pain, headache, insomnia, restlessness, and irritability. Severe toxicity (convulsions, heart rhythm changes, or death) may occur with no warning symptoms. Notify your doctor immediately if you suspect a problem.

Never take or stop medication without your doctor's advice.

Asthma Drug (THEOPHYLLINE)	**Ulcer Drug** (H$_2$ ANTAGONIST)

LIFE-THREATENING

BRAND NAME

Aerolate	Aquaphyllin
Asmalix	Bronkodyl
Elixomin	Elixophyllin
Quibron-T	Respbid
Slo-bid	Slo-Phyllin
Theobid	Theochron
Theoclear	Theo-Dur
Theolair	Theo-24
Theovent	Theo-X
T-Phyl	Uniphyl

BRAND NAME   GENERIC NAME

Tagamet   cimetidine

INSTRUCTIONS

Tagamet is usually taken with meals and/or at bedtime. Antacids may reduce absorption of Tagamet; do not take one for at least two hours after taking Tagamet.

INSTRUCTIONS

Theophylline interacts with food in complex ways, so discuss this issue thoroughly with your doctor and pharmacist. Theophylline may upset the stomach. In some cases this problem can be alleviated by taking the drug with food. See the table of Food and Drug Compatibility on pages 73–91 for more information.

INTERACTION

One common side effect of theophylline is stomach upset, which may in some cases mimic the symptoms of an ulcer or chronic heartburn. If a patient taking theophylline is prescribed Tagamet for symptoms of stomach upset, blood levels of theophylline could reach toxic levels. *This interaction could be life threatening.*

    Tagamet boosts blood levels of theophylline by a third to a half. Patients whose theophylline levels are already a bit high (over 15 mcg/ml) are at highest risk for trouble. Anyone who needs both of these medications should have blood levels of theophylline monitored closely. Notify the physician immediately of any symptoms of theophylline toxicity.

Symptoms of Theophylline Toxicity

Nausea, diarrhea, stomach pain, headache, insomnia, restlessness, and irritability. Severe toxicity (convulsions, heart rhythm changes, or death) may occur with no warning symptoms. Notify your doctor immediately if you suspect a problem.

Never take or stop medication without your doctor's advice.

Asthma Drug	**Antibiotics**
(THEOPHYLLINE)	(MACROLIDES)

DANGEROUS

BRAND NAME

Aerolate	Aquaphyllin
Bronkodyl	Elixomin
Elixophyllin	Quibron-T
Slo-bid	Slo-Phyllin
Theobid	Theochron
Theoclear	Theo-Dur
Theolair	Theo-24
Theovent	Uniphyl

INSTRUCTIONS
Theophylline interacts with food in complex ways, so discuss this issue thoroughly with your doctor and pharmacist. Theophylline may upset the stomach. In some cases this problem can be alleviated by taking the drug with food. See pages 73–91 for more information.

BRAND NAME	GENERIC NAME
Biaxin	clarithromycin
E.E.S.	erythromycin
E-Mycin	erythromycin
ERYC	erythromycin
EryPed	erythromycin
Ery-Tab	erythromycin
Erythrocin	erythromycin
Ilosone	erythromycin
PCE	erythromycin
Pediazole	erythromycin
Tao	troleandomycin

INSTRUCTIONS
Some forms of erythromycin must be taken on an empty stomach; others may be taken with food. See the table of Food and Drug Compatibility on pages 73–91 for specifics. Biaxin can be taken without regard to meals.

INTERACTION
People with asthma are often susceptible to respiratory infections, for which these antibiotics are often prescribed. If both medicines are needed, theophylline levels should be monitored carefully. Oral erythromycin and Tao are both capable of raising blood levels of theophylline. The result could be toxicity. *This interaction is dangerous.*

Because it is similar to erythromycin, Biaxin may also interact with theophylline. People vary greatly in their response to the interaction of theophylline and erythromycin. Those with high theophylline levels (over 15 mcg/ml) may be especially vulnerable. In addition, theophylline may reduce blood levels of erythromycin by as much as 30 percent. If you are on both drugs, stay in close touch with your doctor.
Symptoms of Theophylline Toxicity
Nausea, diarrhea, stomach pain, headache, insomnia, restlessness, and irritability. Severe toxicity (convulsions, heart rhythm changes, or death) may occur with no warning symptoms. Notify your doctor immediately if you suspect a problem.

Never take or stop medication without your doctor's advice.

Asthma Drug
(THEOPHYLLINE)

Anticonvulsant
(CARBAMAZEPINE)

DANGEROUS

BRAND NAME

Aerolate	Aquaphyllin
Asmalix	Bronkodyl
Elixomin	Elixophyllin
Quibron-T	Respbid
Slo-bid	Slo-Phyllin
Theobid	Theochron
Theoclear	Theo-Dur
Theolair	Theo-24
Theovent	Theo-X
T-Phyl	Uniphyl

INSTRUCTIONS

Theophylline interacts with food in complex ways, so discuss this issue thoroughly with your doctor and pharmacist. Theophylline may upset the stomach. In some cases this problem can be alleviated by taking the drug with food. See the table of Food and Drug Compatibility on pages 73–91 for more information.

BRAND NAME   GENERIC NAME

Tegretol   carbamazepine

INSTRUCTIONS

Carbamazepine may upset the stomach; if so, take it with food or milk. Do not stop this drug suddenly; seizures could result. To maintain its strength, it must be stored away from humidity and heat in a tightly closed container.

INTERACTION

This interaction is complex and confusing, because carbamazepine may either increase or decrease blood levels of theophylline. Case reports confirm that both reactions occur.

Increased theophylline levels may lead to toxicity. Diminished levels may be associated with reduced efficacy. In addition, theophylline may reduce carbamazepine levels, leading to a seizure. *This interaction could be dangerous.*

It is important for your physician to check blood levels of both drugs. If you experience symptoms of toxicity, let your doctor know at once.

Symptoms of Theophylline Toxicity

Nausea, diarrhea, stomach pain, headache, insomnia, restlessness, and irritability. Severe toxicity (convulsions, heart rhythm changes, or death) may occur with no warning symptoms. Notify your doctor immediately if you suspect a problem.

Never take or stop medication without your doctor's advice.

Asthma Drug
(THEOPHYLLINE)

Heart/Blood Pressure Drugs
(BETA-BLOCKERS)

DANGEROUS

BRAND NAME

Aerolate	**Aquaphyllin**
Bronkodyl	**Elixomin**
Elixophyllin	**Quibron-T**
Slo-bid	**Slo-Phyllin**
Theobid	**Theochron**
Theoclear	**Theo-Dur**
Theolair	**Theo-24**
Theovent	**Uniphyl**

INSTRUCTIONS
Theophylline interacts with food in complex ways, so discuss this issue thoroughly with your doc tor and pharmacist. Theophylline may upset the stomach. In some cases this problem can be alleviated by taking the drug with food. See pages 73–91 for more information.

BRAND NAME	GENERIC NAME
Blocadren	timolol
Cartrol	carteolol
Inderal	propranolol
Levatol	penbutolol
Timoptic	timolol
Visken	pindolol

INSTRUCTIONS
Cartrol, Levatol, and Visken are taken with or without food. Inderal is best absorbed with meals, but consistency is more important. It should be taken at roughly the same time every day. Ask your eye doctor to show you how to administer Timoptic drops so that their absorption is minimized. Do not stop any of these medicines suddenly except on doctor's orders. Serious side effects could result.

INTERACTION

Because beta-blockers can make breathing difficult, they are not often prescribed for people with asthma. The beta-blockers named above can reduce the body's ability to clear theophylline, resulting in increased blood levels of theophylline, with the potential for theophylline toxicity. *This interaction could be dangerous.*

Neither Corgard nor Tenormin interferes with theophylline clearance. It is uncommon but certainly not unknown for eye drops such as Timoptic to be absorbed into the body and produce systemic side effects. In that case, Timoptic could interact with theophylline.

Symptoms of Theophylline Toxicity
Nausea, diarrhea, stomach pain, headache, insomnia, restlessness, and irritability. Severe toxicity (convulsions, heart rhythm changes, or death) may occur with no warning symptoms. Notify your doctor immediately if you suspect a problem.

Never take or stop medication without your doctor's advice.

Asthma Drug
(THEOPHYLLINE)

Heart/Blood Pressure Drugs
(CALCIUM CHANNEL BLOCKERS)

DANGEROUS

BRAND NAME

Aerolate	**Aquaphyllin**
Asmalix	**Bronkodyl**
Elixomin	**Elixophyllin**
Quibron-T	**Respbid**
Slo-bid	**Slo-Phyllin**
Theobid	**Theochron**
Theoclear	**Theo-Dur**
Theolair	**Theo-24**
Theovent	**Theo-X**
T-Phyl	**Uniphyl**

INSTRUCTIONS
Theophylline interacts with food in complex ways, so discuss this issue thoroughly with your doctor and pharmacist. Theophylline may upset the stomach. In some cases this problem can be alleviated by taking the drug with food. See the table of Food and Drug Compatibility on pages 73–91 for more information.

BRAND NAME	GENERIC NAME
Adalat, Procardia	nifedipine
Calan, Isoptin, Verelan	verapamil
Cardizem, Dilacor XR	diltiazem

INSTRUCTIONS
These drugs come in a variety of doses; follow the doctor's directions carefully. Sustained-release forms, such as Calan SR or Dilacor XR, should not be chewed or crushed and are best taken with food. Avoid taking Adalat or Procardia with grapefruit juice, as this could boost blood levels unexpectedly. See the table on pages 73–91 for specific instructions. Withdrawal symptoms, especially chest pain, may occur if these drugs are stopped suddenly. Follow the doctor's instructions for tapering slowly if the medicine must be discontinued.

INTERACTION
Many medicines, including diltiazem and verapamil, are capable of elevating blood levels of theophylline by interfering with metabolism of the drug. People seem to vary in the degree to which they react to this interaction. *Although the documented increase in circulating theophylline is not large, it could be dangerous for someone whose blood levels were already high.*

Most studies indicate that Procardia has little effect on serum theophylline levels, but there are a few cases of patients who developed toxicity as a result of this interaction.

Symptoms of Theophylline Toxicity
Nausea, diarrhea, stomach pain, headache, insomnia, restlessness, and irritability. Severe toxicity (convulsions, heart rhythm changes, or death) may occur with no warning symptoms. Notify your doctor immediately if you suspect a problem.

Never take or stop medication without your doctor's advice.

Asthma Drug
(THEOPHYLLINE)

Heart Drug
(MEXILETINE)

DANGEROUS

BRAND NAME

Aerolate   **Aquaphyllin**
Asmalix   **Bronkodyl**
Elixomin   **Elixophyllin**
Quibron-T   **Respbid**
Slo-bid   **Slo-Phyllin**
Theobid   **Theochron**
Theoclear   **Theo-Dur**
Theolair   **Theo-24**
Theovent   **Theo-X**
T-Phyl   **Uniphyl**

INSTRUCTIONS
Theophylline interacts with food
in complex ways, so discuss this
issue thoroughly with your doctor and pharmacist. Theophylline
may upset the stomach. In some
cases this problem can be alleviated by taking the drug with food.
See the table of Food and Drug
Compatibility on pages 73–91 for
more information.

BRAND NAME   GENERIC NAME
Mexitil   mexiletine

INSTRUCTIONS
Mexitil may irritate the digestive
tract, so it should be taken with
food or an antacid. Dramatic
changes in diet should be avoided. Notify the doctor immediately if fever, yellow skin and eyes,
sore throat, or unusual tiredness
develop.

INTERACTION
Like many other medicines, Mexitil interferes with the metabolism of
theophylline. Blood levels of theophylline can double, leading to symptoms of toxicity. Because Mexitil is given only to people vulnerable to
heart rhythm changes, there is a possibility of serious heartbeat disturbances. *This interaction could be dangerous.*
Symptoms of Theophylline Toxicity
Nausea, diarrhea, stomach pain, headache, insomnia, restlessness, and
irritability. Severe toxicity (convulsions, heart rhythm changes, or
death) may occur with no warning symptoms. Notify your doctor immediately if you suspect a problem.

Never take or stop medication without your doctor's advice.

Asthma Drug
(THEOPHYLLINE)

Oral Contraceptives

DANGEROUS

BRAND NAME

Aerolate	Aquaphyllin
Asmalix	Bronkodyl
Elixomin	Elixophyllin
Quibron-T	Respbid
Slo-bid	Slo-Phyllin
Theobid	Theochron
Theoclear	Theo-Dur
Theolair	Theo-24
Theovent	Theo-X
T-Phyl	Uniphyl

BRAND NAME	GENERIC NAME
Brevicon	Demulen
Desogen	Genora
Levlen	Loestrin
Lo/Ovral	Modicon
N.E.E.	Nelova
Nordette	Norethin
Norinyl	Norlestrin
Ortho-Cyclen	Ortho-Novum
Ovcon	Ovral
Triphasil	

INSTRUCTIONS

Theophylline interacts with food in complex ways, so discuss this issue thoroughly with your doctor and pharmacist. Theophylline may upset the stomach. In some cases this problem can be alleviated by taking the drug with food. See the table of Food and Drug Compatibility on pages 73–91 for more information.

INSTRUCTIONS

Oral contraceptives should be taken at the same time every day and precisely according to instructions. Missed doses can lead to an unwelcome pregnancy. Additional contraception is needed for at least the first week.

INTERACTION

In clinical studies, oral contraceptives appear to interfere with theophylline metabolism, and to raise blood levels of that drug. *This interaction could result in dangerous theophylline toxicity.*

Although we found no mention in the literature of postmenopausal estrogen therapy interacting with theophylline, theoretically such an interaction might be possible. Stay alert and notify your doctor of any symptoms of theophylline toxicity.

Symptoms of Theophylline Toxicity

Nausea, diarrhea, stomach pain, headache, insomnia, restlessness, and irritability. Severe toxicity (convulsions, heart rhythm changes, or death) may occur with no warning symptoms. Notify your doctor immediately if you suspect a problem.

Never take or stop medication without your doctor's advice.

Asthma Drug
(THEOPHYLLINE)

Alzheimer's Disease Drug

TROUBLESOME

BRAND NAME

Aerolate **Aquaphyllin**
Asmalix **Bronkodyl**
Elixomin **Elixophyllin**
Quibron-T **Respbid**
Slo-bid **Slo-Phyllin**
Theobid **Theochron**
Theoclear **Theo-Dur**
Theolair **Theo-24**
Theovent **Theo-X**
T-Phyl **Uniphyl**

INSTRUCTIONS
Theophylline interacts with food in complex ways, so discuss this issue thoroughly with your doctor and pharmacist. Theophylline may upset the stomach. In some cases this problem can be alleviated by taking the drug with food. See the table of Food and Drug Compatibility on pages 73–91 for more information.

BRAND NAME   GENERIC NAME

Cognex   tacrine

INSTRUCTIONS
The dose must be individualized. Cognex should be taken between meals whenever possible. If it upsets the stomach, it may be taken with food. Liver enzymes should be monitored regularly.

INTERACTION
Cognex interferes with the normal metabolism of theophylline. This can lead to substantial elevations in theophylline levels (double the normal blood level). This might lead to theophylline toxicity. *This interaction could be troublesome.*

If theophylline must be prescribed in combination with Cognex, the doctor may need to adjust the dose of theophylline carefully. Frequent monitoring of blood levels is advisable.

Symptoms of Theophylline Toxicity
Nausea, diarrhea, stomach pain, headache, insomnia, restlessness, and irritability. Severe toxicity (convulsions, heart rhythm changes, or death) may occur with no warning symptoms. Notify your doctor immediately if you suspect a problem.

Never take or stop medication without your doctor's advice.

Asthma Drug	**Anticonvulsants**
(THEOPHYLLINE)	(HYDANTOINS)

TROUBLESOME

BRAND NAME

Aerolate	**Aquaphyllin**
Asmalix	**Bronkodyl**
Elixomin	**Elixophyllin**
Quibron-T	**Respbid**
Slo-bid	**Slo-Phyllin**
Theobid	**Theochron**
Theoclear	**Theo-Dur**
Theolair	**Theo-24**
Theovent	**Theo-X**
T-Phyl	**Uniphyl**

INSTRUCTIONS

Theophylline interacts with food in complex ways, so discuss this issue thoroughly with your doctor and pharmacist. Theophylline may upset the stomach. In some cases this problem can be alleviated by taking the drug with food. See the table of Food and Drug Compatibility on pages 73–91 for more information.

BRAND NAME	GENERIC NAME
Dilantin	phenytoin
Mesantoin	mephenytoin
Peganone	ethotoin

INSTRUCTIONS

Any of these medicines could upset the stomach. This is less likely if they are taken with food. All of them can cause drowsiness or blurred vision and could make driving dangerous.

INTERACTION

This is a double interaction, because both theophylline and the anticonvulsants can lead to lower blood levels of the other drug. The effect of the anticonvulsants, especially Dilantin, is to speed up removal of theophylline from the system by as much as 65 percent. *This interaction could be troublesome, leading to asthma symptoms.*

The interaction may become noticeable within about five days of taking the two drugs together. If both are needed, blood levels of each should be monitored so that doses can be adjusted appropriately by the doctor.

Never take or stop medication without your doctor's advice.

Asthma Drug
(THEOPHYLLINE)

Barbiturates

TROUBLESOME

BRAND NAME

Aerolate	**Aquaphyllin**
Asmalix	**Bronkodyl**
Elixomin	**Elixophyllin**
Quibron-T	**Respbid**
Slo-bid	**Slo-Phyllin**
Theobid	**Theochron**
Theoclear	**Theo-Dur**
Theolair	**Theo-24**
Theovent	**Theo-X**
T-Phyl	**Uniphyl**

BRAND NAME	GENERIC NAME
Alurate	aprobarbital
Amytal	amobarbital
Butisol	butabarbital
Lotusate	talbutal
Mebaral	mephobarbital
Nembutal	pentobarbital
Seconal	secobarbital
Solfoton	phenobarbital
Tuinal	amobarbital/
	secobarbital

INSTRUCTIONS
Theophylline interacts with food in complex ways, so discuss this issue thoroughly with your doctor and pharmacist. Theophylline may upset the stomach. In some cases this problem can be alleviated by taking the drug with food. See the table of Food and Drug Compatibility on pages 73–91 for more information.

INSTRUCTIONS
Any of these medications can cause drowsiness and limit attention. Take them at a time when you will not need to drive or do other complicated tasks.

INTERACTION
Barbiturates stimulate the body to get rid of theophylline more quickly than usual. Laboratory studies show that blood levels of theophylline could drop dramatically. In this event, the previous dose of theophylline might not be enough to allow easy breathing. Blood tests will tell if the dose of theophylline requires adjustment. *This interaction could be troublesome.*

Never take or stop medication without your doctor's advice.

Asthma Drug (THEOPHYLLINE)	**Tuberculosis Drug** (RIFAMPIN)

TROUBLESOME

BRAND NAME		BRAND NAME	GENERIC NAME
Aerolate	**Aquaphyllin**	**Rifadin**	rifampin
Asmalix	**Bronkodyl**	**Rifamate**	isoniazid/
Elixomin	**Elixophyllin**		rifampin
Quibron-T	**Respbid**	**Rimactane**	rifampin
Slo-bid	**Slo-Phyllin**		
Theobid	**Theochron**		
Theoclear	**Theo-Dur**		
Theolair	**Theo-24**		
Theovent	**Theo-X**		
T-Phyl	**Uniphyl**		

Asthma column:

INSTRUCTIONS

Theophylline interacts with food in complex ways, so discuss this issue thoroughly with your doctor and pharmacist. Theophylline may upset the stomach. In some cases this problem can be alleviated by taking the drug with food. See the table of Food and Drug Compatibility on pages 73–91 for more information.

Tuberculosis column:

INSTRUCTIONS

Rifampin should be taken on an empty stomach, at least one hour before or two hours after meals. If you develop fever, chills, unusual tiredness, unusual bleeding or bruising, sore throat, muscle and bone pain, or yellow skin and eyes, contact your physician immediately.

INTERACTION

A person with tuberculosis might very well need both these medications, because the disease could contribute to wheezing and breathing difficulties. Alternatively, theophylline might be prescribed to treat shortness of breath developing as a side effect of rifampin. Rifampin speeds the metabolism of theophylline so that it disappears much more quickly from the body. This takes at least a week and often longer, but as it occurs, theophylline levels drop and asthma may become worse. *This interaction could be troublesome.*

It makes sense for the doctor to check blood levels of theophylline several times when rifampin is added or dropped. These tests will tell if a dosage adjustment is necessary.

Never take or stop medication without your doctor's advice.

Cholesterol Drugs

Mevacor   Pravachol   Zocor

LIFE-THREATENING

Antibiotics (macrolides) Biaxin E.E.S. E-Mycin ERYC
EryPed Ery-Tab Erythrocin Ilosone PCE Pediazole Tao
Cholesterol Drugs Lopid niacin
Transplant Drug Sandimmune

DANGEROUS

Anticoagulant Coumadin

Not every cholesterol drug listed above interacts with each medicine
on this list. See individual summaries for details. Drugs shown here
have the most serious known reactions with this type of cholesterol-
lowering drug, but check with a health professional before taking any
other medicine with one of these agents.

Cholesterol Drugs

Antibiotics
(MACROLIDES)

BRAND NAME	GENERIC NAME
Mevacor	lovastatin
Pravachol	pravastatin
Zocor	simvastatin

INSTRUCTIONS

Mevacor is best taken with the evening meal. Zocor and Pravachol may be taken with or without food before bed. They are most effective in combination with a prudent heart-healthy diet and a sensible exercise program.

BRAND NAME	GENERIC NAME
Biaxin	clarithromycin
E.E.S.	erythromycin
E-Mycin	erythromycin
ERYC	erythromycin
EryPed	erythromycin
Ery-Tab	erythromycin
Erythrocin	erythromycin
Ilosone	erythromycin
PCE	erythromycin
Pediazole	erythromycin
Tao	troleandomycin

INSTRUCTIONS

Some erythromycins must be taken on an empty stomach; others may be taken with food. See the table of Food and Drug Interactions on pages 73–91 for specifics. Biaxin can be swallowed with food or on an empty stomach.

INTERACTION

There is a possibility that erythromycin antibiotics may interact with Mevacor to produce muscle destruction, possibly progressing to kidney failure. *This interaction, if confirmed by further research, could be life threatening, so we alert you to it now.*

Several cases of this reaction, called myopathy or rhabdomyolysis, have been reported when erythromycin was added to Mevacor. Because Mevacor can cause this reaction on its own (although this is rare), experts are uncertain that erythromycin is to blame. If you must take both drugs, however, be alert for signs of muscle weakness, tenderness, or pain, and contact your doctor immediately if they develop. Blood and urine tests will be required to determine if the reaction is serious. It is not known if Biaxin or Tao interacts with Mevacor; nor is it known if Pravachol or Zocor interacts with erythromycin in this way.

Symptoms of Myopathy to Watch For

Muscle weakness, change in gait, muscle pain, and muscles that are tender to the touch.

Never take or stop medication without your doctor's advice.

Cholesterol Drugs | Cholesterol Drugs

BRAND NAME	GENERIC NAME
Mevacor	lovastatin
Pravachol	pravastatin
Zocor	simvastatin

BRAND NAME	GENERIC NAME
Lopid	gemfibrozil
Nicolar	niacin,
	nicotinic acid

INSTRUCTIONS

Mevacor is best taken with the evening meal. Zocor and Pravachol may be taken with or without food before bed. They are most effective in combination with a prudent heart-healthy diet and a sensible exercise program.

INSTRUCTIONS

Lopid is to be taken one-half hour before morning and evening meals. Niacin is best taken with meals. A single aspirin tablet one-half hour before taking niacin may reduce flushing; check with your doctor. Both drugs work best in conjunction with a heart-healthy diet and sensible exercise.

INTERACTION

Some people with high cholesterol have a hard time getting it down with just one drug. Doctors may try a combination of cholesterol-lowering medications in such a case. Both niacin and Lopid have been used together with Mevacor, but there is a risk of serious interaction in both cases. In perhaps 3 or 4 percent of patients, Lopid can interact with Mevacor to produce muscle destruction, possibly progressing to kidney failure. Older women and people with preexisting kidney problems appear especially vulnerable. *Although we are aware of no deaths, this interaction could be life threatening.*

Several cases of this reaction, called myopathy or rhabdomyolysis, have also been reported with niacin and Mevacor. If you must take either drug with Mevacor, be alert for signs of muscle weakness, tenderness, or pain, and contact your doctor immediately if they develop. Blood and urine tests will be required to determine if the reaction is serious.

Zocor and Pravachol may also interact dangerously with Lopid.

Symptoms of Myopathy to Watch For

Muscle weakness, change in gait, muscle pain, and muscles that are tender to the touch.

Never take or stop medication without your doctor's advice.

Cholesterol Drugs | # Transplant Drug
(CYCLOSPORINE)

LIFE-THREATENING

BRAND NAME | GENERIC NAME
Mevacor | lovastatin
Pravachol | pravastatin
Zocor | simvastatin

INSTRUCTIONS

Mevacor is best taken with the evening meal. Zocor and Pravachol may be taken with or without food before bed. They are most effective in combination with a prudent heart-healthy diet and a sensible exercise program.

BRAND NAME | GENERIC NAME
Sandimmune cyclosporine

INSTRUCTIONS

Sandimmune comes as an oral solution with a taste reminiscent of castor oil. It should be mixed in a glass with milk, chocolate milk, or orange juice at room temperature and drunk at once. Then the glass (no plastic) should be rinsed and the rinsing fluid drunk to get the full dose. Do not take Sandimmune with grapefruit juice unless the physician is monitoring blood levels of the drug closely. (See page 53.)

Due to a possible interaction between cyclosporine and oral contraceptives, barrier methods of contraception should be used while taking this drug.

Regular monitoring is important. Do not stop this medicine unless your doctor so directs.

INTERACTION

Although we are aware of no fatalities, the combination of Sandimmune and one of these cholesterol-lowering drugs could lead to a syndrome of muscle destruction (resulting in weakness and pain) and consequent kidney failure. This reaction, known as rhabdomyolysis, can occur with Mevacor alone, but adding Sandimmune increases the risk substantially. Some reports estimate that up to 30 percent of patients on this combination of drugs may experience muscle wasting. If you need both medications, stay alert and notify your doctor immediately of any symptoms of muscle problems. Blood and urine tests may be needed. *This interaction could be life threatening.*

Symptoms of Myopathy to Watch For

Muscle weakness, change in gait, muscle pain, and muscles that are tender to the touch.

Never take or stop medication without your doctor's advice.

Cholesterol Drugs

Anticoagulant
(WARFARIN)

DANGEROUS

BRAND NAME   GENERIC NAME
Mevacor   lovastatin

BRAND NAME   GENERIC NAME
Coumadin   warfarin

INSTRUCTIONS
Mevacor is best taken with the evening meal. It is most effective in combination with a prudent heart-healthy diet and a sensible exercise program.

INSTRUCTIONS
Warfarin tablets can be swallowed with food or on an empty stomach. Try to avoid large variations in the quantity of vitamin-K–containing vegetables—such as broccoli, cabbage, or spinach—that you eat each day. Consuming much more or less than usual could change the action of the drug.

INTERACTION
Mevacor appears to increase the effects of warfarin in some patients. Two middle-aged men requiring warfarin were later put on Mevacor for elevated cholesterol. Each of them developed unexpected bleeding and prolonged prothrombin times. *This interaction could be dangerous.* If Mevacor and warfarin are both needed, frequent blood tests will guide warfarin dose adjustment. There is no evidence that·the other cholesterol-lowering drugs, Pravachol (generic: pravastatin) or Zocor (generic: simvastatin), interact with warfarin in the same fashion. Because they are similar to Mevacor, however, caution is probably advisable.

Symptoms of Warfarin Overdose
There may be no early warning signs of danger. Blood tests are essential. Symptoms include any unusual bleeding, including rectal or urinary tract bleeding, excessive menstrual bleeding, nosebleeds, bleeding around gums, bruising, red or tar-black stools, vomiting blood, and red or dark-brown urine. Notify your doctor immediately if you suspect a problem.

Never take or stop medication without your doctor's advice.

Diabetes Drugs

DiaBeta	Diabinese	Dymelor	Glucotrol
Glynase	Micronase	Orinase	Tolinase

LIFE-THREATENING

Phenylbutazone Azolid Butazolidin

DANGEROUS

Alcohol

Antibiotics (co-trimoxazole) Bactrim Septra etc.

Antidepressant (MAO inhibitor) Nardil

TROUBLESOME

Antidepressants (tricyclic) Adapin Aventyl Elavil
Endep Norpramin Pamelor Pertofrane Sinequan
Tofranil etc.

Antifungal Drug Diflucan

Aspirin and Arthritis Drugs (salicylates)

Cholesterol Drug Lopid

Cortisonelike Drugs Aristocort Cortef cortisone
Decadron Kenacort etc.

Diuretics Dyazide HydroDIURIL etc.

Heart/Blood Pressure Drugs (ACE inhibitors)
Accupril Capoten Lotensin Prinivil Vasotec Zestril etc.

Oral Contraceptives

Tuberculosis Drug (rifampin) Rifadin Rifamate
Rimactane

Not every diabetes drug interacts with each drug on this list. See the
interaction summaries for details. Diabetes drugs also interact with
other medications. Be sure to check with your physician and pharmacist if you must take any other drugs in combination with diabetes
medicines.

Diabetes Drugs | Phenylbutazone

LIFE-THREATENING

BRAND NAME	GENERIC NAME
Diabinese	chlorpropamide
Dymelor	acetohexamide
Orinase	tolbutamide

INSTRUCTIONS
These diabetes drugs may be taken with food if they upset the stomach. Blood glucose monitoring is important. Notify the doctor immediately if you experience rash, fever, sore throat, or unusual bleeding or bruising.

BRAND NAME	GENERIC NAME
Azolid,	
Butazolidin	phenylbutazone

INSTRUCTIONS
Phenylbutazone should be taken with food to minimize digestive upset. Notify the doctor immediately if you experience sore throat, mouth sores, unusual bleeding or bruising, swollen legs and feet, rash, blurred vision, fever, abdominal pain, black tarry stools, or sudden weight gain.

INTERACTION

Phenylbutazone can raise blood levels or lengthen the time that several of the oral diabetes drugs spend circulating in the body. The consequence of this can be unexpectedly low blood sugar, potentially leading to hypoglycemic coma. A person needing both medications should definitely monitor blood sugar more closely than usual. *This interaction could be lethal.* **At least one death has been reported.**

There have been no reports of interactions between phenylbutazone and the oral diabetes drugs DiaBeta and Glucotrol; nevertheless, it would be wise to monitor blood sugar closely if you take this combination of drugs.

Symptoms of Hypoglycemia (Low Blood Sugar)
Shaking, sweating, tiredness, low temperature, faintness, palpitations, hunger, headache, confusion, irritability, visual disturbances, and coma. Close observation (preferably in the hospital) is recommended for two or three days after such a reaction.

Never take or stop medication without your doctor's advice.

Diabetes Drugs

Alcohol

DANGEROUS

BRAND NAME	GENERIC NAME
Diabinese	chlorpropamide
Glucotrol	glipizide
Orinase	tolbutamide

NAME
beer
liquor
wine
medicines that contain alcohol

INSTRUCTIONS
Glucotrol should be taken 15 minutes to half an hour before meals.
The others may be taken with
food, especially if they upset the
stomach. Daily blood glucose
monitoring is important. Notify
the doctor immediately if you
experience rash, fever, sore
throat, or unusual bleeding or
bruising.

INSTRUCTIONS
The absorption and effects of
alcohol are magnified if you
drink on an empty stomach. Fatty food can delay alcohol absorption. If you drink, do so in moderation, and never drive.

INTERACTION
*The interaction between alcohol and oral diabetes drugs is compli-
cated, and some aspects of this interaction are potentially dangerous.* If patients taking Diabinese drink alcohol, they may experience an
unpleasant reaction, with symptoms of nausea and vomiting, flushing,
sweating, and throbbing headache. Alcohol may have other effects
upon diabetes drugs. The person who drinks regularly may not be able
to control blood sugar with the usual dose of Orinase (tolbutamide).
On the other hand, if a person who doesn't often drink alcohol has several drinks, he or she may have a longer-than-expected effect from
Glucotrol, with possible hypoglycemic symptoms. It is suggested that
patients taking any of these oral diabetes drugs generally avoid alcohol. Remember that some liquid medicines contain alcohol (see page
203 for a list).

Symptoms of Hypoglycemia (Low Blood Sugar)
Shaking, sweating, tiredness, low temperature, faintness, palpitations,
hunger, headache, confusion, irritability, visual disturbances, and
coma. Close observation (preferably in the hospital) is recommended
for two or three days after such a reaction.

Never take or stop medication without your doctor's advice.

Diabetes Drugs	**Antibiotic**
	(CO-TRIMOXAZOLE)

DANGEROUS

BRAND NAME	GENERIC NAME
DiaBeta, Glynase,	
Micronase	glyburide
Diabinese	chlorpropamide
Dymelor	acetohexamide
Glucotrol	glipizide
Orinase	tolbutamide
Tolinase	tolazamide

INSTRUCTIONS

DiaBeta, Glucotrol, and Micronase should be taken 15 minutes to half an hour before meals. The others may be taken with food if they upset the stomach. Blood glucose monitoring is important. Notify the doctor immediately if you experience rash, fever, sore throat, or unusual bleeding or bruising.

BRAND NAME
Bactrim,
Cotrim,
Septra,
SMZ-TMP,
Sulfatrim,
Uroplus
(All co-trimoxazole, formerly known as trimethoprim-sulfamethoxazole)

INSTRUCTIONS

This drug is best absorbed when taken on an empty stomach, at least one hour before or two hours after a meal. It may be taken with food if it upsets the stomach. Drink at least eight cups of water a day to help keep the drug from crystallizing in the kidney, and avoid large doses of vitamin C.

INTERACTION

These oral diabetes drugs last longer in the body when a person also takes a sulfa antibiotic such as Bactrim or Septra. Some patients have experienced hypoglycemia as a consequence. Orinase and Diabinese have been implicated most frequently, but there is one case report of this interaction causing hypoglycemia in a patient on Glucotrol. *This interaction could be dangerous.* DiaBeta, Glynase, and Micronase do not appear to interact with co-trimoxazole to cause hypoglycemia. Still, if you are on any oral diabetes drug and need to take this antibiotic, monitor your blood sugar carefully and be alert for hypoglycemia.

Symptoms of Hypoglycemia (Low Blood Sugar)

Shaking, sweating, tiredness, low temperature, faintness, palpitations, hunger, headache, confusion, irritability, visual disturbances, and coma. Close observation (preferably in the hospital) is recommended for two or three days after such a reaction.

Never take or stop medication without your doctor's advice.

Diabetes Drugs	Antidepressant
	(MAO INHIBITOR)

DANGEROUS

BRAND NAME	GENERIC NAME
DiaBeta, Glynase,	
Micronase	glyburide
Diabinese	chlorpropamide
Glucotrol	glipizide
Orinase	tolbutamide
Tolinase	tolazamide

INSTRUCTIONS

DiaBeta, Glucotrol, and Micronase should be taken 15 minutes to half an hour before meals. The others may be taken with food if they upset the stomach. Blood glucose monitoring is important. Notify the doctor immediately if you experience rash, fever, sore throat, or unusual bleeding or bruising.

BRAND NAME	GENERIC NAME
Nardil	phenelzine

INSTRUCTIONS

MAO inhibitors can interact in dangerous ways with tyramine-containing foods and beverages. See page 59. Consult your doctor before taking other prescription or over-the-counter drugs. Notify him or her if you notice a skin rash, severe headache, yellow eyes or skin, or dark urine. Do not stop this medicine unless your doctor so advises.

INTERACTION

Nardil, an MAO inhibitor, can increase the glucose-lowering effects of the oral diabetes drugs and also of insulin. *Since severe hypoglycemia could result, this interaction may be dangerous.*

If you need both medications, monitor blood sugar more carefully so that the doctor can help you adjust the dose of medication if necessary. This is not a do-it-yourself project. Notify your doctor if you develop hypoglycemia. The MAO inhibitor Parnate does not appear to lower blood sugar in the same way.

Symptoms of Hypoglycemia (Low Blood Sugar)

Shaking, sweating, tiredness, low temperature, faintness, palpitations, hunger, headache, confusion, irritability, visual disturbances, and coma. Close observation (preferably in the hospital) is recommended for two or three days after such a reaction.

Never take or stop medication without your doctor's advice.

Diabetes Drugs	Antidepressants
	(TRICYCLIC)

TROUBLESOME

BRAND NAME	GENERIC NAME
DiaBeta, Glynase,	
Micronase	glyburide
Diabinese	chlorpropamide
Glucotrol	glipizide
Orinase	tolbutamide
Tolinase	tolazamide

INSTRUCTIONS
DiaBeta, Glucotrol, and Micronase should be taken 15 minutes to half an hour before meals. The others may be taken with food if they upset the stomach. Blood glucose monitoring is important. Notify the doctor immediately if you experience rash, fever, sore throat, or unusual bleeding or bruising.

BRAND NAME	GENERIC NAME
Adapin,	
Sinequan	doxepin
Aventyl,	
Pamelor	nortriptyline
Elavil, Endep	amitriptyline
Norpramin,	
Pertofrane	desipramine
Tofranil	imipramine
etc.	

INSTRUCTIONS
Usually these medications are better taken with food, in the evening to avoid daytime drowsiness. A high-fiber diet may interfere with absorption, however. Sinequan Concentrate should be mixed with four ounces of milk, water, or juice just before taking, not ahead of time. Do not stop taking any of these drugs suddenly; if they must be discontinued, your doctor will supervise gradual phaseout.

INTERACTION

This interaction has been deduced from case reports and needs confirmation from clinical studies. Tricyclic antidepressants are apparently capable of increasing the effects of oral diabetes drugs, so that a person might experience severe hypoglycemia. *This interaction could be troublesome.*

If you must take an antidepressant together with your oral diabetes drug, measure your blood sugar more frequently. Let your doctor know if you have an episode of low blood sugar.

Symptoms of Hypoglycemia (Low Blood Sugar)
Shaking, sweating, tiredness, low temperature, faintness, palpitations, hunger, headache, confusion, irritability, visual disturbances, and coma. Close observation (preferably in the hospital) is recommended for two or three days after such a reaction.

Never take or stop medication without your doctor's advice.

Diabetes Drug	**Antifungal Drug**

TROUBLESOME

BRAND NAME	GENERIC NAME	BRAND NAME	GENERIC NAME
Orinase	tolbutamide	**Diflucan**	fluconazole

INSTRUCTIONS
Tolbutamide may be taken with food, especially if it upsets the stomach. Daily blood glucose monitoring is important. Notify the doctor immediately if you experience rash, fever, sore throat, or unusual bleeding or bruising.

INSTRUCTIONS
Ask your doctor for precise instructions on how to take Diflucan. Doses are individualized, depending on the infection treated, and the first dose is often higher than the rest.

INTERACTION

Diflucan can boost blood levels of Orinase or generic tolbutamide. In the study that established this interaction, none of the healthy young men experienced dangerous changes in blood sugar level. However, diabetics might discover that this antifungal could make their Orinase more effective than expected. Hypoglycemia is theoretically possible. *This interaction could be troublesome.*

There is no indication that Diflucan interacts with other diabetes drugs, but it was not tested to rule out such an interaction. If you must take both medications, monitor your blood sugar carefully and notify your doctor if it is low.

Symptoms of Hypoglycemia (Low Blood Sugar)
Shaking, sweating, tiredness, low temperature, faintness, palpitations, hunger, headache, confusion, irritability, visual disturbances, and coma. Close observation (preferably in the hospital) is recommended for two or three days after such a reaction.

Never take or stop medication without your doctor's advice.

Diabetes Drugs

Aspirin and Arthritis Drugs
(SALICYLATES)

TROUBLESOME

BRAND NAME	GENERIC NAME
DiaBeta, Glynase,	
Micronase	glyburide
Diabinese	chlorpropamide
Glucotrol	glipizide
Orinase	tolbutamide
Tolinase	tolazamide

INSTRUCTIONS

DiaBeta, Glucotrol, and Micronase should be taken 15 minutes to half an hour before meals. The others may be taken with food if they upset the stomach. Blood glucose monitoring is important. Notify the doctor immediately if you experience rash, fever, sore throat, or unusual bleeding or bruising.

BRAND NAME	GENERIC NAME
Alka-Seltzer	acetylsalicylic acid
Anacin	acetylsalicylic acid
Arthropan	choline salicylate
Ascriptin	acetylsalicylic acid
aspirin	acetylsalicylic acid
Bayer	acetylsalicylic acid
Bufferin	acetylsalicylic acid
Disalcid	salsalate
Ecotrin	acetylsalicylic acid
Uracel 5	sodium salicylate

INSTRUCTIONS

Aspirin may be taken with food or milk to reduce stomach upset, always with a full eight ounces of liquid. Pregnant women should take aspirin only under the doctor's supervision. Children with flu or chicken pox must avoid aspirin as it increases the risk of Reye's Syndrome.

INTERACTION

Aspirin and some related medicines, such as Arthropan and Disalcid, can lower blood sugar by themselves. In combination with the diabetes drugs, they may lower blood sugar more than expected. *This interaction could be troublesome.*

If you need aspirin or another salicylate as well as one of these diabetes drugs, monitor blood sugar and be alert for symptoms of hypoglycemia. If you notice any, your doctor may wish to adjust the dose of the diabetes drug.

Symptoms of Hypoglycemia (Low Blood Sugar)

Shaking, sweating, tiredness, low temperature, faintness, palpitations, hunger, headache, confusion, irritability, visual disturbances, and coma. Close observation (preferably in the hospital) is recommended for two or three days after such a reaction.

Never take or stop medication without your doctor's advice.

Diabetes Drug	**Cholesterol Drug**

TROUBLESOME

BRAND NAME   GENERIC NAME
DiaBeta, Glynase,
  Micronase glyburide

INSTRUCTIONS
DiaBeta, Glucotrol, and Micronase should be taken 15 minutes to half an hour before meals. Daily blood glucose monitoring is important. Notify the doctor immediately if you experience rash, fever, sore throat, or unusual bleeding or bruising.

BRAND NAME   GENERIC NAME
Lopid   gemfibrozil

INSTRUCTIONS
Lopid is to be taken one-half hour before morning and evening meals. It works best in conjunction with a heart-healthy diet and sensible exercise.

INTERACTION

Diabetics are at higher risk of heart disease than the population in general, and many non-insulin-dependent diabetics have high cholesterol levels. It is certainly logical that such a person might end up taking both DiaBeta (or another brand of glyburide) and Lopid. The cholesterol drug can increase the blood-sugar-lowering power of DiaBeta, and the result may be hypoglycemia. *This interaction could be troublesome.*

   If you must take both medications, monitor your blood sugar carefully and notify your doctor if it is low. The dose of DiaBeta may need to be adjusted.

Symptoms of Hypoglycemia (Low Blood Sugar)
Shaking, sweating, tiredness, low temperature, faintness, palpitations, hunger, headache, confusion, irritability, visual disturbances, and coma. Close observation (preferably in the hospital) is recommended for two or three days after such a reaction.

Never take or stop medication without your doctor's advice.

Diabetes Drugs | Cortisone-like Drugs

TROUBLESOME

BRAND NAME	GENERIC NAME
DiaBeta, Glynase, Micronase	glyburide
Diabinese	chlorpropamide
Glucotrol	glipizide
Orinase	tolbutamide
Tolinase	tolazamide

INSTRUCTIONS

DiaBeta, Glucotrol, and Micronase should be taken 15 minutes to half an hour before meals. The others may be taken with food if they upset the stomach. Blood glucose monitoring is important. Notify the doctor immediately if you experience rash, fever, sore throat, or unusual bleeding or bruising.

BRAND NAME	GENERIC NAME
Aristocort, Kenacort	triamcinolone
Celestone	betamethasone
Cortef	hydrocortisone
Cortisone	cortisone
Decadron	dexamethasone
Deltasone	prednisone
etc.	

INSTRUCTIONS

Any of these medicines could upset the stomach, so they should be taken with food. These medications should not be stopped suddenly, but rather tapered off with gradually decreasing doses as the doctor instructs.

INTERACTION

Cortisone and other drugs in its class can raise blood sugar noticeably. As many as 14 percent of patients taking these drugs for several weeks or more will experience this side effect.

As a consequence, blood sugar control may be affected. Monitor blood sugar carefully when starting or stopping any cortisonelike drug so that the dose of the diabetes medicine can be adjusted if necessary.

Never take or stop medication without your doctor's advice.

Diabetes Drugs | Diabetes Drugs

Diabetes Drugs	Diuretics

TROUBLESOME

BRAND NAME	GENERIC NAME
DiaBeta, Glynase, Micronase	glyburide
Diabinese	chlorpropamide
Glucotrol	glipizide
Orinase	tolbutamide
Tolinase	tolazamide

INSTRUCTIONS

DiaBeta, Glucotrol, and Micronase should be taken 15 minutes to half an hour before meals. The others may be taken with food if they upset the stomach. Blood glucose monitoring is important. Notify the doctor immediately if you experience rash, fever, sore throat, or unusual bleeding or bruising.

BRAND NAME	GENERIC NAME
Aquatensen, Enduron	methyclothiazide
Diachlor, Diuril	chlorothiazide
Diucardin, aluron	hydroflumethiazide
Dyazide, Maxzide	hydrochlorothiazide and triamterene
Dyrenium	triamterene
Esidrix, HydroDIURIL	hydrochlorothiazide
Hygroton, Hylidone	chlorthalidone
Lozol	indapamide
etc.	

INSTRUCTIONS

Diuretics should be taken early in the day to reduce the number of times you have to get up at night to urinate. They may be taken with food or milk if they cause stomach upset.

INTERACTION

Diuretics can raise blood sugar in susceptible people, especially diabetics. Such medicine can also make oral diabetes drugs less effective. *This interaction could be troublesome, leading to hyperglycemia.*

The interaction may become noticeable within a few days of taking the two drugs together, or it may not show up for a few months. If both drugs are needed, blood sugar levels should be monitored so that the the doctor can adjust the dose of the diabetes medicine appropriately. Electrolyte levels and kidney function should also be checked; an excessive loss of potassium or even sodium is possible. The latter is especially problematic if Diabinese is prescribed with triamterene (Dyrenium, Dyazide, Maxzide).

Never take or stop medication without your doctor's advice.

Diabetes Drugs	Heart/Blood Pressure Drugs (ACE INHIBITORS)

TROUBLESOME

BRAND NAME	GENERIC NAME
DiaBeta, Glynase, Micronase	glyburide
Diabinese	chlorpropamide
Dymelor	acetohexamide
Glucotrol	glipizide
Orinase	tolbutamide
Tolinase	tolazamide

INSTRUCTIONS
DiaBeta, Glucotrol, and Micronase should be taken 15 minutes to half an hour before meals. The others may be taken with food if they upset the stomach. Blood glucose monitoring is important. Notify the doctor immediately if you experience rash, fever, sore throat, or unusual bleeding or bruising.

BRAND NAME	GENERIC NAME
Accupril	quinapril
Altace	ramipril
Capoten	captopril
Lotensin	benazepril
Monopril	fosinopril
Prinivil, Zestril	lisinopril
Vasotec	enalapril

INSTRUCTIONS
Capoten should be taken one hour before meals. High-fat meals may reduce absorption of Accupril. Food does not affect the other drugs in this class.

INTERACTION

Like many other drugs, ACE blood pressure medicines may increase the effectiveness of the oral diabetes medications. This could cause a greater drop in blood sugar than expected, with possible symptoms of hypoglycemia. Check with the doctor if you notice a change in blood sugar after starting Capoten, Vasotec, or one of the other drugs in this class. Stay alert for symptoms of hypoglycemia. *This interaction could be troublesome.*

Symptoms of Hypoglycemia (Low Blood Sugar)
Shaking, sweating, tiredness, low temperature, faintness, palpitations, hunger, headache, confusion, irritability, visual disturbances, and coma. Close observation (preferably in the hospital) is recommended for two or three days after such a reaction.

Never take or stop medication without your doctor's advice.

Diabetes Drugs	**Oral Contraceptives**

TROUBLESOME

BRAND NAME	GENERIC NAME		BRAND NAME	GENERIC NAME
DiaBeta, Glynase,			**Brevicon**	**Demulen**
Micronase	glyburide		**Desogen**	**Genora**
Diabinese	chlorpropamide		**Levlen**	**Loestrin**
Glucotrol	glipizide		**Lo/Ovral**	**Modicon**
Orinase	tolbutamide		**N.E.E.**	**Nelova**
Tolinase	tolazamide		**Nordette**	**Norethin**
			Norinyl	**Norlestrin**
			Ortho-Cyclen	**Ortho-Novum**
			Ovcon	**Ovral**
			Triphasil	

INSTRUCTIONS

DiaBeta, Glucotrol, and Micronase should be taken 15 minutes to half an hour before meals. The others may be taken with food if they upset the stomach. Blood glucose monitoring is important. Notify the doctor immediately if you experience rash, fever, sore throat, or unusual bleeding or bruising.

INSTRUCTIONS

For maximum effectiveness, oral contraceptives should be taken at the same time every day and precisely according to instructions. Missed doses can lead to an unwelcome pregnancy. Additional contraception is needed for at least the first week.

INTERACTION

Oral contraceptives can raise blood sugar, but this effect is less likely with the lower-dose oral contraceptives. If you use an oral contraceptive together with a diabetes drug, measure your blood sugar regularly to make sure it is well controlled. *This interaction could be troublesome.*

Never take or stop medication without your doctor's advice.

Diabetes Drugs	**Tuberculosis Drug** (RIFAMPIN)

TROUBLESOME

BRAND NAME	GENERIC NAME
DiaBeta, Glynase, Micronase	glyburide
Diabinese	chlorpropamide
Glucotrol	glipizide
Orinase	tolbutamide
Tolinase	tolazamide

INSTRUCTIONS

DiaBeta, Glucotrol, and Micronase should be taken 15 minutes to half an hour before meals. The others may be taken with food if they upset the stomach. Blood glucose monitoring is important. Notify the doctor immediately if you experience rash, fever, sore throat, or unusual bleeding or bruising.

BRAND NAME	GENERIC NAME
Rifadin	rifampin
Rifamate	isoniazid/ rifampin
Rimactane	rifampin

INSTRUCTIONS

Rifampin should be taken on an empty stomach, at least one hour before or two hours after meals. If you develop fever, chills, unusual tiredness, unusual bleeding or bruising, sore throat, muscle and bone pain, or yellow skin and eyes, contact your physician immediately.

INTERACTION

Rifampin revs up the body's machinery for processing these oral diabetes drugs, so they are eliminated more quickly and circulate at lower levels. Studies in healthy people have established this interaction, although they did not have higher blood sugar as a result. Several case reports concern diabetics who required higher doses of their diabetes drug to keep blood sugar under control after starting on the tuberculosis treatment. Monitor blood sugar carefully when starting or stopping rifampin, because the dose of the diabetes drug may need adjustment. *This interaction could be troublesome.*

Never take or stop medication without your doctor's advice.

Diuretics (POTASSIUM-SPARING)

Aldactazide   Aldactone   Dyazide   Dyrenium
Maxzide   Midamor   Moduretic

LIFE-THREATENING

Heart/Blood Pressure Drugs (ACE inhibitors)
Accupril Altace Capoten Lotensin Monopril Prinivil
Vasotec Zestril etc.
Potassium Kaon-C Kay Ciel K-Dur Klor-Con Klorvess
Klotrix K-Lyte K-Norm K-Tab Micro-K Slow-K Ten-K
etc.

DANGEROUS

Arthritis Drugs (NSAIDs) Advil Aleve aspirin
Indocin Lodine Motrin Naprosyn Relafen Toradol
Voltaren etc.
Lithium Cibalith-S Eskalith Lithobid Lithonate
Lithotabs

TROUBLESOME

Diabetes Drugs DiaBeta Diabinese Glucotrol Glynase
Micronase Orinase Tolinase
Heart Drug Lanoxin
Laxatives

Not every potassium-saving diuretic interacts with each drug listed.
See the individual summaries for details. We have tried to list the most
significant interactions, but other medications may also interact.
Be sure to check with your physician and pharmacist if you must take
other drugs in combination with potassium-sparing diuretics.

Diuretics
(POTASSIUM-SPARING)

Heart/Blood Pressure Drugs
(ACE INHIBITORS)

LIFE-THREATENING

BRAND NAME	GENERIC NAME
Aldactazide	spironolactone, HCTZ
Aldactone	spironolactone
Dyazide	triamterene, HCTZ
Dyrenium	triamterene
Maxzide	triamterene, HCTZ
Midamor	amiloride
Moduretic	amiloride, HCTZ

INSTRUCTIONS
Midamor and Dyrenium may upset the stomach, so they are best taken right after meals. Maxzide can be taken without regard to meals. Midamor and Aldactone may interfere with the alertness and coordination necessary for driving. Periodic blood tests for magnesium and potassium are advisable.

BRAND NAME	GENERIC NAME
Accupril	quinapril
Altace	ramipril
Capoten	captopril
Lotensin	benazepril
Monopril	fosinopril
Prinivil,	
Zestril	lisinopril
Vasotec	enalapril

INSTRUCTIONS
Capoten should be taken one hour before meals. High-fat meals may reduce absorption of Accupril. Food does not affect the other drugs in this class.

INTERACTION
Capoten, Vasotec, and other drugs in this category may increase potassium levels in susceptible patients. When these drugs are combined with potassium-sparing diuretics, serum potassium levels could rise into the dangerous range. *This situation could be life threatening. Irregular heart rhythms and cardiac arrest might occur.* **Deaths have been reported.** Elderly patients and those with kidney problems appear to be at the highest risk of this interaction. Diabetes may also contribute to the danger. Otherwise healthy patients may have no trouble and some with very low potassium levels may actually benefit from such a combination with careful medical supervision. However, if a potassium-sparing diuretic is prescribed together with an ACE inhibitor blood pressure drug, potassium levels should be monitored very closely. This may also be true of combination diuretics such as Dyazide or Maxzide.
Normal Serum Potassium Levels: 3.5 to 5 mEq/L

Never take or stop medication without your doctor's advice.

Diuretics (POTASSIUM-SPARING)		**Potassium**	
LIFE-THREATENING			
BRAND NAME	GENERIC NAME	BRAND NAME	GENERIC NAME
Aldactazide	spironolactone, HCTZ	**Kaon-Cl**	**Kay Ciel**
Aldactone	spironolactone	**K-Dur**	**Klor-Con**
Dyazide	triamterene, HCTZ	**Klorvess**	**Klotrix**
		K-Lyte	**K-Norm**
Dyrenium	triamterene	**K-Tab**	**Micro-K**
Maxzide	triamterene, HCTZ	**Slow-K**	**Ten-K**
Midamor	amiloride	etc.	
Moduretic	amiloride, HCTZ		

INSTRUCTIONS

Midamor and Dyrenium may upset the stomach, so they are best taken right after meals. Maxzide can be taken without regard to meals. Midamor and Aldactone may interfere with the alertness and coordination necessary for driving. Periodic blood tests for magnesium and potassium are advisable.

INSTRUCTIONS

These supplements may upset the stomach. They are best taken right after meals, with a full glass of water. Tell the doctor immediately if you have nausea, vomiting, abdominal pain, or black stools.

INTERACTION

Potassium-sparing diuretics are capable of increasing potassium levels, particularly in susceptible patients. When these drugs are combined with potassium supplements or salt substitutes that contain potassium, serum potassium levels could rise into the dangerous range. *This situation could be life threatening. Irregular heart rhythms and cardiac arrest might occur.* **Deaths have been reported.**

Elderly patients and those with kidney problems appear to be at the highest risk for this interaction. Diabetes may also contribute to the danger. Patients with very low potassium levels may sometimes be prescribed a potassium-sparing diuretic together with a potassium supplement. In this case potassium levels must be monitored very carefully. *Extreme caution is called for.*

Normal Serum Potassium Levels: 3.5 to 5 mEq/L

Never take or stop medication without your doctor's advice.

Diuretics	Arthritis Drugs
(POTASSIUM-SPARING)	(NSAIDS)

DANGEROUS

BRAND NAME	GENERIC NAME
Aldactazide	spironolactone, HCTZ
Aldactone	spironolactone
Dyazide	triamterene, HCTZ
Dyrenium	triamterene
Maxzide	triamterene, HCTZ
Midamor	amiloride
Moduretic	amiloride, HCTZ

BRAND NAME	GENERIC NAME
Advil, Motrin, Nuprin	ibuprofen
Aleve, Naprosyn	naproxen
Ansaid	flurbiprofen
Aspirin	aspirin
Indocin	indomethacin
Lodine	etodolac
Relafen	nabumetone
Voltaren	diclofenac
etc.	

INSTRUCTIONS

Midamor and Dyrenium may upset the stomach, so they are best taken right after meals. Maxzide can be taken without regard to meals. Midamor and Aldactone may interfere with the alertness and coordination necessary for driving. Periodic blood tests for magnesium and potassium are advisable.

INSTRUCTIONS

Take with food to reduce the risk of stomach irritation. (See table on pages 73–91.) Aspirin and OTC ibuprofen or naproxen should not be mixed with prescription NSAIDs or each other.

INTERACTION

Some arthritis drugs may reduce the effectiveness of diuretics. Fluid may build up, posing a serious problem for patients with heart trouble. Thiazide diuretics such as hydrochlorothiazide may be less effective in lowering blood pressure. If diuretics and arthritis drugs are taken simultaneously, blood pressure should be monitored carefully. Indocin may raise potassium levels to dangerous levels when combined with potassium-sparing diuretics like Moduretic. Measure potassium levels periodically. Potassium-sparing diuretics containing triamterene (Dyazide, Dyrenium, Maxzide) may interact badly with ibuprofen, Indocin, or Voltaren. Kidney damage has been reported. Other arthritis drugs may also interact.

Symptoms of Heart and Kidney Problems

Notify your doctor of sudden weight gain, swollen legs and feet, change in the color of the urine, unusual back pain, fatigue, cough, or breathlessness. Elevated serum creatinine may mean kidney trouble. Monitor blood pressure frequently.

Never take or stop medication without your doctor's advice.

Diuretics
(POTASSIUM-SPARING)

Lithium

DANGEROUS

BRAND NAME	GENERIC NAME
Aldactazide	spironolactone, HCTZ
Aldactone	spironolactone
Dyazide	triamterene, HCTZ
Dyrenium	triamterene
Maxzide	triamterene, HCTZ
Midamor	amiloride
Moduretic	amiloride, HCTZ

INSTRUCTIONS
Midamor and Dyrenium may upset the stomach, so they are best taken right after meals. Maxzide can be taken without regard to meals. Midamor and Aldactone may interfere with the alertness and coordination necessary for driving. Periodic blood tests for magnesium and potassium are advisable.

BRAND NAME
Cibalith-S
Eskalith
Lithobid
Lithonate
Lithotabs

INSTRUCTIONS
Lithium should be taken immediately after meals or with food or milk to reduce stomach upset. It is essential to drink 8 to 12 glasses of water or other fluid each day while on lithium. This medication can affect alertness, so activities such as driving or operating machinery can be dangerous for people on lithium.

INTERACTION
A number of cases have been reported in which diuretics, when taken in conjunction with lithium, have precipitated symptoms of lithium toxicity. Lithium blood levels may be raised into the danger zone. This interaction is somewhat murky and more research is needed to understand the clinical significance. *Nonetheless, this interaction could be dangerous.*

Lithium levels should be monitored periodically. Notify the doctor of any symptoms of lithium toxicity.

Symptoms of Lithium Toxicity
Drowsiness, incoordination, unsteady gait, dizziness, tremor, muscle twitching, blurred vision, ringing in the ears, slurred speech, confusion, seizures, and coma.

Never take or stop medication without your doctor's advice.

Diuretics	Diabetes Drugs
(POTASSIUM-SPARING)	

TROUBLESOME

BRAND NAME	GENERIC NAME	BRAND NAME	GENERIC NAME
Aldactazide	spironolactone, HCTZ	**DiaBeta, Glynase, Micronase**	glyburide
Aldactone	spironolactone		
Dyazide	triamterene, HCTZ	**Diabinese**	chlorpropamide
Dyrenium	triamterene	**Glucotrol**	glipizide
Maxzide	triamterene, HCTZ	**Orinase**	tolbutamide
Midamor	amiloride	**Tolinase**	tolazamide
Moduretic	amiloride, HCTZ		

INSTRUCTIONS

Midamor and Dyrenium may upset the stomach, so they are best taken right after meals. Maxzide can be taken without regard to meals. Midamor and Aldactone may interfere with the alertness and coordination necessary for driving. Periodic blood tests for magnesium and potassium are advisable.

INSTRUCTIONS

DiaBeta, Glucotrol, and Micronase should be taken 15 minutes to half an hour before meals. The others may be taken with food if they upset the stomach. Blood glucose monitoring is important. Notify your doctor immediately if you experience rash, fever, sore throat, or unusual bleeding or bruising.

INTERACTION

Diuretics can raise blood sugar in susceptible people, especially diabetics. Such medicine can also make oral diabetes drugs less effective. *This interaction could be troublesome, leading to hyperglycemia.*

The interaction may become noticeable within a few days of taking the two drugs together, or it may not show up for a few months. If both drugs are needed, blood sugar levels should be monitored so that the the doctor can adjust the dose of the diabetes medicine appropriately. Electrolyte levels and kidney function should also be checked; an excessive loss of potassium or even sodium is possible. The latter is especially problematic if Diabinese is prescribed with triamterene (Dyrenium, Dyazide, Maxzide).

Never take or stop medication without your doctor's advice.

Diuretics
(POTASSIUM-SPARING)

Heart Drug
(DIGOXIN)

TROUBLESOME

BRAND NAME	GENERIC NAME
Aldactazide	spironolactone, HCTZ
Aldactone	spironolactone
Midamor	amiloride
Moduretic	amiloride, HCTZ

INSTRUCTIONS
Midamor may upset the stomach, so it is best taken right after meals. Midamor and Aldactone may interfere with the alertness and coordination necessary for driving. Periodic blood tests for magnesium and potassium are advisable.

BRAND NAME	GENERIC NAME
Lanoxin	digoxin

INSTRUCTIONS
Digoxin should be taken in a consistent fashion, preferably with food but not with a meal high in fiber. Bran may limit the absorption of this drug.

Do not stop this medicine unless your doctor so directs.

INTERACTION

This is an incredibly complicated interaction that could create considerable confusion. Aldactone and Aldactazide may produce falsely elevated readings of standard tests of serum digoxin levels. In other words, because of inaccurate test results, a physician might think patients were getting too much digoxin when in fact they were getting the right amount. But there is also evidence that these diuretics may actually boost digoxin levels, thereby increasing the risk of side effects. Be vigilant for signs of digoxin toxicity.

Midamor and Moduretic may also increase digoxin levels, especially in patients with reduced kidney function. But these diuretics may partially interfere with the effectiveness of digoxin. If such drugs are combined it is very important to monitor digoxin reaction and heart function.

Symptoms of Digoxin Toxicity
Nausea, vomiting, loss of appetite, diarrhea, stomach pain, visual disturbances (green or yellow tint and a halo around lights), weakness, drowsiness, depression, confusion, palpitations, rash, headaches, and hallucinations. Notify the doctor immediately if you experience any of these symptoms.

Never take or stop medication without your doctor's advice.

Diuretics	Laxatives
(POTASSIUM-SPARING)	

TROUBLESOME

BRAND NAME   GENERIC NAME

Dyazide   triamterene, HCTZ

Dyrenium   triamterene

Maxzide   triamterene, HCTZ

(other diuretics may also be affected)

INSTRUCTIONS
Dyrenium may upset the stomach, so it is best taken right after meals. Maxzide can be taken without regard to meals. Periodic blood tests for magnesium and potassium are advisable.

INSTRUCTIONS
Try to avoid regular use of any laxative. A high-fiber diet that incorporates bran, fruits, and vegetables and includes lots of liquids can often eliminate the need for laxatives. If a laxative is needed, bulk-forming products are believed to be the safest.

INTERACTION

The manufacturers of Dyazide offer the following caution: "Chronic or overuse of laxatives may reduce serum potassium levels by promoting excessive potassium loss from the intestinal tract; laxatives may interfere with the potassium-retaining effects of triamterene." What this means is that Dyazide, Dyrenium, and Maxzide may not work as well as expected in preserving potassium when they are taken in combination with a laxative. Monitor potassium levels if laxatives are a part of your routine.

Normal Serum Potassium Levels: 3.5 to 5 mEq/L

Never take or stop medication without your doctor's advice.

Diuretics (POTASSIUM-WASTING)

Bumex	Diuril	Edecrin	HydroDIURIL
Lasix	Lozol	etc.	

DANGEROUS

Arthritis Drugs Advil Aleve aspirin Clinoril Indocin Lodine Motrin Naprosyn Nuprin Relafen Voltaren etc.
Blood Pressure Drug (emergency treatment) Hyperstat IV
Heart Drug Lanoxin
Lithium

TROUBLESOME

Calcium
Cholesterol Drugs Colestid Questran
Diabetes Drugs DiaBeta Diabinese Dymelor Glucotrol Glynase Micronase Orinase Tolinase
Heart/Blood Pressure Drugs (ACE inhibitors) Accupril Capoten Lotensin Prinivil Vasotec Zestril etc.
Laxatives

Not every potassium-wasting diuretic interacts with each drug listed. See the descriptions for details. We have tried to list the most significant interactions but other medications may also interact. Be sure to check with your physician and pharmacist if you must take other drugs in combination with potassium-wasting diuretics.

Diuretics (POTASSIUM-WASTING)		**Arthritis Drugs** (NSAIDS)	
DANGEROUS			
BRAND NAME	GENERIC NAME	BRAND NAME	GENERIC NAME
Bumex	bumetanide	**Advil,**	
Diachlor,		**Motrin,**	
Diuril,	chlorothiazide	**Nuprin**	ibuprofen
Diucardin,		**Aleve,**	
Saluron	hydroflumethiazide	**Naprosyn**	naproxen
Edecrin	ethacrynic acid	Aspirin	aspirin
Enduron	methyclothiazide	**Clinoril**	sulindac
Esidrix,		**Indocin**	indomethacin
HydroDIURIL	hydrochlorothiazide	**Lodine**	etodolac
Hygroton	chlorthalidone	**Relafen**	nabumetone
Lasix	furosemide	**Voltaren**	diclofenac
Lozol	indapamide	(Other NSAIDs may also interact.)	

INSTRUCTIONS

Taking a diuretic early in the day may reduce nighttime urination. If it causes stomach upset, the drug may be taken with food or milk. See the Food and Drug Compatibility Table on pages 73–91 for specifics.

INSTRUCTIONS

Take with food to reduce the risk of stomach irritation. (See table on pages 73–91.) Aspirin and OTC ibuprofen or naproxen should not be mixed with prescription NSAIDs or each other.

INTERACTION

NSAIDs such as ibuprofen and Indocin appear to reduce the effectiveness of diuretics such as Bumex and Lasix. (Clinoril may also affect Bumex). Fluid may build up and symptoms of heart failure could become worse. This is a very serious situation for people with heart trouble. Thiazide diuretics such as chlorthalidone, chlorothiazide, and hydrochlorothiazide may be less effective in lowering blood pressure, but this interaction does not seem so serious. Blood pressure should be monitored to make sure adequate control is maintained.

Symptoms of Heart Problems

Fluid retention, fatigue, cough, and breathlessness are possible signs of congestive heart failure. Monitor blood pressure frequently. Notify the physician immediately of symptoms.

Never take or stop medication without your doctor's advice.

Diuretics (POTASSIUM-WASTING)	**Blood Pressure Drug** (EMERGENCY TREATMENT)

DANGEROUS

BRAND NAME	GENERIC NAME
Bumex	bumetanide
Diachlor, **Diuril**	chlorothiazide
Diucardin, **Saluron**	hydroflumethiazide
Edecrin	ethacrynic acid
Enduron	methyclothiazide
Esidrix, **HydroDIURIL**	hydrochlorothiazide
Hygroton	chlorthalidone
Lasix	furosemide
Lozol	indapamide

INSTRUCTIONS

Taking a diuretic early in the day may reduce nighttime urination. If it causes stomach upset, the drug may be taken with food or milk. See the Food and Drug Compatibility Table on pages 73–91 for specifics.

BRAND NAME	GENERIC NAME
Hyperstat I.V.	diazoxide

INSTRUCTIONS

This drug will be administered by appropriate hospital personnel during an emergency blood pressure situation. If a patient has been taking a thiazide diuretic, make sure health professionals are aware of this potentially serious interaction.

INTERACTION

This combination can lead to very high levels of blood sugar (glucose), creating symptoms of diabetes. Acidosis (a buildup of acid) can have serious consequences. It can take weeks for this effect to wear off. If someone must receive Hyperstat I.V. to control hypertension while they have been on one of these diuretics, it is essential that glucose levels be carefully monitored.

Normal Blood Glucose Levels: 70 to 110 mg/dl

Never take or stop medication without your doctor's advice.

Diuretics	Heart Drug
(POTASSIUM-WASTING)	(DIGOXIN)

DANGEROUS

BRAND NAME	GENERIC NAME
Bumex	bumetanide
Diachlor,	
Diuril	chlorothiazide
Diucardin,	
Saluron	hydroflumethiazide
Edecrin	ethacrynic acid
Enduron	methyclothiazide
Esidrix,	
HydroDIURIL	hydrochlorothiazide
Hygroton	chlorthalidone
Lasix	furosemide
Lozol	indapamide

INSTRUCTIONS

Taking a diuretic early in the day may reduce nighttime urination. If it causes stomach upset, the drug may be taken with food or milk. See the Food and Drug Compatibility Table on pages 73–91 for specifics.

BRAND NAME	GENERIC NAME
Lanoxin	digoxin

INSTRUCTIONS

Digoxin should be taken in a consistent fashion, preferably with food but not with a meal high in fiber. Bran may limit the absorption of this drug.

Do not stop this medicine unless your doctor so directs.

INTERACTION

Physicians may prescribe diuretics in combination with digoxin to rid the body of excess fluid. There is rarely a problem, but electrolytes must be monitored carefully to avoid the danger of loss of potassium or magnesium. When these minerals are too low, digoxin might cause dangerous heart rhythm irregularities. *This interaction could be very dangerous.*

Regular blood tests are crucial. If levels of potassium and magnesium drop below the normal range, the doctor will probably prescribe supplements. Keep a diary of your potassium and magnesium levels.

Symptoms of Too Little Potassium: Muscle cramps, weakness, difficulty breathing, lethargy, and irregular heart rhythms.

Symptoms of Low Magnesium: Hard to diagnose. Be alert for loss of appetite, nausea, vomiting, weakness, fatigue, personality change, tremor, and muscle twitches.

Normal Electrolyte Values: Potassium: 3.5 to 5 mEq/L. Magnesium: 1.8 to 3 mEq/L

Never take or stop medication without your doctor's advice.

Diuretics (POTASSIUM-WASTING)		**Lithium**	
DANGEROUS			
BRAND NAME	GENERIC NAME	BRAND NAME	GENERIC NAME
Bumex	bumetanide	**Cibalith-S**	
Diachlor,		**Eskalith**	
Diuril	chlorothiazide	**Lithobid**	
Diucardin,		**Lithonate**	
Saluron	hydroflumethiazide	**Lithotabs**	
Edecrin	ethacrynic acid		
Enduron	methyclothiazide		
Esidrix,			
HydroDIURIL	hydrochlorothiazide		
Hygroton	chlorthalidone		
Lasix	furosemide		
Lozol	indapamide		

Lithium (INSTRUCTIONS):

INSTRUCTIONS

Taking a diuretic early in the day may reduce nighttime urination. If it causes stomach upset, the drug may be taken with food or milk. See the Food and Drug Compatibility Table on pages 73– 91 for specifics.

INSTRUCTIONS

Lithium should be taken immediately after meals or with food or milk to reduce stomach upset. It is essential to drink 8 to 12 glasses of water or other fluid each day while on lithium. This medication can affect alertness, so activities such as driving or operating machinery can be dangerous for people on lithium.

INTERACTION

A number of cases have been reported in which diuretics, when taken in combination with lithium, have precipitated symptoms of lithium toxicity. Lithium blood levels may be raised into the danger zone. This interaction is somewhat murky and more research is needed to understand the clinical significance. Lithium may be taken with diuretics as long as potassium levels are carefully monitored. *Nonetheless, this interaction could be dangerous.* Notify your doctor of any symptoms of lithium toxicity.

Symptoms of Lithium Toxicity

Drowsiness, incoordination, unsteady gait, dizziness, tremor, muscle twitching, blurred vision, ringing in the ears, slurred speech, confusion, seizures, and coma.

Never take or stop medication without your doctor's advice.

Diuretics (POTASSIUM-WASTING)		**Calcium**	
TROUBLESOME			

BRAND NAME	GENERIC NAME
Diachlor, Diuril	chlorothiazide
Diucardin, Saluron	hydroflumethiazide
Enduron	methyclothiazide
Esidrix, HydroDIURIL	hydrochloro-thiazide
Hygroton	chlorthalidone
Lozol	indapamide
Naqua	trichlor-methiazide
Naturetin	bendroflu-methiazide

BRAND NAME	GENERIC NAME
Citracal	calcium citrate
Caltrate 600	calcium carbonate
Os-Cal	calcium carbonate
Posture	calcium phosphate
Rolaids-Calcium Rich	calcium carbonate
Titralac	calcium carbonate
Tums	calcium carbonate
etc.	

INSTRUCTIONS

Taking a diuretic early in the day may reduce nighttime urination. If it causes stomach upset, the drug may be taken with food or milk. See the Food and Drug Compatibility Table on pages 73–91 for specifics.

INSTRUCTIONS

Generally, calcium supplements should be taken with meals for best absorption, but not with iron supplements. Calcium carbonate may be constipating in some people, but other calcium salts are less likely to cause this problem.

INTERACTION

Thiazide diuretics such as those listed on this page conserve calcium by modifying the way the kidneys eliminate this mineral. This action might be beneficial against osteoporosis and fractures. A problem may arise, however, if someone also took large amounts of calcium and vitamin D. Too much calcium could build up in the bloodstream, leading to toxicity. If this condition is allowed to progress, it can lead to kidney damage. *This troublesome interaction, if ignored, could become dangerous.*

Symptoms of Calcium Toxicity

Nausea, vomiting, loss of appetite, constipation, pain in the lower stomach, weakness, and headache. Notify the physician of any symptoms. Serum calcium should be monitored.

Normal Serum Calcium Values: 8.8 to 10.3 mg/dl.

Never take or stop medication without your doctor's advice.

Diuretics	Cholesterol Drugs
(POTASSIUM-WASTING)	

TROUBLESOME

BRAND NAME	GENERIC NAME
Diachlor, Diuril	chlorothiazide
Diucardin, Saluron	hydroflumethiazide
Enduron	methyclothiazide
Esidrix, HydroDIURIL	hydrochloro-thiazide
Hygroton	chlorthalidone
Lozol	indapamide
Naqua	trichlor-methiazide
Naturetin	bendroflu-methiazide

INSTRUCTIONS

Taking a diuretic early in the day may reduce nighttime urination. If it causes stomach upset, the drug may be taken with food or milk. See the Food and Drug Compatibility Table on pages 73–91 for specifics.

BRAND NAME	GENERIC NAME
Colestid	colestipol
Questran	cholestyramine

INSTRUCTIONS

Questran and Colestid come in powder form and need to be mixed with a glassful of water. Questran should not be taken with carbonated beverages. These medications are usually taken before meals, but check with a physician or pharmacist for specific instructions.

INTERACTION

These cholesterol-lowering drugs may interfere with proper absorption of diuretics. Some studies have shown that Questran can reduce hydrochlorothiazide levels by roughly one third. This could decrease the effectiveness of diuretics. For people with high blood pressure or congestive heart failure such a reaction could be quite serious. If one of these cholesterol-lowering drugs must be used in conjunction with a thiazide diuretic, they should be taken at least four hours apart. This is no guarantee of safety, though, so careful monitoring is essential.

Symptoms of Too Little Diuretic: Blood pressure may increase, fluid could be retained, and symptoms of heart failure might get worse. Measure blood pressure and heart function frequently. Notify the physician of any symptoms.

Never take or stop medication without your doctor's advice.

Diuretics
(POTASSIUM-WASTING)

Diabetes Drugs

TROUBLESOME

BRAND NAME	GENERIC NAME
Diachlor, Diuril	chlorothiazide
Diucardin, Saluron	hydro-flumethiazide
Enduron	methyclothiazide
Esidrix, HCTZ, HydroDIURIL	hydro-chlorothiazide
Hygroton, Hylidone	chlorthalidone
Lozol	indapamide
Naturetin	bendro-flumethiazide

BRAND NAME	GENERIC NAME
DiaBeta, Glynase, Micronase	glyburide
Diabinese	chlorpropamide
Glucotrol	glipizide
Orinase	tolbutamide
Tolinase	tolazamide

INSTRUCTIONS
Taking a diuretic early in the day may reduce nighttime urination. If it causes stomach upset, the drug may be taken with food or milk. See the Food and Drug Compatibility Table on pages 73–91 for specifics.

INSTRUCTIONS
DiaBeta, Glucotrol, and Micronase should be taken 15 minutes to half an hour before meals. The others may be taken with food if they upset the stomach. Blood glucose monitoring is important. Notify the doctor immediately if you experience rash, fever, sore throat, or unusual bleeding or bruising.

INTERACTIONS
Diuretics can raise blood sugar in susceptible people, especially diabetics. Such medicine can also make oral diabetes drugs less effective. *This interaction could be troublesome, leading to hyperglycemia.*

The interaction may become noticeable within a few days of taking the two drugs together, or it may not show up for a few months. If both drugs are needed, blood sugar levels should be monitored so that the doctor can adjust the dose of the diabetes medicine appropriately. Electrolyte levels and kidney function should also be checked; an excessive loss of potassium or even sodium is possible.

Never take or stop medication without your doctor's advice.

Diuretics
(LOOP)

Heart/Blood Pressure Drugs
(ACE INHIBITORS)

TROUBLESOME

BRAND NAME	GENERIC NAME
Bumex	bumetanide
Edecrin	ethacrynic acid
Lasix	furosemide

INSTRUCTIONS

Taking a diuretic early in the day may reduce nighttime urination. If it causes stomach upset, the drug may be taken with food or milk. See the Food and Drug Compatibility Table on pages 73–91 for specifics.

BRAND NAME	GENERIC NAME
Accupril	quinapril
Altace	ramipril
Capoten	captopril
Lotensin	benazepril
Monopril	fosinopril
Prinivil,	
Zestril	lisinopril
Vasotec	enalapril

INSTRUCTIONS

Capoten should be taken one hour before meals. High-fat meals may reduce absorption of Accupril. Food does not affect the other drugs in this class.

INTERACTIONS

Often when blood pressure is not completely controlled by the initial medication, the doctor will prescribe a second medicine in addition. As a result, a patient may need to take both an ACE inhibitor blood pressure drug and a strong diuretic. Some patients have experienced problems when ACE inhibitor drugs were added to a high-dose loop diuretic regimen. Starting either Capoten or Vasotec in conjunction with high doses of diuretics may contribute to excessively low blood pressure. People may feel faint. There also have been a few cases reported in which this combination resulted in serious kidney problems. *Blood pressure and kidney function should be monitored in people on a loop diuretic together with an ACE blood pressure drug.* Serum electrolytes (sodium, potassium, etc.) should also be monitored.

Never take or stop medication without your doctor's advice.

Diuretics
(POTASSIUM-WASTING)

Laxatives

TROUBLESOME

BRAND NAME	GENERIC NAME
Aquatensen, Enduron	methyclothiazide
Bumex	bumetanide
Diachlor, Diuril	chlorothiazide
Diucardin, Saluron	hydroflumethiazide
Edecrin	ethacrynic acid
Esidrix, HydroDIURIL	hydrochloro-thiazide
Hygroton, Hylidone	chlorthalidone
Lasix	furosemide
Lozol	indapamide

INSTRUCTIONS
Taking a diuretic early in the day may reduce nighttime urination. If it causes stomach upset, the drug may be taken with food or milk. See the Food and Drug Compatibility Table on pages 73–91 for specifics.

INSTRUCTIONS
Try to avoid regular use of any laxative. A high-fiber diet that incorporates bran, fruits, and vegetables and includes lots of liquids can often eliminate the need for laxatives. If a laxative is needed, bulk-forming products are believed to be the safest.

INTERACTIONS
Regular use of laxatives can lead to loss of potassium from the body. Since diuretics can also deplete the body of potassium, such a combination can create serious potassium disturbances. This could be life threatening, especially if a person were also taking a digitalis-type heart medicine (see page 369). DO NOT make laxatives a part of your routine if you are also on a potassium-wasting diuretic!
Normal Serum Potassium Levels: 3.5 to 5 mEq/L

Never take or stop medication without your doctor's advice.

Heart Drug (DIGOXIN)

Lanoxin

LIFE-THREATENING

Heart Drug Cordarone
Heart Drug Rythmol
Heart Drug (quinidine) Cardioquin Quinaglute
Quinalan Quinidex Quinora
Transplant Drug Sandimmune

DANGEROUS

Antibiotics (macrolides) Biaxin E.E.S. E-Mycin
ERYC EryPed Ery-Tab Erythrocin Ilosone PCE
Pediazole etc.
Antibiotics (tetracyclines) Achromycin V Declomycin
Minocin Sumycin Terramycin Vibramycin etc.
Diuretics (potassium-wasting) Bumex Diuril
Edecrin HydroDIURIL Lasix Lozol etc.
Heart/Blood Pressure Drugs (calcium blockers)
Calan Cardizem Dilacor XR Isoptin Plendil Procardia
Vascor Verelan

TROUBLESOME

Anti-Anxiety Drugs (benzodiazepines) Valium
Xanax
Cholesterol Drugs Colestid Questran
Diuretics (potassium-sparing) Aldactazide
Aldactone Dyazide Maxzide Midamor Moduretic

See individual summaries for details. Be sure to check with your physician and pharmacist if you must take any other drugs in combination with this heart medicine.

Heart Drug (DIGOXIN)	**Heart Drug** (AMIODARONE)

LIFE-THREATENING

BRAND NAME	GENERIC NAME	BRAND NAME	GENERIC NAME
Lanoxin	digoxin	**Cordarone**	amiodarone

INSTRUCTIONS
Digoxin should be taken in a consistent fashion, preferably with food but not with a meal high in fiber. Bran may limit the absorption of this drug.

Do not stop this medicine unless your doctor so directs.

INSTRUCTIONS
Follow the physician's directions carefully. Tell your doctor if you notice shortness of breath or changes in vision, or if your skin turns blue.

INTERACTION

A patient who needs both these medications should be under the doctor's watchful eye almost all the time. They would be prescribed together only in the case of very serious heart problems. *The interaction is potentially lethal.*

Cordarone can greatly increase levels of the heart drug digoxin, leading to toxicity. In most studies, digoxin levels doubled when Cordarone was added. In some instances, digoxin levels increased as much as 800 percent. At levels this high, a patient is likely to be feeling very sick. Very close monitoring and dose adjustment is essential.

Because Cordarone can last a long time in the body, the problems may continue for some time even if the drug is discontinued. Digoxin levels will probably need close monitoring during that time until they restabilize. If your doctor prescribes this combination, frequent blood tests to check your digoxin levels are essential. Notify your physician immediately if you experience any of the symptoms of digoxin overdose.

Symptoms of Digoxin Toxicity

Nausea, vomiting, loss of appetite, diarrhea, stomach pain, visual disturbances (green or yellow tint and a halo around lights), weakness, drowsiness, depression, confusion, palpitations, rash, headaches, and hallucinations. Notify your doctor immediately if you experience any of these symptoms.

Never take or stop medication without your doctor's advice.

Heart Drug (DIGOXIN)	**Heart Drug** (PROPAFENONE)
LIFE-THREATENING	

BRAND NAME	GENERIC NAME	BRAND NAME	GENERIC NAME
Lanoxin	digoxin	**Rythmol**	propafenone

INSTRUCTIONS

Digoxin should be taken in a consistent fashion, preferably with food but not with a meal high in fiber. Bran may limit the absorption of this drug.

Do not stop this medicine unless your doctor so directs.

INSTRUCTIONS

These tablets are best taken with food every eight hours. Alert the doctor if you develop symptoms of toxicity such as unusual sleepiness, low blood pressure, slower heart rate, or abnormal heartbeats. Do not stop this medicine unless your doctor tells you to.

INTERACTION

A patient with complicated heart problems may require this combination of potent medications together with very careful monitoring. Both of these heart medicines are used to control irregular heartbeats. This is a relatively new interaction, but it seems well documented. Digoxin levels may become dangerously high. *This situation could be lethal.*

To avoid digoxin toxicity, make sure your physician monitors your serum digoxin levels very closely. The dose may have to be adjusted to keep the digoxin level normal. Notify your physician instantly if you experience any symptoms of toxicity.

Symptoms of Digoxin Toxicity

Nausea, vomiting, loss of appetite, diarrhea, stomach pain, visual disturbances (green or yellow tint and a halo around lights), weakness, drowsiness, depression, confusion, palpitations, rash, headaches, and hallucinations. Notify your doctor immediately if you experience any of these symptoms.

Never take or stop medication without your doctor's advice.

Heart Drug	**Heart Drug**
(DIGOXIN)	(QUINIDINE)

LIFE-THREATENING

BRAND NAME	GENERIC NAME
Lanoxin	digoxin

INSTRUCTIONS

Digoxin should be taken in a consistent fashion, preferably with food but not with a meal high in fiber. Bran may limit the absorption of this drug.

Do not stop this medicine unless your doctor so directs.

BRAND NAME	GENERIC NAME
Cardioquin	quinidine
Quinaglute	quinidine
Quinalan	quinidine
Quinidex	quinidine
Quinora	quinidine

INSTRUCTIONS

Quinidine may upset the stomach. Taking it with food may help alleviate this problem. Sustained-release tablets (Quinaglute Dura-Tabs, Quinalan, Quinidex Extentabs) should not be chewed or crushed.

Quinidine may provoke visual disturbances, ringing in the ears, headache, dizziness, nausea, skin rash, or breathing difficulties. Notify your doctor if you develop any of these symptoms. Do not stop this medicine unless your doctor so directs.

INTERACTION

These drugs may both be needed for treating atrial flutter or atrial fibrillation, or in some other situations. Unfortunately, quinidine increases and may even double blood levels of digoxin. *This interaction could result in serious or life-threatening digitalis toxicity.*

It took 60 years before doctors discovered how dangerous these two heart drugs can be in combination. If both drugs are needed, the cardiologist should monitor you closely so the dose can be adjusted properly. Measuring serum levels of digoxin may not be enough to ensure safety. It is necessary but not sufficient, since electrocardiogram changes may occur even when blood levels of digoxin are within the "normal" range (0.5 to 2 ng/ml). Stay in close touch with your doctor and let him or her know of any symptoms.

Symptoms of Digoxin Toxicity

Nausea, vomiting, loss of appetite, diarrhea, stomach pain, visual disturbances (green or yellow tint and a halo around lights), weakness, drowsiness, depression, confusion, palpitations, rash, headaches, and hallucinations. Notify your doctor immediately if you experience any of these symptoms.

Never take or stop medication without your doctor's advice.

Heart Drug (DIGOXIN)	**Transplant Drug** (CYCLOSPORINE)

LIFE-THREATENING

BRAND NAME	GENERIC NAME	BRAND NAME	GENERIC NAME
Lanoxin	digoxin	**Sandimmune**	cyclosporine

INSTRUCTIONS

Digoxin should be taken in a consistent fashion, preferably with food but not with a meal high in fiber. Bran may limit the absorption of this drug.

Do not stop this medicine unless your doctor so directs.

INSTRUCTIONS

Sandimmune comes as an oral solution with a taste reminiscent of castor oil. It should be mixed in a glass with milk, chocolate milk, or orange juice at room temperature and drunk at once. Then the glass (no plastic) should be rinsed and the rinsing fluid drunk to get the full dose. Do not take Sandimmune with grapefruit juice unless the physician is monitoring blood levels of the drug closely. (See page 53.) Due to a possible interaction between cyclosporine and oral contraceptives, barrier methods of contraception should be used while taking this drug.

Regular monitoring is important. Do not stop this medicine unless your doctor so directs.

INTERACTION

This interaction could be life threatening. It was discovered when people awaiting heart transplant were given the immune-suppressing drug Sandimmune in addition to the heart drug digoxin. The result was a significant rise in digoxin levels and severe digoxin toxicity. When patients require both these medications, they are usually seriously ill and under close medical supervision. Physicians will need to monitor digoxin blood levels closely and adjust the dose carefully. *Be alert for signs of toxicity and notify your doctor if you experience any.*

Symptoms of Digoxin Toxicity

Nausea, vomiting, loss of appetite, diarrhea, stomach pain, visual disturbances (green or yellow tint and a halo around lights), weakness, drowsiness, depression, confusion, palpitations, rash, headaches, and hallucinations. Notify the doctor immediately if you experience any of these symptoms.

Never take or stop medication without your doctor's advice.

Heart Drug (DIGOXIN)	**Antibiotics** (MACROLIDES)

DANGEROUS

BRAND NAME   GENERIC NAME
Lanoxin   digoxin

INSTRUCTIONS
Digoxin should be taken in a consistent fashion, preferably with food but not with a meal high in fiber. Bran may limit the absorption of this drug.

Do not stop this medicine unless your doctor so directs.

E.E.S.	**E-Mycin**
ERYC	**EryPed**
Ery-Tab	**Erythrocin**
Eryzole	**Ilosone**
Ilotycin	**Pediazole**
PCE	**Robimycin**

INSTRUCTIONS
Some forms of erythromycin must be taken on an empty stomach; others may be taken with food. See pages 73–91 for specifics. Liquid suspensions should be stored in the refrigerator and shaken well before each dose. Finish the entire prescription unless your doctor tells you to stop.

INTERACTION

This is a strange interaction that affects only a small percentage of those who take the heart medicine digoxin. No one knows why one in ten people reacts differently to digoxin than the rest of us. These individuals depend on bacteria in their digestive tract to help eliminate this heart medicine from their system. If bacteria in the gut are killed off by the antibiotic erythromycin, digoxin levels can climb, possibly to toxic levels. *In susceptible people, erythromycin boosts blood levels of digoxin; this interaction could prove dangerous.*

There is no simple way to tell if you are among the 10 percent who depend on bacteria in the GI tract to metabolize digoxin. To avoid toxicity, ask your physician to monitor your serum digoxin levels carefully and adjust the dose accordingly. This reaction can persist for weeks or months after erythromycin has been stopped. That is because it can take a long time for the good bacteria in your gut to reestablish a normal balance. Tell your doctor if you have symptoms of digoxin overdose.

Symptoms of Digoxin Toxicity
Nausea, vomiting, loss of appetite, diarrhea, stomach pain, visual disturbances (green or yellow tint and a halo around lights), weakness, drowsiness, depression, confusion, palpitations, rash, headaches, and hallucinations. Notify your doctor immediately if you experience any of these symptoms.

Never take or stop medication without your doctor's advice.

Heart Drug (DIGOXIN)	**Antibiotics** (TETRACYCLINES)

DANGEROUS

BRAND NAME	GENERIC NAME
Lanoxin	digoxin

INSTRUCTIONS

Digoxin should be taken in a consistent fashion, preferably with food but not with a meal high in fiber. Bran may limit the absorption of this drug.

Do not stop this medicine unless your doctor so directs.

BRAND NAME	GENERIC NAME
Achromycin V	tetracycline
Declomycin	demeclocycline
Doryx	doxycycline
Minocin	minocycline
Rondomycin	methacycline
Sumycin	tetracycline
Terramycin	oxytetracycline
Uri-Tet	oxytetracycline
Vibramycin	doxycycline

INSTRUCTIONS

Take most forms of tetracycline on an empty stomach. See pages 73–91 for specifics. Do not take these drugs with antacids, calcium or iron supplements, or dairy products. Never take outdated tetracycline, which may be toxic to the kidneys.

INTERACTION

This strange interaction affects only a small portion of those who take the heart medicine digoxin. No one knows why one in ten people depends on bacteria in their digestive tracts to help eliminate this heart medicine. If bacteria in the gut are killed off by tetracycline antibiotics, digoxin levels can climb, possibly to toxic levels. *In susceptible people, tetracycline boosts blood levels of digoxin; this interaction could prove dangerous.*

It's hard to tell if you are among the 10 percent who depend on bacteria to metabolize digoxin. To avoid toxicity, ask your physician to monitor your serum digoxin levels carefully and adjust the dose accordingly. It can take a long time for the bacteria in your gut to reestablish a normal balance after tetracycline has been stopped, so this reaction can persist for weeks or months. Tell your doctor if you have symptoms of digoxin toxicity.

Symptoms of Digoxin Toxicity

Nausea, vomiting, loss of appetite, diarrhea, stomach pain, visual disturbances (green or yellow tint and a halo around lights), weakness, drowsiness, depression, confusion, palpitations, rash, headaches, and hallucinations. Notify the doctor immediately if you experience any of these symptoms.

Never take or stop medication without your doctor's advice.

Heart Drug
(DIGOXIN)

Diuretics
(POTASSIUM-WASTING)

DANGEROUS

BRAND NAME	GENERIC NAME
Lanoxin	digoxin

INSTRUCTIONS

Digoxin should be taken in a consistent fashion, preferably with food but not with a meal high in fiber. Bran may limit the absorption of this drug.

Do not stop this medicine unless your doctor so directs.

BRAND NAME	GENERIC NAME
Bumex	bumetanide
Diachlor,	
Diuril	chlorothiazide
Diucardin,	
Saluron	hydroflumethiazide
Edecrin	ethacrynic acid
Enduron	methyclothiazide
Esidrix,	
HydroDIURIL	hydrochlorothiazide
Hygroton	chlorthalidone
Lasix	furosemide
Lozol	indapamide

INSTRUCTIONS

Taking a diuretic early in the day may reduce nighttime urination. If it causes stomach upset, the drug may be taken with food or milk.

INTERACTION

Physicians may prescribe diuretics in combination with digoxin to rid the body of excess fluid. There is rarely a problem, but electrolytes must be monitored carefully to avoid the danger of loss of potassium or magnesium. When these minerals are too low, digoxin might cause dangerous heart rhythm irregularities. *This interaction could be very dangerous.*

Regular blood tests are crucial. If levels of potassium and magnesium drop below the normal range, your doctor will probably prescribe supplements. Keep a diary of your potassium and magnesium levels.

Symptoms of Too Little Potassium: Muscle cramps, weakness, difficulty breathing, lethargy, and irregular heart rhythms.

Symptoms of Low Magnesium: Hard to diagnose. Be alert for loss of appetite, nausea, vomiting, weakness, fatigue, personality change, tremor, and muscle twitches.

Normal Electrolyte Values: Potassium: 3.5 to 5 mEq/L. Magnesium: 1.8 to 3 mEq/L .

Never take or stop medication without your doctor's advice.

Heart Drug (DIGOXIN)	**Heart/Blood Pressure Drugs** (CALCIUM CHANNEL BLOCKERS)

DANGEROUS

BRAND NAME	GENERIC NAME
Lanoxin	digoxin

INSTRUCTIONS

Digoxin should be taken in a consistent fashion, preferably with food but not with a meal high in fiber. Bran may limit the absorption of this drug.

Do not stop this medicine unless your doctor so directs.

BRAND NAME	GENERIC NAME
Adalat, Procardia	nifedipine
Calan, Isoptin, Verelan	verapamil
Cardizem, Dilacor XR	diltiazem
Plendil	felodipine
Vascor	bepridil

INSTRUCTIONS

These drugs come in a variety of doses; follow the doctor's directions. Sustained-release forms should not be chewed or crushed. Taking Adalat, Plendil, or Procardia with grapefruit juice could boost blood levels of the drug unexpectedly. See the table of Food and Drug Compatibility on pages 73–91. If the drug must be discontinued, follow the doctor's instructions for gradual tapering.

INTERACTION

Patients with certain heart rhythm problems may require this combination of medicines. Others might be taking both drugs to treat different conditions. In either event, this interaction could be a problem, resulting in higher than expected digoxin levels. Be alert for signs of toxicity. The doctor should monitor blood levels of digoxin and also the electrocardiogram. Verapamil can raise serum digoxin levels as much as 75 percent, enough to result in toxicity in some cases. Diltiazem also seems to raise digoxin levels in the blood, although the studies do not agree on this effect. Bepridil, a relatively new blood pressure medicine, interacts with digoxin to slow heartbeat and modify the electrocardiogram. *This interaction could be dangerous.*

Symptoms of Digoxin Toxicity

Nausea, vomiting, loss of appetite, diarrhea, stomach pain, visual disturbances (green or yellow tint and a halo around lights), weakness, drowsiness, depression, confusion, palpitations, rash, headaches, and hallucinations. Notify your doctor immediately if you experience any of these symptoms.

Never take or stop medication without your doctor's advice.

Heart Drug (DIGOXIN)	**Anti-Anxiety Drugs** (BENZODIAZEPINES)

TROUBLESOME

BRAND NAME	GENERIC NAME
Lanoxin	digoxin

INSTRUCTIONS

Digoxin should be taken in a consistent fashion, preferably with food but not with a meal high in fiber. Bran may limit the absorption of this drug.

Do not stop this medicine unless your doctor so directs.

BRAND NAME	GENERIC NAME
Valium	diazepam
Xanax	alprazolam

INSTRUCTIONS

These drugs may be taken with food, especially if they upset the digestive tract.

INTERACTION

Valium (diazepam) has been shown to raise the blood levels of digoxin. One woman had a dramatic jump in digoxin after she started taking Xanax at bedtime for insomnia. She experienced symptoms of digoxin toxicity, including digestive tract upset, fatigue, and "head pressure." This Xanax and digoxin interaction remains unconfirmed in a more scientific study, however. Other benzodiazepines have not been adequately tested. Until such research is completed, people should have their digoxin levels monitored frequently if they need to take a benzodiazepine-type drug simultaneously.

Symptoms of Digoxin Toxicity

Nausea, vomiting, loss of appetite, diarrhea, stomach pain, visual disturbances (green or yellow tint and a halo around lights), weakness, drowsiness, depression, confusion, palpitations, rash, headaches, and hallucinations. Notify your doctor immediately if you experience any of these symptoms.

Never take or stop medication without your doctor's advice.

Heart Drug (DIGOXIN)	**Cholesterol Drugs**

TROUBLESOME

BRAND NAME | GENERIC NAME
Lanoxin | digoxin

INSTRUCTIONS
Digoxin should be taken in a consistent fashion, preferably with food but not with a meal high in fiber. Bran may limit the absorption of this drug.

Do not stop this medicine unless your doctor so directs.

BRAND NAME | GENERIC NAME
Colestid | colestipol
Questran | cholestyramine

INSTRUCTIONS
These drugs are to be taken before meals and washed down with plenty of fluids. Vitamin supplements may be advisable. If used, the supplements should be taken at least one hour before or six hours after the cholesterol medicine.

INTERACTION
It is entirely possible a person could have irregular heartbeats and high cholesterol, and so need both these medicines. Unfortunately, Colestid and Questran bind not only to bile acids, but also to other drugs. They can reduce the absorption of digoxin by 20 to 40 percent, leading to lowered digoxin levels. *For patients with irregular heart rhythms or congestive heart failure who depend on digoxin, this interaction is worrisome.*

It is usually possible to overcome this drug interaction by taking the cholesterol-lowering drugs at a different time of day from digoxin. Allow at least eight hours either before or after taking digoxin to prevent interference with its absorption.

The best way to determine if this interaction is causing trouble is to monitor serum digoxin levels carefully. Ask your physician for periodic tests. If digoxin levels drop too low, your doctor will want to adjust the dosage.

Never take or stop medication without your doctor's advice.

Heart Drug (DIGOXIN)	**Diuretics** (POTASSIUM-SPARING)

TROUBLESOME

BRAND NAME	GENERIC NAME
Lanoxin	digoxin

INSTRUCTIONS

Digoxin should be taken in a consistent fashion, preferably with food but not with a meal high in fiber. Bran may limit the absorption of this drug.

Do not stop this medicine unless your doctor so directs.

BRAND NAME	GENERIC NAME
Aldactazide	spironolactone, HCTZ
Aldactone	spironolactone
Dyazide	triamterene, HCTZ
Maxzide	triamterene, HCTZ
Midamor	amiloride
Moduretic	amiloride, HCTZ

INSTRUCTIONS

Midamor may upset the stomach, so it is best taken right after meals. Midamor and Aldactone may interfere with the alertness and coordination necessary for driving. Periodic blood tests for magnesium and potassium are advisable.

INTERACTION

This is an incredibly complicated interaction that could create considerable confusion. Aldactone and Aldactazide may produce falsely elevated readings of standard tests of serum digoxin levels. In other words, because of inaccurate test results, a physician might think patients were getting too much digoxin when in fact they were getting the right amount of digoxin. But there is also evidence that these diuretics may actually boost digoxin levels, thereby increasing the risk of side effects. Be vigilant for signs of digoxin toxicity.

Midamor and Moduretic may also increase digoxin levels, especially in patients with reduced kidney function. But these diuretics may partially interfere with the effectiveness of digoxin. If such drugs are combined, it is very important to monitor digoxin reaction and heart function.

Symptoms of Digoxin Toxicity

Nausea, vomiting, loss of appetite, diarrhea, stomach pain, visual disturbances (green or yellow tint and a halo around lights), weakness, drowsiness, depression, confusion, palpitations, rash, headaches, and hallucinations. Notify your doctor immediately if you experience any of these symptoms.

Never take or stop medication without your doctor's advice.

Heart/Blood Pressure Drugs (ACE INHIBITORS)

Accupril	Altace	Capoten	Lotensin
Monopril	Prinvil	Vasotec	Zestril

LIFE-THREATENING

Diuretics (potassium-sparing) Aldactazide
Aldactone Dyazide Dyrenium Maxzide Midamor
Moduretic

Potassium Kaon-Cl Kay Ciel K-Dur Klor-Con
Klorvess Klotrix K-Lyte K-Norm K-Tab Micro-K
Slow-K Ten-K etc.

DANGEROUS

Arthritis Drugs and Aspirin
Gout Medicine Zyloprim
Lithium Cibalith-S Eskalith Lithobid Lithonate
Lithotabs
Transplant Drug Sandimmune

TROUBLESOME

Diabetes Drugs DiaBeta Diabinese Dymelor
Glucotrol Glynase Micronase Orinase Tolinase
Diuretics (loop) Bumex Edecrin Lasix
Tuberculosis Drug (rifampin) Rifadin Rifamate
Rimactane

Not every ACE inhibitor blood pressure drug interacts with each drug listed here. See individual descriptions for details. Be sure to check with your physician and pharmacist if you must take any other drugs in combination with any of these blood pressure pills.

Heart/Blood Pressure Drugs
(ACE INHIBITORS)

Diuretics
(POTASSIUM-SPARING)

LIFE-THREATENING

BRAND NAME	GENERIC NAME
Accupril	quinapril
Altace	ramipril
Capoten	captopril
Lotensin	benazepril
Monopril	fosinopril
Prinivil,	
Zestril	lisinopril
Vasotec	enalapril

BRAND NAME	GENERIC NAME
Aldactazide	spironolactone, HCTZ
Aldactone	spironolactone
Dyazide	triamterene, HCTZ
Dyrenium	triamterene
Maxzide	triamterene, HCTZ
Midamor	amiloride
Moduretic	amiloride, HCTZ

INSTRUCTIONS

Capoten should be taken one hour before meals. High-fat meals may reduce absorption of Accupril. Food does not affect the other drugs in this class.

INSTRUCTIONS

Midamor and Dyrenium may upset the stomach, so they are best taken right after meals. Maxzide can be taken without regard to meals. Midamor and Aldactone may interfere with the alertness and coordination necessary for driving. Periodic blood tests for magnesium and potassium are advisable.

INTERACTION

Capoten, Vasotec, and other drugs in this category may increase potassium levels in susceptible patients. When these drugs are combined with potassium-sparing diuretics, serum potassium levels could rise into the dangerous range. *This situation could be life threatening. Irregular heart rhythms and cardiac arrest might occur.* **Deaths have been reported.** Elderly patients and those with kidney problems appear to be at the highest risk of this interaction. Diabetes may also contribute to the danger. Otherwise healthy patients may have no trouble and some with very low potassium levels may actually benefit from such a combination with careful medical supervision. However, if a potassium-sparing diuretic is prescribed together with an ACE inhibitor blood pressure drug, potassium levels should be monitored very closely. This may also be true of combination diuretics such as Dyazide and Maxzide.

Normal Serum Potassium Levels: 3.5 to 5 mEq/L

Never take or stop medication without your doctor's advice.

Heart/Blood Pressure Drugs (ACE INHIBITORS)

Potassium

LIFE-THREATENING

BRAND NAME	GENERIC NAME
Accupril	quinapril
Altace	ramipril
Capoten	captopril
Lotensin	benazepril
Monopril	fosinopril
Prinivil,	
Zestril	lisinopril
Vasotec	enalapril

BRAND NAME	
Kaon-Cl	**Kay Ciel**
K-Dur	**Klor-Con**
Klorvess	**Klotrix**
K-Lyte	**K-Norm**
K-Tab	**Micro-K**
Slow-K	**Ten-K**
etc.	

INSTRUCTIONS

Capoten should be taken one hour before meals. High-fat meals may reduce absorption of Accupril. Food does not affect the other drugs in this class.

INSTRUCTIONS

These supplements may upset the stomach. They are best taken right after meals, with a full glass of water. Tell your doctor immediately if you have nausea, vomiting, abdominal pain, or black stools.

INTERACTION

Capoten, Vasotec, and other drugs in this category may increase potassium levels, particularly in susceptible patients. Without frequent blood tests to monitor serum potassium levels, the combination of potassium supplements and one of these ACE inhibitors can lead to excessive levels of the mineral (over 5.5 mEq/L). *This interaction could lead to irregular heart rhythms and cardiac arrest.* **Deaths have been reported.**

Elderly patients and those with kidney problems appear at highest risk from this interaction. Diabetes may also contribute to the danger. Otherwise healthy patients may have no trouble. However, if a potassium supplement is prescribed together with an ACE blood pressure drug, potassium levels should be monitored closely.

Salt substitutes, many containing potassium, are often recommended for people with high blood pressure. If you are taking one of these blood pressure medicines, do not use a commercial salt substitute unless you have regular blood tests for serum potassium.

Normal Serum Potassium Levels: 3.5 to 5 mEq/L

Never take or stop medication without your doctor's advice.

Heart/Blood Pressure Drugs (ACE INHIBITORS)		Arthritis Drugs (NSAIDS)	
DANGEROUS			
BRAND NAME	GENERIC NAME	BRAND NAME	GENERIC NAME
Accupril	quinapril	**Advil,**	
Altace	ramipril	**Motrin,**	
Capoten	captopril	**Nuprin**	ibuprofen
Lotensin	benazepril	**Aleve,**	
Monopril	fosinopril	**Naprosyn**	naproxen
Prinivil,		**Ansaid**	flurbiprofen
Zestril	lisinopril	Aspirin	aspirin
Vasotec	enalapril	**Indocin**	indomethacin
		Lodine	etodolac
		Relafen	nabumetone
		Toradol	ketorolac
		etc.	

INSTRUCTIONS

Capoten should be taken one hour before meals. High-fat meals may reduce absorption of Accupril. Food does not affect the other drugs in this class.

INSTRUCTIONS

Take with food to reduce the risk of stomach irritation. (See table on pages 73–91.) Aspirin and OTC ibuprofen or naproxen should not be mixed with prescription NSAIDs or each other.

INTERACTION

Some of the arthritis drugs on this list can drastically diminish the effectiveness of blood pressure medicines such as Capoten or Vasotec. Indocin can wipe out the blood-pressure-lowering power of these drugs; ibuprofen can interact similarly with Capoten. Even aspirin given with or before Vasotec can reduce that drug's benefit for treating congestive heart failure. Although some people do not react badly to this combination, it makes sense to assume that any arthritis medicine could interfere with any ACE medication, and keep careful tabs on blood pressure and cardiac function if both drugs are needed. *This interaction could be dangerous.*

Kidney problems are a rare but serious reaction to both these classes of drugs. Taking them in combination may increase the risk of this problem. *Notify the doctor immediately of sudden weight gain, swollen legs and feet, change in the color of the urine, or unusual back pain.* A kidney function test may be in order. **Monitor blood pressure regularly.**

Never take or stop medication without your doctor's advice.

Heart/Blood Pressure Drugs (ACE INHIBITORS)	Gout Medicine (ALLOPURINOL)

DANGEROUS

BRAND NAME	GENERIC NAME
Accupril	quinapril
Altace	ramipril
Capoten	captopril
Lotensin	benazepril
Monopril	fosinopril
Prinivil,	
Zestril	lisinopril
Vasotec	enalapril

INSTRUCTIONS

Capoten should be taken one hour before meals. High-fat meals may reduce absorption of Accupril. Food does not affect the other drugs in this class.

BRAND NAME	GENERIC NAME
Lopurin	allopurinol
Zurinol	allopurinol
Zyloprim	allopurinol

INSTRUCTIONS

Allopurinol may upset the stomach less if it is taken with food or milk. While on this drug, drink at least ten full glasses of fluid daily. Because allopurinol may cause drowsiness, try to avoid driving or other complex tasks while taking this medicine.

INTERACTION

If gout and high blood pressure are both problems, the doctor may want to prescribe both these medications. There are several cases reported of serious hypersensitivity reactions when Zyloprim and Capoten are combined. This reaction may begin as a rash and progress to a potentially fatal syndrome called Stevens-Johnson. Joint pain and fever may accompany this reaction. Although researchers cannot be sure that the cases were due to the interaction rather than to either drug alone, it is suspected that a person on both medicines may be more susceptible. *This interaction could be dangerous. At least one death has been reported.*

Patients with kidney failure are likely to be at greatest risk of this problem. There are no reports of Zyloprim interacting with other ACE medications, and experts speculate that an interaction with Vasotec may be unlikely. If you take both allopurinol and an ACE inhibitor, notify your doctor at the earliest hint of a rash.

Symptoms to notice: Rash, joint pain, fever.

Never take or stop medication without your doctor's advice.

Heart/Blood Pressure Drugs (ACE INHIBITORS)	Lithium

DANGEROUS

BRAND NAME	GENERIC NAME
Accupril	quinapril
Altace	ramipril
Capoten	captopril
Lotensin	benazepril
Monopril	fosinopril
Prinivil, Zestril	lisinopril
Vasotec	enalapril

INSTRUCTIONS
Capoten should be taken one hour before meals. High-fat meals may reduce absorption of Accupril. Food does not affect the other drugs in this class.

BRAND NAME
Cibalith-S
Eskalith
Lithobid
Lithonate
Lithotabs

INSTRUCTIONS
Lithium should be taken immediately after meals or with food or milk to reduce stomach upset. It is essential to drink 8 to 12 glasses of water or other fluid each day while on lithium. This medication can affect alertness, so activities such as driving or operating machinery can be dangerous for people on lithium.

INTERACTION
A number of cases have been reported in which one of these blood pressure drugs added to a previously stable lithium regimen precipitated symptoms of lithium toxicity. Lithium blood levels were raised into the danger zone. This interaction did not occur in an experiment with ten healthy volunteers, so there may be other factors at play. *Nonetheless, this interaction could be dangerous.*

If both lithium and an ACE blood pressure drug are needed, lithium levels should be monitored.
Symptoms of Lithium Toxicity
Nausea, diarrhea, incoordination, muscle weakness, and difficulty walking may be signs of toxicity. Ringing in the ears, visual problems, dizziness, slurred speech, confusion, agitation, and incontinence are more serious. Notify the physician promptly of any such symptoms.

Never take or stop medication without your doctor's advice.

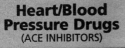

| **Heart/Blood Pressure Drugs** (ACE INHIBITORS) | **Transplant Drug** (CYCLOSPORINE) |

DANGEROUS

BRAND NAME	GENERIC NAME
Accupril	quinapril
Altace	ramipril
Capoten	captopril
Lotensin	benazepril
Monopril	fosinopril
Prinivil,	
Zestril	lisinopril
Vasotec	enalapril

INSTRUCTIONS

Capoten should be taken one hour before meals. High-fat meals may reduce absorption of Accupril. Food does not affect the other drugs in this class.

BRAND NAME	GENERIC NAME
Sandimmune	cyclosporine

INSTRUCTIONS

Sandimmune comes as an oral solution with a taste reminiscent of castor oil. It should be mixed in a glass with milk, chocolate milk, or orange juice at room temperature and drunk at once. Then the glass (no plastic) should be rinsed and the rinsing fluid drunk to get the full dose. Do not take Sandimmune with grapefruit juice unless the physician is monitoring blood levels of the drug closely. (See page 53.)

Due to a possible interaction between cyclosporine and oral contraceptives, barrier methods of contraception should be used while taking this drug.

Regular monitoring is important. Do not stop this medicine unless your doctor so directs.

INTERACTION

Experts are not sure if Sandimmune really interacts with the ACE blood pressure medicines, but at least two cases have been reported. In these cases, kidney failure developed after Vasotec was added to the patients' medications, and cleared up when Vasotec was withdrawn. There is no reason to believe that Vasotec would be different from other ACE inhibitor drugs in this respect. If one of these medications is needed for a patient taking Sandimmune, kidney function should be monitored closely for at least the first several months. *This interaction could be dangerous.*

Never take or stop medication without your doctor's advice.

Heart/Blood Pressure Drugs (ACE INHIBITORS)	Diabetes Drugs

TROUBLESOME

BRAND NAME	GENERIC NAME	BRAND NAME	GENERIC NAME
Accupril	quinapril	**DiaBeta,**	
Altace	ramipril	**Glynase,**	
Capoten	captopril	**Micronase**	glyburide
Lotensin	benazepril	**Diabinese**	chlorpropamide
Monopril	fosinopril	**Dymelor**	acetohexamide
Prinivil,		**Glucotrol**	glipizide
Zestril	lisinopril	**Orinase**	tolbutamide
Vasotec	enalapril	**Tolinase**	tolazamide

INSTRUCTIONS

Capoten should be taken one hour before meals. High-fat meals may reduce absorption of Accupril. Food does not affect the other drugs in this class.

INSTRUCTIONS

DiaBeta, Glucotrol, and Micronase should be taken 15 minutes to half an hour before meals. The others may be taken with food if they upset the stomach. Blood glucose monitoring is important. Notify your doctor immediately if you experience rash, fever, sore throat, or unusual bleeding or bruising.

INTERACTION

Like many other drugs, ACE blood pressure medicines may increase the effectiveness of the oral diabetes medications. This could cause a greater drop in blood sugar than expected, with possible symptoms of hypoglycemia. Check with your doctor if you notice a change in blood sugar after starting Capoten, Vasotec, or one of the other drugs in this class. Stay alert for symptoms of hypoglycemia. *This interaction could be troublesome.*

Symptoms of Hypoglycemia (Low Blood Sugar)

Shaking, sweating, tiredness, low temperature, faintness, palpitations, hunger, headache, confusion, irritability, visual disturbances, coma. Close observation (preferably in the hospital) is recommended for two or three days after such a reaction.

Never take or stop medication without your doctor's advice.

Heart/Blood Pressure Drugs (ACE INHIBITORS)	**Diuretics** (LOOP)

TROUBLESOME

BRAND NAME	GENERIC NAME	BRAND NAME	GENERIC NAME
Accupril	quinapril	**Bumex**	bumetanide
Altace	ramipril	**Edecrin**	ethacrynic acid
Capoten	captopril	**Lasix**	furosemide
Lotensin	benazepril		
Monopril	fosinopril		
Prinivil,			
Zestril	lisinopril		
Vasotec	enalapril		

INSTRUCTIONS

Capoten should be taken one hour before meals. High-fat meals may reduce absorption of Accupril. Food does not affect the other drugs in this class.

INSTRUCTIONS

Taking a diuretic early in the day may reduce nighttime urination. If it causes stomach upset, the drug may be taken with food or milk. See the Food and Drug Compatibility Table on pages 73–91 for specifics.

INTERACTION

Often when blood pressure is not completely controlled by the initial medication, the doctor will prescribe a second medicine in addition. As a result, a patient may need to take both an ACE inhibitor blood pressure drug and a strong diuretic. Some patients have experienced problems when ACE inhibitor drugs are added to a high-dose loop diuretic regimen. Starting either Capoten and Vasotec in conjunction with high doses of diuretics may contribute to excessively low blood pressure. People may feel faint. There are also a few cases reported in which this combination resulted in serious kidney problems. *Blood pressure and kidney function should be monitored in people on a loop diuretic together with an ACE blood pressure drug.* Serum electrolytes (sodium, potassium, etc.) should also be monitored.

Never take or stop medication without your doctor's advice.

Heart/Blood Pressure Drugs (ACE INHIBITORS)	**Tuberculosis Drug** (RIFAMPIN)

TROUBLESOME

BRAND NAME   GENERIC NAME

Accupril   quinapril
Altace   ramipril
Capoten   captopril
Lotensin   benazepril
Monopril   fosinopril
Prinivil,
   Zestril   lisinopril
Vasotec   enalapril

INSTRUCTIONS
Capoten should be taken one hour before meals. High-fat meals may reduce absorption of Accupril. Food does not affect the other drugs in this class.

BRAND NAME   GENERIC NAME

Rifadin   rifampin
Rifamate   isoniazid/
         rifampin
Rimactane   rifampin

INSTRUCTIONS
Rifampin should be taken on an empty stomach, at least one hour before or two hours after meals. If you develop fever, chills, unusual tiredness, unusual bleeding or bruising, sore throat, muscle and bone pain, or yellow skin and eyes, contact your physician immediately.

INTERACTION
The tuberculosis medication may counteract the ACE blood pressure drugs, although evidence for this interaction is weak. One 35-year-old man with high blood pressure and tuberculosis was treated with this combination of medicines (together with several others). Vasotec was controlling his blood pressure well, but when rifampin was added, his blood pressure rose. Rifampin was discontinued, and his blood pressure returned to normal. When the antituberculosis agent was given again, his blood pressure soared again.

No one knows if the interaction was peculiar to this individual, or if it may occur more commonly. If both rifampin and an ACE inhibitor drug are needed, blood pressure should be monitored carefully. *This interaction could be troublesome.*
Monitor blood pressure regularly.

Never take or stop medication without your doctor's advice.

Heart/Blood Pressure Drugs (BETA-BLOCKERS)

Blocadren   Cartrol   Corgard   Inderal   Lopressor
Normodyne   Tenormin   Timoptic   Toprol XL   Trandate
Visken

LIFE-THREATENING

Blood Pressure Drug Catapres
Epinephrine Adrenalin

DANGEROUS

Antibiotic Ampicillin
Arthritis Drugs (NSAIDs) Advil Aleve aspirin
Indocin Lodine Motrin Naprosyn Relafen Toradol
Voltaren etc.
Asthma Drug (theophylline) Elixophyllin Quibron-T
Respbid Slo-bid Slo-Phyllin Theobid Theochron
Theoclear Theo-Dur Theolair Theo-24 Theovent etc.
Barbiturates Amytal Butisol Mebaral Nembutal
phenobarbital Seconal Tuinal
Drugs for Migraine Cafergot D.H.E. 45 Ergomar
Sansert
Drugs for Schizophrenia Mellaril Thorazine
Heart Drugs Cardioquin Cordarone quinidine
Quinora Rythmol Tambocor
**Heart/Blood Pressure Drugs (calcium channel
blockers)** Calan Cardene Cardizem Dilacor XR
Isoptin Procardia Verelan

TROUBLESOME

Anti-Anxiety Drugs (benzodiazepines) Centrax
Dalmane Halcion Librium Tranxene Valium
Blood Pressure Drugs Apresoline Minipress
Calcium
Cholesterol Drugs Colestid Questran
Oral Contraceptives
Tuberculosis Drug (rifampin) Rifadin Rifamate
Rimactane
Ulcer Drug Tagamet

Not every beta-blocker interacts with each drug on this list. See
individual summaries for details. Check with your physician and
pharmacist if you must take any other drugs in combination with a
beta-blocker.

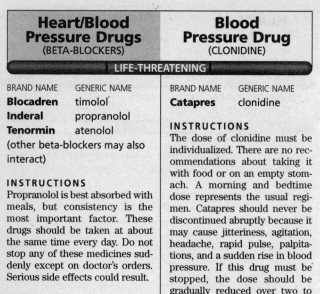

Heart/Blood Pressure Drugs
(BETA-BLOCKERS)

Blood Pressure Drug
(CLONIDINE)

LIFE-THREATENING

BRAND NAME	GENERIC NAME
Blocadren	timolol
Inderal	propranolol
Tenormin	atenolol

(other beta-blockers may also interact)

INSTRUCTIONS
Propranolol is best absorbed with meals, but consistency is the most important factor. These drugs should be taken at about the same time every day. Do not stop any of these medicines suddenly except on doctor's orders. Serious side effects could result.

BRAND NAME	GENERIC NAME
Catapres	clonidine

INSTRUCTIONS
The dose of clonidine must be individualized. There are no recommendations about taking it with food or on an empty stomach. A morning and bedtime dose represents the usual regimen. Catapres should never be discontinued abruptly because it may cause jitteriness, agitation, headache, rapid pulse, palpitations, and a sudden rise in blood pressure. If this drug must be stopped, the dose should be gradually reduced over two to four days under careful medical supervision.

INTERACTION
There are confusing reports that simultaneous administration of Inderal and Catapres may reduce the antihypertensive action of one or both drugs. This has not been confirmed. What does appear clear, however, is that no one who is taking both a beta-blocker and clonidine should ever discontinue either drug suddenly. There have been life-threatening sudden increases in blood pressure when Catapres was stopped while someone was also taking a beta-blocker. *This situation is potentially lethal.*

The manufacturer recommends that "if therapy is to be discontinued in patients receiving beta-blockers and clonidine concurrently, beta-blockers should be discontinued several days before the gradual withdrawal of Catapres."

Symptoms of Rebound Hypertension
Sudden discontinuation of Catapres could lead to anxiety, agitation, headache, palpitations, rapid pulse, nausea, flushing, vomiting, or rapid increase in blood pressure. Notify the physician immediately of any of these symptoms.

Never take or stop medication without your doctor's advice.

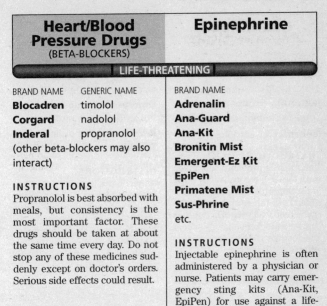

| **Heart/Blood Pressure Drugs** (BETA-BLOCKERS) | **Epinephrine** |

LIFE-THREATENING

BRAND NAME   GENERIC NAME

Blocadren   timolol
Corgard   nadolol
Inderal   propranolol
(other beta-blockers may also interact)

INSTRUCTIONS
Propranolol is best absorbed with meals, but consistency is the most important factor. These drugs should be taken at about the same time every day. Do not stop any of these medicines suddenly except on doctor's orders. Serious side effects could result.

BRAND NAME

Adrenalin
Ana-Guard
Ana-Kit
Bronitin Mist
Emergent-Ez Kit
EpiPen
Primatene Mist
Sus-Phrine
etc.

INSTRUCTIONS
Injectable epinephrine is often administered by a physician or nurse. Patients may carry emergency sting kits (Ana-Kit, EpiPen) for use against a life-threatening allergic reaction.

INTERACTION

People taking a beta-blocker may experience an extremely dangerous elevation in blood pressure if epinephrine is injected. There are a number of cases in the medical literature of people who went in for plastic surgery while taking propranolol. Shortly after an injection of the local anesthetic Xylocaine combined with epinephrine, systolic blood pressure skyrocketed—in some cases to over 200. One woman went to the emergency room with a bad case of hives. When she arrived her blood pressure was 120/70. Two minutes after an injection of epinephrine she complained of a bad headache and her blood pressure zoomed to 220/110. She experienced a stroke. *This interaction can be life threatening.*

We have found no cases of hypertensive crisis due to the aerosol form of epinephrine interacting with beta-blockers, but a physician should supervise such a combination.

Symptoms of Hypertensive Crisis
Headache, rapid increase in blood pressure, palpitations, chest pain, chills, nausea, anxiety, and perspiration. Stroke is a risk. Notify your physician immediately of any of these symptoms.

Never take or stop medication without your doctor's advice.

Heart/Blood Pressure Drugs (BETA-BLOCKERS)	**Antibiotic** (PENICILLIN-TYPE)

DANGEROUS

BRAND NAME	GENERIC NAME
Tenormin	atenolol

(other beta-blockers may also interact)

INSTRUCTIONS
Tenormin is probably best taken with meals, but consistency is the most important factor. Tenormin should be taken at roughly the same time every day. Do not stop any beta-blocker suddenly except on doctor's orders. Serious side effects could result.

BRAND NAME	GENERIC NAME
Omnipen	ampicillin
Polycillin	ampicillin
Principen	ampicillin
Totacillin	ampicillin

INSTRUCTIONS
Ampicillin, like most penicillin-type antibiotics, is best taken with a full eight-ounce glass of water on an empty stomach (one hour before meals or two hours after eating). Successful therapy requires completing all pills to prevent reinfection.

INTERACTION
Ampicillin may reduce the absorption of Tenormin. Blood levels of this beta-blocker may reach only one fourth to one half of those expected when the antihypertensive agent is taken by itself. This might diminish the blood-pressure-lowering and anti-anginal benefits of the beta-blocker. Such an effect could be disastrous for certain patients. If an antibiotic such as penicillin must be given to someone taking a beta-blocker such as Tenormin, it is critical to monitor blood pressure and heart function frequently.

People allergic to penicillin may be in far greater danger if they are also taking a beta-blocker. Deaths are reported in cases in which people taking Inderal or Corgard developed anaphylactic shock after exposure to penicillin. Beta-blockers may make severe allergic reactions (anaphylactic shock) worse and may make treatment more difficult (see epinephrine, page 387).

Symptoms of Beta-Blocker Undertreatment
Blood pressure may climb and heart symptoms might appear. Notify your physician promptly of any symptoms such as chest pain or palpitations.

Never take or stop medication without your doctor's advice.

| **Heart/Blood Pressure Drugs** (BETA-BLOCKERS) | | **Arthritis Drugs** (NSAIDS) | |

BRAND NAME	GENERIC NAME	BRAND NAME	GENERIC NAME
Blocadren	timolol	**Advil, Motrin,**	
Corgard	nadolol	**Nuprin**	ibuprofen
Inderal	propranolol	**Aleve,**	
Lopressor,		**Naprosyn**	naproxen
Toprol XL	metoprolol	**Ansaid**	flurbiprofen
Tenormin	atenolol	Aspirin	aspirin
Visken	pindolol	**Indocin**	indomethacin
(Other beta-blockers may also		**Lodine**	etodolac
interact.)		**Relafen**	nabumetone
		etc.	

INSTRUCTIONS

Inderal and Lopressor are best taken with meals, but consistency is the most important factor. These drugs should be taken at about the same time every day. Do not stop any of these medicines except on doctor's orders. Serious side effects could result.

INSTRUCTIONS

Take with food to reduce the risk of stomach irritation. (See table on pages 73–91.) Aspirin and OTC ibuprofen or naproxen should not be mixed with prescription NSAIDs or each other.

INTERACTION

This combination is of concern because so many people take beta-blockers for high blood pressure and heart problems. Millions rely on NSAIDs for pain relief. NSAIDs may reduce the effectiveness of blood-pressure-lowering beta-blockers. People may not realize a beta-blocker is not working as efficiently as it should to control hypertension. Experts warn doctors to avoid this combination if possible. The arthritis drug Clinoril (sulindac) may be less likely to interact with beta-blockers, but no matter which arthritis drug is used, people taking an arthritis drug in combination with a beta-blocker will need to have blood pressure monitored frequently. If hypertension becomes a problem, the physician should adjust the dose of beta-blocker or reconsider treatment options.

Symptoms of Beta-Blocker Undertreatment

Blood pressure may climb and heart symptoms might appear. Be alert for chest pain or palpitations and notify your doctor immediately. Monitor blood pressure carefully.

Never take or stop medication without your doctor's advice.

Heart/Blood Pressure Drugs
(BETA-BLOCKERS)

Asthma Drug
(THEOPHYLLINE)

DANGEROUS

BRAND NAME	GENERIC NAME
Blocadren	timolol
Cartrol	carteolol
Inderal	propranolol
Levatol	penbutolol
Timoptic	timolol
Visken	pindolol

INSTRUCTIONS

Cartrol, Levatol, and Visken are taken with or without food. Inderal is best absorbed with meals, but consistency is more important. It should be taken at roughly the same time every day. Ask your eye doctor to show you how to administer Timoptic drops so that their absorption is minimized. Do not stop any of these medicines suddenly except on doctor's orders. Serious side effects could result.

BRAND NAME	
Aerolate	**Aquaphyllin**
Asmalix	**Bronkodyl**
Elixomin	**Elixophyllin**
Quibron-T	**Respbid**
Slo-bid	**Slo-Phyllin**
Theobid	**Theochron**
Theoclear	**Theo-Dur**
Theolair	**Theo-24**
Theovent	**Theo-X**
T-Phyl	**Uniphyl**

INSTRUCTIONS

Theophylline interacts with food in complex ways, so discuss this issue thoroughly with your doctor and pharmacist. Theophylline may upset the stomach. In some cases this problem can be alleviated by taking the drug with food. See the table of Food and Drug Interactions on pages 73–91 for more information.

INTERACTION

Because beta-blockers can make breathing difficult, they are not often prescribed for people with asthma. The beta-blockers named above can reduce the body's ability to clear theophylline, resulting in increased blood levels of theophylline, with the potential for theophylline toxicity. *This interaction could be dangerous.*

Neither Corgard nor Tenormin interferes with theophylline clearance. It is uncommon but certainly not unknown for eye drops such as Timoptic to be absorbed into the body and produce systemic side effects. In that case, Timoptic could interact with theophylline.

Symptoms of Theophylline Toxicity

Nausea, diarrhea, stomach pain, headache, insomnia, restlessness, and irritability. Severe toxicity (convulsions, heart rhythm changes, or death) may occur with no warning symptoms. Notify your doctor immediately if you suspect a problem.

Never take or stop medication without your doctor's advice.

Heart/Blood Pressure Drugs (BETA-BLOCKERS)	**Barbiturates**

DANGEROUS

BRAND NAME	GENERIC NAME
Inderal	propranolol
Lopressor,	
Toprol XL	metoprolol

(other beta-blockers may also interact)

INSTRUCTIONS

Propranolol and metoprolol are best taken with meals, but consistency is the most important factor. These drugs should be taken at about the same time every day. Do not stop any of these medicines suddenly except on doctor's orders. Serious side effects could result.

BRAND NAME	GENERIC NAME
Alurate	aprobarbital
Amytal	amobarbital
Butisol	butabarbital
Fiorinal	butalbital/ aspirin/caffeine
Lotusate	talbutal
Mebaral	mephobarbital
Nembutal	pentobarbital
Seconal	secobarbital
Solfoton	phenobarbital
Tuinal	combination

INSTRUCTIONS

Any of these medications can cause drowsiness and should not be used if you must drive or operate machinery. Never drink alcohol if you are taking a barbiturate.

INTERACTION

Because barbiturates accelerate drug metabolism, many medications become less effective if they are taken in combination with barbiturates. Birth control pills, acetaminophen (Tylenol, etc.), and beta-blockers are just some of the drugs that are affected. Physicians and patients may not realize a beta-blocker is not working as efficiently as it should to control hypertension or maintain heart health. Anyone taking a beta-blocker such as Inderal or Lopressor should have blood pressure and heart function monitored carefully. If problems develop, a physician may need to change the dose of the beta-blocker or reevaluate treatment options.

Symptoms of Beta-Blocker Undertreatment

Blood pressure may climb and heart symptoms might appear. Be alert for chest pain or palpitations. Monitor blood pressure carefully. Notify the physician promptly of any symptoms.

Never take or stop medication without your doctor's advice.

Heart/Blood Pressure Drugs (BETA-BLOCKERS)	Drugs for Migraine (ERGOT-BASED)

DANGEROUS

BRAND NAME	GENERIC NAME	BRAND NAME	GENERIC NAME
Blocadren	timolol	**Cafergot**	ergotamine
Corgard	nadolol	**Cafetrate**	ergotamine
Inderal	propranolol	**D.H.E. 45**	dihydroergotamine
Levatol	penbutolol	**Ercaf**	ergotamine
Visken	pindolol	**Ergomar**	ergotamine
(other beta-blockers may also interact)		**Ergostat**	ergotamine
		Sansert	methysergide

INSTRUCTIONS

Inderal is best absorbed with meals, but consistency is most important. Take these drugs at approximately the same time every day. Do not stop any of these medicines suddenly because serious side effects could result.

INSTRUCTIONS

Sansert is best taken with food to reduce digestive upset. Ergotamine is to be taken at the very first signs of a migraine attack. Never take more than three tablets per 24 hours, or more than 10 mg per week.

INTERACTION

This interaction is quite controversial. Physicians have been arguing about its likelihood and significance for more than 20 years. We do worry about it, though, because beta-blockers such as propranolol are often prescribed to prevent migraine headaches. Such patients may also take ergotamine to treat a severe migraine attack. Consequently, this interaction could occur quite frequently. The fear is that such a combination may increase constriction in blood vessels in the extremities. This could lead to reduced blood flow and even gangrene. One person had his leg amputated below the knee because of such a reaction. Physicians should be very cautious about prescribing beta-blockers and ergotamine simultaneously. Dosage should be adjusted carefully and people monitored for adequate circulation.

Symptoms of Ergotamine Toxicity

Pale, cold fingers or toes; a feeling of numbness, tingling, or pain in extremities; weakness in arms or legs, especially after exercise. Such symptoms require emergency treatment.

Never take or stop medication without your doctor's advice.

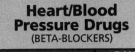

| **Heart/Blood Pressure Drugs** (BETA-BLOCKERS) | **Drugs for Schizophrenia** |

DANGEROUS

BRAND NAME	GENERIC NAME
Inderal	propranolol
Visken	pindolol

(other beta-blockers may also interact)

INSTRUCTIONS
Inderal is best absorbed with meals, but consistency is the most important factor. These drugs should be taken at the same time and in the same way every day. Do not stop any of these medicines suddenly except on doctor's orders. Serious side effects could result.

BRAND NAME	GENERIC NAME
Mellaril	thioridazine
Thorazine	chlorpromazine

INSTRUCTIONS
Mellaril and Thorazine are best taken with food. The dose is highly variable and must be individualized for each patient. These drugs can make skin more sensitive to sunburn; avoid exposure or use appropriate protection. Notify your doctor of vision problems, yellow skin or eyes, or muscle twitching.

INTERACTION

This is a very complex interaction. Each drug may affect metabolism of the other to increase blood levels. This could lead to increased side effects from either or both. In one study, blood levels of Thorazine were five times higher in many patients while they also took propranolol.

Other beta-blockers may also interact with the drugs for schizophrenia. For example, Visken (pindolol) boosted Mellaril levels by more than one-third.

Mellaril and Thorazine can also increase blood levels of beta-blockers. Be alert for increased side effects. Anyone on such a combination should be monitored carefully. *This interaction could be dangerous.*

Symptoms of Beta-Blocker Toxicity
If beta-blocker blood levels get too high, people may experience side effects such as low blood pressure, very slow heart rate, breathing difficulties, or heart failure.

Symptoms of Chlorpromazine Toxicity
Delirium, agitation, drowsiness, low blood pressure, supersensitivity to sun, grand mal seizure. Notify the physician promptly of any symptoms of toxicity of either drug.

Never take or stop medication without your doctor's advice.

Heart/Blood Pressure Drugs (BETA-BLOCKERS)	Heart Drugs

DANGEROUS

BRAND NAME	GENERIC NAME
Inderal	propranolol
Lopressor,	
Toprol XL	metoprolol
Tenormin	atenolol

INSTRUCTIONS
Propranolol and metoprolol are best taken with meals, but consistency is the most important factor. These drugs should be taken at about the same time every day. Do not stop any of these medicines suddenly except on doctor's orders. Serious side effects could result.

BRAND NAME	GENERIC NAME
Cardioquin	quinidine
Cordarone	amiodarone
Quinaglute	quinidine
Quinidex	quinidine
Quinora	quinidine
Rythmol	propafenone
Tambocor	flecaininde

INSTRUCTIONS
Quinidine is best taken with food to reduce stomach upset. Tambocor can also be taken with meals. Check with your physician and pharmacist on proper dosing for all these drugs because the dose must be individualized and timed carefully.

INTERACTION
Cordarone, quinidine, Rythmol, and Tambocor may alter the metabolism of some beta-blockers. Blood levels of propranolol, metoprolol, and atenolol have been increased, sometimes substantially. This has occasionally lead to an exaggerated effect of the beta-blocker and produced symptoms such as dizziness, low blood pressure, nightmares, and cardiac failure. If such drugs are prescribed together, it is important that a physician monitor cardiac function quite carefully and modify dosage if side effects become a problem. Cordarone may not interact with Tenormin.

Symptoms of Beta-Blocker Toxicity
If beta-blocker blood levels get too high, people may experience side effects such as low blood pressure, dizziness, very slow heart rate, breathing difficulties, or heart failure. Notify your physician promptly of any symptoms.

Never take or stop medication without your doctor's advice.

Heart/Blood Pressure Drugs
(BETA-BLOCKERS)

Heart/Blood Pressure Drugs
(CALCIUM CHANNEL BLOCKERS)

DANGEROUS

BRAND NAME	GENERIC NAME
Blocadren	timolol
Inderal	propranolol
Lopressor,	
Toprol XL	metoprolol
Tenormin	atenolol
Timoptic	timolol
Visken	pindolol

INSTRUCTIONS
Inderal and Lopressor are best taken with meals, but consistency is most important. Take these drugs at roughly the same time every day. Ask your eye doctor to show you how to instill Timoptic drops to minimize absorption. Do not stop any of these medicines suddenly because serious side effects could result.

BRAND NAME	GENERIC NAME
Adalat,	
Procardia	nifedipine
Calan, Isoptin,	
Verelan	verapamil
Cardene	nicardipine
Cardizem,	
Dilacor XR	diltiazem
DynaCirc	isradipine
Plendil	felodipine

INSTRUCTIONS
Sustained-release forms, such as Calan SR and Dilacor XR, should not be chewed or crushed. Taking Adalat, Plendil, or Procardia with grapefruit juice could boost blood levels of the drug unexpectedly. See pages 73–91 for more information. If the drug must be discontinued, follow your doctor's instructions for gradual tapering.

INTERACTION
Many people with high blood pressure or unstable angina need a combination of drugs to control their symptoms. Often, a calcium channel blocker and a beta-blocker will work together. Some people, however, experience serious heart problems as a result of an interaction. *This interaction could be dangerous.*

A person who needs both a beta-blocker and a calcium channel blocker should have cardiac function monitored carefully. The doctor may need to adjust the dose of one or both drugs. Nifedipine may be somewhat less likely than other calcium channel blockers to interact with beta-blockers, but serious problems have been reported. Even Timoptic eye drops are capable of interacting with verapamil and, presumably, other calcium blockers.

Notify the doctor if you experience irregular heartbeat or palpitations, worsening of angina, swelling of hands and feet, shortness of breath, hives, rash, or unusual bleeding.

Never take or stop medication without your doctor's advice.

Heart/Blood Pressure Drugs
(BETA-BLOCKERS)

Anti-Anxiety Drugs
(BENZODIAZEPINES)

TROUBLESOME

BRAND NAME	GENERIC NAME
Inderal	propranolol
Lopressor,	
Toprol XL	metoprolol

INSTRUCTIONS
Propranolol and metoprolol are best absorbed with meals, but consistency is the most important factor. These drugs should be taken at about the same time every day. Do not stop any of these medicines suddenly except on doctor's orders. Serious side effects could result.

BRAND NAME	GENERIC NAME
Dalmane	flurazepam
Halcion	triazolam
Librium	chlordiazepoxide
Tranxene	clorazepate
Valium	diazepam

INSTRUCTIONS
These drugs may be taken with food, especially if they upset the digestive tract.

INTERACTION

Blood levels of diazepam may be slightly increased by beta-blockers such as metoprolol and propranolol. The anti-anxiety agent also appears to persist longer in the body. People may find they are less alert when on such a combination and their visual acuity and reaction time might be affected. Serax does not seem to be impacted by propranolol. Be sensitive for any change in consciousness.

Symptoms of Benzodiazepine Overdose:
This interaction could lead to symptoms of overdose such as disorientation, unsteadiness, confusion, slurred speech, drowsiness, dizziness, amnesia, and loss of motor coordination. Contact your physician if such symptoms occur.

Never take or stop medication without your doctor's advice.

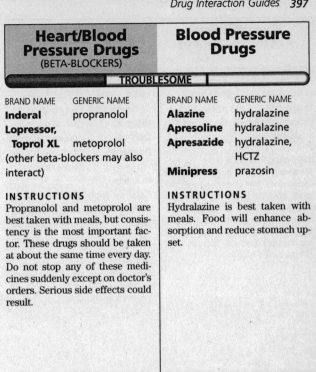

Heart/Blood Pressure Drugs (BETA-BLOCKERS)		Blood Pressure Drugs	
TROUBLESOME			
BRAND NAME	GENERIC NAME	BRAND NAME	GENERIC NAME
Inderal	propranolol	**Alazine**	hydralazine
Lopressor,		**Apresoline**	hydralazine
Toprol XL	metoprolol	**Apresazide**	hydralazine, HCTZ
(other beta-blockers may also interact)		**Minipress**	prazosin

INSTRUCTIONS

Propranolol and metoprolol are best taken with meals, but consistency is the most important factor. These drugs should be taken at about the same time every day. Do not stop any of these medicines suddenly except on doctor's orders. Serious side effects could result.

INSTRUCTIONS

Hydralazine is best taken with meals. Food will enhance absorption and reduce stomach upset.

INTERACTION

Physicians prescribe beta-blockers and hydralazine with some regularity so this is not an interaction that causes great concern. Nevertheless, the potential exists for each of these drugs to increase blood levels of the other compound and magnify the antihypertensive effect. Beta-blockers also seem to exaggerate the dizziness that occurs when people stand up suddenly while taking prazosin. Blood pressure response should be carefully monitored for people combining beta-blockers and hydralazine or prazosin. If dizziness or low blood pressure becomes a problem, the doctor may need to modify the dose.

Symptoms of Hydralazine Toxicity

Be vigilant for low blood pressure, dizziness, rapid pulse, headache, flushing, and palpitations. With prazosin, be very careful about standing suddenly, as this may lead to dizziness or fainting. Notify your physician of any symptoms.

Never take or stop medication without your doctor's advice.

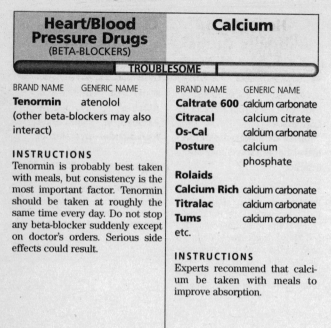

Heart/Blood Pressure Drugs
(BETA-BLOCKERS)

Calcium

TROUBLESOME

BRAND NAME	GENERIC NAME
Tenormin	atenolol

(other beta-blockers may also interact)

INSTRUCTIONS
Tenormin is probably best taken with meals, but consistency is the most important factor. Tenormin should be taken at roughly the same time every day. Do not stop any beta-blocker suddenly except on doctor's orders. Serious side effects could result.

BRAND NAME	GENERIC NAME
Caltrate 600	calcium carbonate
Citracal	calcium citrate
Os-Cal	calcium carbonate
Posture	calcium phosphate
Rolaids	
Calcium Rich	calcium carbonate
Titralac	calcium carbonate
Tums	calcium carbonate
etc.	

INSTRUCTIONS
Experts recommend that calcium be taken with meals to improve absorption.

INTERACTION
This is probably not a particularly dangerous interaction, but because Tenormin is prescribed so frequently and because so many people are taking calcium-based antacids or supplements, it is an interaction that may occur more frequently than physicians or pharmacists realize. There is data to suggest that calcium reduces blood levels of Tenormin by 30 to 50 percent. Whether this is clinically significant is yet to be determined. There is no agreement in this regard. At the very least people who take atenolol should monitor blood pressure before and after the addition of calcium to their regimen. That way they should be able to determine if calcium supplementation in any way reduces the anti-hypertensive benefits of this beta-blocker.

Symptoms of Beta-Blocker Undertreatment
Blood pressure may climb and heart symptoms might appear. Be alert for chest pain or palpitations. Monitor blood pressure carefully. Notify your physician of any symptoms.

Never take or stop medication without your doctor's advice.

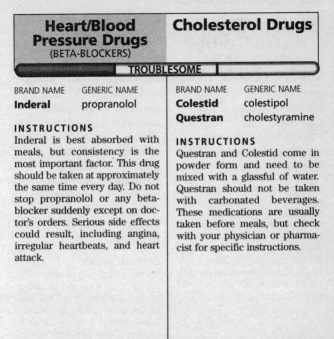

Heart/Blood Pressure Drugs
(BETA-BLOCKERS)

Cholesterol Drugs

TROUBLESOME

BRAND NAME   GENERIC NAME
Inderal   propranolol

INSTRUCTIONS
Inderal is best absorbed with meals, but consistency is the most important factor. This drug should be taken at approximately the same time every day. Do not stop propranolol or any beta-blocker suddenly except on doctor's orders. Serious side effects could result, including angina, irregular heartbeats, and heart attack.

BRAND NAME   GENERIC NAME
Colestid   colestipol
Questran   cholestyramine

INSTRUCTIONS
Questran and Colestid come in powder form and need to be mixed with a glassful of water. Questran should not be taken with carbonated beverages. These medications are usually taken before meals, but check with your physician or pharmacist for specific instructions.

INTERACTION
The absorption of many drugs may be reduced by these common cholesterol-lowering agents. Acetaminophen (Tylenol, etc.), cortisone-type medications, Coumadin, digitalis drugs, arthritis compounds, diuretics, thyroid hormone, and propranolol seem to be affected. Levels of propranolol could be reduced substantially but experts are still debating the significance of this effect. There is some contradictory data with regard to Colestid; one study actually showed an increase in the blood levels of propranolol when it was taken in combination with Colestid. The recommendation is to monitor blood pressure to see if there is lowered effectiveness. An added precaution to reduce the likelihood of an interaction would be to take propranolol at least one hour before—or four to five hours after—swallowing this cholesterol-lowering drink.

Symptoms of Beta-Blocker Undertreatment
Blood pressure may climb and heart symptoms might appear. Be alert for chest pain or palpitations. Monitor blood pressure carefully. Notify your physician of any symptoms.

Never take or stop medication without your doctor's advice.

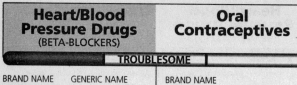

Heart/Blood Pressure Drugs (BETA-BLOCKERS)	Oral Contraceptives

TROUBLESOME

BRAND NAME	GENERIC NAME
Inderal	propranolol
Lopressor,	
Toprol XL	metoprolol

(other beta-blockers may also interact)

INSTRUCTIONS
Propranolol and metoprolol are best taken with meals, but consistency is the most important factor. These drugs should be taken at about the same time every day. Do not stop any of these medicines suddenly except on doctor's orders. Serious side effects could result.

BRAND NAME

Brevicon	**Demulen**
Desogen	**Genora**
Levlen	**Loestrin**
Lo/Ovral	**Modicon**
N.E.E.	**Nelova**
Nordette	**Norethin**
Norinyl	**Norlestrin**
Ortho-Cyclen	**Ortho-Novum**
Ovcon	**Ovral**
Triphasil	

INSTRUCTIONS
For maximum effectiveness, oral contraceptives should be taken at the same time every day and precisely according to instructions. Missed doses can lead to an unwelcome pregnancy. Additional contraception is needed for at least the first week.

INTERACTION
There are several reports that birth control pills can increase blood levels of metoprolol and propranolol. The significance of this interaction is somewhat murky. There may be no cause for concern, but the possibility exists that the effects of these beta-blockers could be magnified. Blood pressure and pulse should be monitored carefully and if the drugs produce side effects, the prescribing physician may choose to reevaluate the dose of beta-blocker.

Symptoms of Beta-Blocker Toxicity
Low blood pressure, dizziness, very slow heart rate, breathing difficulties, and heart failure. Notify your physician of any symptoms.

Never take or stop medication without your doctor's advice.

| **Heart/Blood Pressure Drugs** (BETA-BLOCKERS) | **Tuberculosis Drug** (RIFAMPIN) |

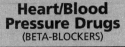

TROUBLESOME

BRAND NAME	GENERIC NAME
Inderal	propranolol
Lopressor,	
Toprol XL	metoprolol

(other beta-blockers may also interact)

INSTRUCTIONS

Propranolol and metoprolol are best taken with meals, but consistency is the most important factor. These drugs should be taken at about the same time every day. Do not stop any of these medicines suddenly except on doctor's orders. Serious side effects could result.

BRAND NAME	GENERIC NAME
Rifadin	rifampin
Rifamate	isoniazid/ rifampin
Rimactane	rifampin

INSTRUCTIONS

Rifampin should be taken on an empty stomach, at least one hour before or two hours after meals. If you develop fever, chills, unusual tiredness, unusual bleeding or bruising, sore throat, muscle and bone pain, or yellow skin and eyes, contact your physician immediately.

INTERACTION

Rifampin stimulates the liver to metabolize other drugs more efficiently. This means that blood levels of other medications may be reduced along with their effectiveness. Acetaminophen (Tylenol, etc.), oral contraceptives, and beta-blockers are just some of the compounds that can be affected. The clinical significance of this interaction remains controversial. At the time of this writing all we can say is that careful monitoring of blood pressure before and after initiation of tuberculosis treatment is crucial. If blood pressure climbs, your physician will have to reevaluate the beta-blocker dosage or treatment regimen.

Symptoms of Beta-Blocker Undertreatment

Blood pressure may climb and heart symptoms might appear. Be alert for chest pain or palpitations. Monitor blood pressure carefully. Notify your physician of any symptoms.

Never take or stop medication without your doctor's advice.

Heart/Blood Pressure Drugs
(BETA-BLOCKERS)

Ulcer Drug
(H₂ ANTAGONIST)

TROUBLESOME

BRAND NAME	GENERIC NAME
Inderal	propranolol
Lopressor	metoprolol
Normodyne	labetalol
Trandate	labetalol

INSTRUCTIONS
Inderal and Lopressor are best taken with meals, but consistency is the most important factor. They should be taken at roughly the same time every day. Do not stop these medicines suddenly except on doctor's orders. Serious side effects could result.

BRAND NAME	GENERIC NAME
Tagamet	cimetidine

INSTRUCTIONS
Tagamet is usually taken with meals and/or at bedtime. Antacids may reduce absorption of Tagamet; do not take one for at least two hours after taking Tagamet.

INTERACTION
Tagamet appears to affect the liver's ability to metabolize certain beta-blockers such as Inderal and Lopressor. These drugs may not be eliminated as efficiently as expected, leading to increased blood levels. One study noted a doubling or even tripling impact on propranolol. The effect on metoprolol is more complicated. Some research has shown increased blood levels while other data show there is no problem. With such contradictory information, all we can suggest is prudent caution.

When blood levels of beta-blockers are substantially increased, there could be unwanted side effects. There have been reports of very slow heart rate and low blood pressure. If there is a compelling reason to take both Tagamet and Inderal or Lopressor simultaneously, blood pressure and pulse should be closely monitored. A physician may wish to reevaluate the standard dose of beta-blocker as well.

Symptoms of Beta-Blocker Toxicity
If beta-blocker blood levels get too high, people may experience side effects such as low blood pressure, dizziness, very slow heart rate, breathing difficulties, or heart failure. Notify your physician promptly of any symptoms.

Never take or stop medication without your doctor's advice.

Heart/Blood Pressure Drugs
(CALCIUM CHANNEL BLOCKERS)

Adalat	Isoptin	Calan	Cardene
Procardia	Cardizem	Verelan	etc.

LIFE-THREATENING

Heart Drug (quinidine) Cardioquin Quinaglute
Quinalan Quinidex Quinora

DANGEROUS

Anticonvulsant Tegretol
Asthma Drug (theophylline) Elixophyllin Quibron-T
Respbid Slo-bid Slo-Phyllin Theobid Theochron
Theoclear Theo-Dur Theolair Theo-24 Theovent etc.
Heart Drug Lanoxin
Heart/Blood Pressure Drugs (beta-blockers)
Blocadren Inderal Lopressor Tenormin Timoptic
Toprol XL Visken
Transplant Drug Sandimmune
Tuberculosis Drug (rifampin) Rifadin Rifamate
Rimactane

TROUBLESOME

Alcohol
Antidepressant (serotonin-based) Prozac
Antidepressants (tricyclic) Janimine Tofranil
Barbiturates Amytal Butisol Mebaral Nembutal
phenobarbital Seconal Tuinal
Blood Pressure Minipress
Calcium
Grapefruit Juice
Ulcer Drug Tagamet

Never take or stop medication without your doctor's advice.

Heart/Blood Pressure Drugs
(CALCIUM CHANNEL BLOCKERS)

Heart Drug
(QUINIDINE)

LIFE-THREATENING

BRAND NAME	GENERIC NAME
Adalat,	
Procardia	nifedipine
Calan, Isoptin,	
Verelan	verapamil

BRAND NAME	GENERIC NAME
Cardioquin	quinidine
Quinaglute	quinidine
Quinidex	quinidine
Quinora	quinidine

INSTRUCTIONS
Sustained-release forms such as Calan SR should not be chewed or crushed. Taking Adalat or Procardia with grapefruit juice could boost blood levels of the drug unexpectedly. See pages 73–91. If the drug must be discontinued, follow the doctor's instructions for gradual tapering.

INSTRUCTIONS
This drug may upset the stomach and should be taken with food. Sustained-release tablets should not be chewed or crushed.

Quinidine may provoke visual disturbances, ringing in the ears, headache, dizziness, nausea, skin rash, or breathing difficulties. Notify your doctor if you develop any of these symptoms. Do not stop this medicine unless your doctor so directs.

INTERACTION
This interaction is extremely complicated. Both of these medicines are used to control irregular heartbeats, and some patients do well on this combination. Others may experience very low blood pressure, very slow heart rate, or serious changes in heart rhythm. *Although no deaths have been reported, in theory this interaction could be lethal.* Verapamil can apparently lead to higher quinidine levels and potentially to toxicity. Nifedipine, on the other hand, has been reported to lower quinidine levels, although this seems to be rare. Quinidine, however, may increase circulating nifedipine. Evidence on other calcium channel blockers is lacking.

The doctor should probably monitor cardiac function carefully for at least several months after a patient starts taking quinidine together with any calcium channel blocker.

Symptoms of Quinidine Toxicity
Nausea, diarrhea, vomiting, headache, lethargy, confusion, palpitations, blurred vision, ringing in the ears, slowed breathing. Notify your doctor immediately of such symptoms.

Symptoms of Calcium Channel Blocker Toxicity
Headaches, facial flushing, low blood pressure, dizziness, fluid retention, nervousness, weakness, sleep problems, rapid or irregular heartbeat, palpitations. Notify the doctor promptly.

Never take or stop medication without your doctor's advice.

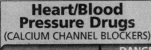

Heart/Blood Pressure Drugs (CALCIUM CHANNEL BLOCKERS)	**Anticonvulsant** (CARBAMAZEPINE)

DANGEROUS

BRAND NAME	GENERIC NAME
Calan, Isoptin,	
Verelan	verapamil
Cardizem,	
Dilacor XR	diltiazem
Plendil	felodipine

INSTRUCTIONS

These drugs come in a variety of doses; follow the doctor's directions. Sustained-release forms, such as Calan SR and Dilacor XR, should not be chewed or crushed. Taking Plendil with grapefruit juice could boost blood levels of the drug unexpectedly. See the table of Food and Drug Compatibility on pages 73–91. If the drug must be discontinued, follow the doctor's instructions for gradual tapering.

BRAND NAME	GENERIC NAME
Tegretol	carbamazepine

INSTRUCTIONS

Carbamazepine may upset the stomach; if so, take it with food or milk. Do not stop this drug suddenly; seizures could result. To maintain its strength, it must be stored away from humidity and heat in a tightly closed container.

INTERACTION

Both verapamil and diltiazem have been associated with elevated blood levels of carbamazepine, with the possibility of toxicity. *This interaction could be dangerous.*

Carbamazepine concentrations should be monitored closely if this drug is taken with a calcium channel blocker. Nifedipine may not interact, but the dose of carbamazepine may need to be reduced by as much as 50 percent when combined with verapamil. Monitoring is crucial if a patient on Tegretol stops taking a calcium channel blocker.

If a patient on Plendil takes carbamazepine, blood pressure may not be controlled with the normal dose of Plendil. One study found that patients on Tegretol had only about 6 percent the amount of Plendil in their bloodstreams as people taking Plendil alone. In such a case, the doctor may want to adjust the dose of Plendil.

Symptoms of Carbamazepine Toxicity

Nausea, vomiting, drowsiness, unsteadiness, incoordination, dizziness, muscle twitching or tremor, irregular breathing, rapid heartbeat, changes in blood pressure, changes in urination, and impaired consciousness. Notify the physician immediately of any such symptoms.

Never take or stop medication without your doctor's advice.

Heart/Blood Pressure Drugs
(CALCIUM CHANNEL BLOCKERS)

Asthma Drug
(THEOPHYLLINE)

DANGEROUS

BRAND NAME	GENERIC NAME
Adalat,	
Procardia	nifedipine
Calan, Isoptin,	
Verelan	verapamil
Cardizem,	
Dilacor XR	diltiazem

INSTRUCTIONS
These drugs come in a variety of doses; follow the doctor's directions carefully. Sustained-release forms, such as Calan SR and Dilacor XR, should not be chewed or crushed and are best taken with food. Avoid taking Adalat or Procardia with grapefruit juice, as this could boost blood levels unexpectedly. See the table on pages 73–91 for specific instructions. Withdrawal symptoms, especially chest pain, may occur if these drugs are stopped suddenly. Follow your doctor's instructions for tapering slowly if the medicine must be discontinued.

BRAND NAME	
Aerolate	**Aquaphyllin**
Asmalix	**Bronkodyl**
Elixomin	**Elixophyllin**
Quibron-T	**Respbid**
Slo-bid	**Slo-Phyllin**
Theobid	**Theochron**
Theoclear	**Theo-Dur**
Theolair	**Theo-24**
Theovent	**Theo-X**
T-Phyl	**Uniphyl**

INSTRUCTIONS
Theophylline interacts with food in complex ways, so discuss this issue thoroughly with your doctor and pharmacist. Theophylline may upset the stomach. In some cases this problem can be alleviated by taking the drug with food. See the table of Food and Drug Compatibility on pages 73–91 for more information.

INTERACTION
Many medicines, including diltiazem and verapamil, are capable of elevating blood levels of theophylline by interfering with metabolism of the drug. People seem to vary in the degree to which they react to this interaction. *Although the documented increase in circulating theophylline is not large, it could be dangerous for someone whose blood levels were already high.*

Most studies indicate that Procardia has little effect on serum theophylline levels, but there are a few cases of patients who developed toxicity as a result of this interaction.

Symptoms of Theophylline Toxicity
Nausea, diarrhea, stomach pain, headache, insomnia, restlessness, and irritability. Severe toxicity (convulsions, heart rhythm changes, or death) may occur with no warning symptoms. Notify your doctor immediately if you suspect a problem.

Never take or stop medication without your doctor's advice.

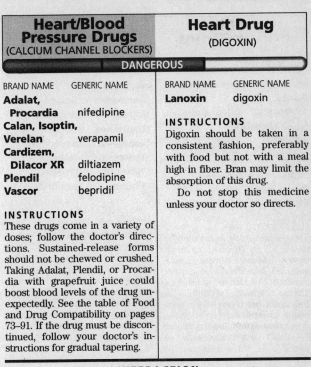

Heart/Blood Pressure Drugs (CALCIUM CHANNEL BLOCKERS)	**Heart Drug** (DIGOXIN)
DANGEROUS	

BRAND NAME	GENERIC NAME
Adalat, Procardia	nifedipine
Calan, Isoptin, Verelan	verapamil
Cardizem, Dilacor XR	diltiazem
Plendil	felodipine
Vascor	bepridil

INSTRUCTIONS

These drugs come in a variety of doses; follow the doctor's directions. Sustained-release forms should not be chewed or crushed. Taking Adalat, Plendil, or Procardia with grapefruit juice could boost blood levels of the drug unexpectedly. See the table of Food and Drug Compatibility on pages 73–91. If the drug must be discontinued, follow your doctor's instructions for gradual tapering.

BRAND NAME	GENERIC NAME
Lanoxin	digoxin

INSTRUCTIONS

Digoxin should be taken in a consistent fashion, preferably with food but not with a meal high in fiber. Bran may limit the absorption of this drug.

Do not stop this medicine unless your doctor so directs.

INTERACTION

Patients with certain heart rhythm problems may require this combination of medicines. Others might be taking both drugs to treat different conditions. In either event, this interaction could be a problem, resulting in higher than expected digoxin levels. Be alert for signs of toxicity. The doctor should monitor blood levels of digoxin and also the electrocardiogram. Verapamil can raise serum digoxin levels as much as 75 percent, enough to result in toxicity in some cases. Diltiazem also seems to raise digoxin levels in the blood, although the studies do not agree on this effect. Bepridil, a relatively new blood pressure medicine, interacts with digoxin to slow heart beat and modify the electrocardiogram. *This interaction could be dangerous.*

Symptoms of Digoxin Toxicity

Nausea, vomiting, loss of appetite, diarrhea, stomach pain, visual disturbances (green or yellow tint and a halo around lights), weakness, drowsiness, depression, confusion, palpitations, rash, headaches, and hallucinations. Notify your doctor immediately if you experience any of these symptoms.

Never take or stop medication without your doctor's advice.

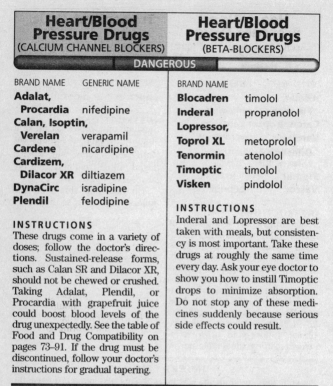

Heart/Blood Pressure Drugs
(CALCIUM CHANNEL BLOCKERS)

Heart/Blood Pressure Drugs
(BETA-BLOCKERS)

DANGEROUS

BRAND NAME	GENERIC NAME
Adalat,	
Procardia	nifedipine
Calan, Isoptin,	
Verelan	verapamil
Cardene	nicardipine
Cardizem,	
Dilacor XR	diltiazem
DynaCirc	isradipine
Plendil	felodipine

BRAND NAME	
Blocadren	timolol
Inderal	propranolol
Lopressor,	
Toprol XL	metoprolol
Tenormin	atenolol
Timoptic	timolol
Visken	pindolol

INSTRUCTIONS
These drugs come in a variety of doses; follow the doctor's directions. Sustained-release forms, such as Calan SR and Dilacor XR, should not be chewed or crushed. Taking Adalat, Plendil, or Procardia with grapefruit juice could boost blood levels of the drug unexpectedly. See the table of Food and Drug Compatibility on pages 73–91. If the drug must be discontinued, follow your doctor's instructions for gradual tapering.

INSTRUCTIONS
Inderal and Lopressor are best taken with meals, but consistency is most important. Take these drugs at roughly the same time every day. Ask your eye doctor to show you how to instill Timoptic drops to minimize absorption. Do not stop any of these medicines suddenly because serious side effects could result.

INTERACTION
Many people with high blood pressure or unstable angina need a combination of drugs to control their symptoms. Often, a calcium channel blocker and a beta-blocker will work together. Some people, however, experience serious heart problems as a result of an interaction. *This interaction could be dangerous.*

A person who needs both a beta-blocker and a calcium channel blocker should have cardiac function monitored carefully. The doctor may need to adjust the dose of one or both drugs. Nifedipine may be somewhat less likely than other calcium channel blockers to interact with beta-blockers, but serious problems have been reported. Even Timoptic eye drops are capable of interacting with verapamil and, presumably, other calcium blockers.

Notify your doctor if you experience irregular heartbeat or palpitations, worsening of angina, swelling of hands and feet, shortness of breath, hives, rash, or unusual bleeding.

Never take or stop medication without your doctor's advice.

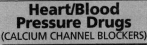

Heart/Blood Pressure Drugs
(CALCIUM CHANNEL BLOCKERS)

Transplant Drug

DANGEROUS

BRAND NAME	GENERIC NAME
Calan, Isoptin,	
Verelan	verapamil
Cardene	nicardipine
Cardizem,	
Dilacor XR	diltiazem

INSTRUCTIONS
These drugs come in a variety of doses; follow the doctor's directions. Sustained-release forms such as Calan SR should not be chewed or crushed. See the table of Food and Drug Compatibility on pages 73–91. If the drug must be discontinued, follow your doctor's instructions for gradual tapering.

BRAND NAME	GENERIC NAME
Sandimmune	cyclosporine

INSTRUCTIONS
Sandimmune comes as an oral solution with a taste reminiscent of castor oil. It should be mixed in a glass with milk, chocolate milk, or orange juice at room temperature and drunk at once. Then the glass (no plastic) should be rinsed and the rinsing fluid drunk to get the full dose. Do not take Sandimmune with grapefruit juice unless the physician is monitoring blood levels of the drug closely. (See page 53.)

Due to a possible interaction between cyclosporine and oral contraceptives, barrier methods of contraception should be used while taking this drug.

Regular monitoring is important. Do not stop this medicine unless your doctor so directs.

INTERACTION
The potential interaction is complicated, because patients receiving a kidney or heart transplant may be given a calcium channel blocker such as diltiazem or verapamil first before Sandimmune. When given in this manner, these medications seem to help protect the kidney from possible damage due to Sandimmune.

If Sandimmune is already being taken, however, both verapamil and diltiazem can raise blood levels of this transplant drug to potentially toxic levels, usually within a week. Whenever the dose of one of these drugs is changed, cyclosporine levels should be monitored carefully so that the dose may be adjusted if necessary. *This interaction could be dangerous.*

Cardene has also been reported to interact with Sandimmune, while the calcium channel blocker Procardia does not seem to.

Signs of Cyclosporine Toxicity
Kidney problems, changes in liver or kidney function. Close monitoring of blood and urine is essential.

Never take or stop medication without your doctor's advice.

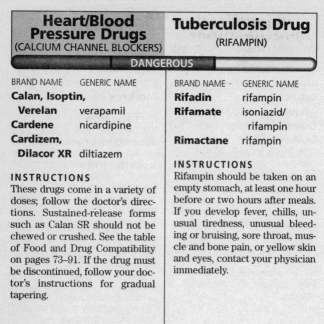

Heart/Blood Pressure Drugs
(CALCIUM CHANNEL BLOCKERS)

Tuberculosis Drug
(RIFAMPIN)

DANGEROUS

BRAND NAME	GENERIC NAME
Calan, Isoptin,	
Verelan	verapamil
Cardene	nicardipine
Cardizem,	
Dilacor XR	diltiazem

INSTRUCTIONS
These drugs come in a variety of doses; follow the doctor's directions. Sustained-release forms such as Calan SR should not be chewed or crushed. See the table of Food and Drug Compatibility on pages 73–91. If the drug must be discontinued, follow your doctor's instructions for gradual tapering.

BRAND NAME	GENERIC NAME
Rifadin	rifampin
Rifamate	isoniazid/ rifampin
Rimactane	rifampin

INSTRUCTIONS
Rifampin should be taken on an empty stomach, at least one hour before or two hours after meals. If you develop fever, chills, unusual tiredness, unusual bleeding or bruising, sore throat, muscle and bone pain, or yellow skin and eyes, contact your physician immediately.

INTERACTION
Tuberculosis medicines containing rifampin can dramatically reduce the effectiveness of verapamil, leading to a potentially dangerous rise in blood pressure or increase in angina symptoms. A similar interaction has been reported with nifedipine and may be expected with Cardene. Injected (IV) verapamil does not appear to be much affected by rifampin. If rifampin is needed, the doctor will want to monitor the patient closely to make sure the calcium channel blocker is working properly. In some cases, an alternate medication may be needed.

Never take or stop medication without your doctor's advice.

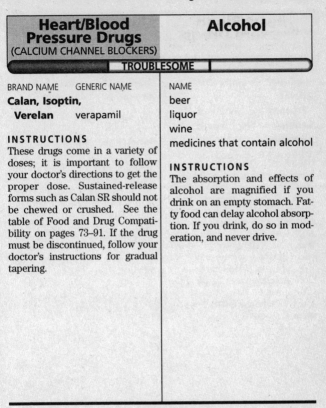

Heart/Blood Pressure Drugs (CALCIUM CHANNEL BLOCKERS)	Alcohol

TROUBLESOME

BRAND NAME   GENERIC NAME
Calan, Isoptin,
  Verelan   verapamil

INSTRUCTIONS
These drugs come in a variety of doses; it is important to follow your doctor's directions to get the proper dose. Sustained-release forms such as Calan SR should not be chewed or crushed. See the table of Food and Drug Compatibility on pages 73–91. If the drug must be discontinued, follow your doctor's instructions for gradual tapering.

NAME
beer
liquor
wine
medicines that contain alcohol

INSTRUCTIONS
The absorption and effects of alcohol are magnified if you drink on an empty stomach. Fatty food can delay alcohol absorption. If you drink, do so in moderation, and never drive.

INTERACTION

People taking Calan, Isoptin, or Verelan may get more of a bang from their booze than they bargained for. A study of healthy young men showed that verapamil can increase blood alcohol concentrations by an average of 17 percent, and keep the alcohol in the bloodstream about 30 percent longer. This drug interferes with the body's ability to eliminate alcohol and can prolong the effects of alcohol intoxication. Remember that some liquid medicines contain alcohol (see page 203 in the discussion on alcohol for a list). *This interaction between alcohol and verapamil could be troublesome.*

Symptoms of Alcohol Overdose
This interaction may lead to alcohol toxicity. Disorientation, unsteadiness, or loss of motor coordination would be symptoms to watch for.

Never take or stop medication without your doctor's advice.

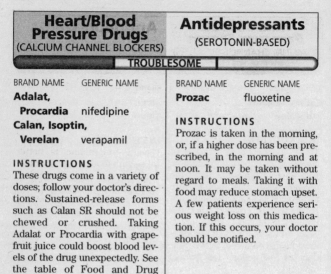

Heart/Blood Pressure Drugs (CALCIUM CHANNEL BLOCKERS)	**Antidepressants** (SEROTONIN-BASED)

TROUBLESOME

BRAND NAME	GENERIC NAME
Adalat,	
Procardia	nifedipine
Calan, Isoptin,	
Verelan	verapamil

INSTRUCTIONS

These drugs come in a variety of doses; follow your doctor's directions. Sustained-release forms such as Calan SR should not be chewed or crushed. Taking Adalat or Procardia with grapefruit juice could boost blood levels of the drug unexpectedly. See the table of Food and Drug Compatibility, pages 73–91. If the drug must be discontinued, follow your doctor's instructions for gradual tapering.

BRAND NAME	GENERIC NAME
Prozac	fluoxetine

INSTRUCTIONS

Prozac is taken in the morning, or, if a higher dose has been prescribed, in the morning and at noon. It may be taken without regard to meals. Taking it with food may reduce stomach upset. A few patients experience serious weight loss on this medication. If this occurs, your doctor should be notified.

INTERACTION

There are a few case reports of increased toxicity of calcium channel blockers such as Calan and Procardia due to this combination. *This interaction could be troublesome.*

Side Effects of Calcium Channel Blockers

Nausea, constipation, skin rash, dizziness, headache, drowsiness, insomnia, shortness of breath, fluid retention, and changes in heart rate or rhythm. Contact your physician promptly if any such adverse effects appear while you are on Prozac and one of the calcium channel blockers.

Never take or stop medication without your doctor's advice.

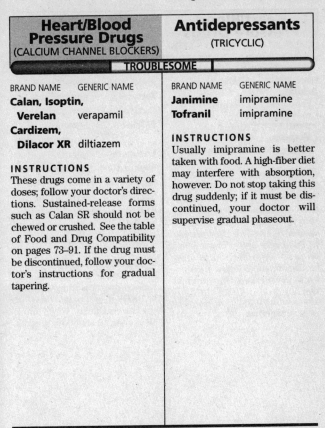

Heart/Blood Pressure Drugs
(CALCIUM CHANNEL BLOCKERS)

Antidepressants
(TRICYCLIC)

TROUBLESOME

BRAND NAME   GENERIC NAME

Calan, Isoptin,
   Verelan   verapamil

Cardizem,
   Dilacor XR   diltiazem

INSTRUCTIONS
These drugs come in a variety of doses; follow your doctor's directions. Sustained-release forms such as Calan SR should not be chewed or crushed. See the table of Food and Drug Compatibility on pages 73–91. If the drug must be discontinued, follow your doctor's instructions for gradual tapering.

BRAND NAME   GENERIC NAME

Janimine   imipramine
Tofranil   imipramine

INSTRUCTIONS
Usually imipramine is better taken with food. A high-fiber diet may interfere with absorption, however. Do not stop taking this drug suddenly; if it must be discontinued, your doctor will supervise gradual phaseout.

INTERACTION

Diltiazem and verapamil may raise blood levels of the antidepressant imipramine. The clinical significance of this interaction remains murky. For some people this might lead to imipramine toxicity. It would be a good idea to have serum imipramine levels monitored periodically.

Symptoms of Antidepressant Toxicity
People vary in their response to higher doses of tricyclics. Side effects may include sedation, confusion, dilated pupils, flushing, dry mouth, hallucinations, heart palpitations, and agitation. Older people may be especially vulnerable. Notify your physician of symptoms.

Never take or stop medication without your doctor's advice.

| **Heart/Blood Pressure Drugs** (CALCIUM CHANNEL BLOCKERS) | **Barbiturates** |

TROUBLESOME

BRAND NAME	GENERIC NAME
Adalat, Procardia	nifedipine
Calan, Isoptin Verelan	verapamil
Cardizem, Dilacor XR	diltiazem

INSTRUCTIONS
These drugs come in a variety of doses; follow your doctor's directions. Sustained-release forms such as Calan SR should not be chewed or crushed. See the table of Food and Drug Compatibility on pages 73–91. If the drug must be discontinued, follow the doctor's instructions for gradual tapering.

BRAND NAME	GENERIC NAME
Amytal	amobarbital
Butisol	butabarbital
Fiorinal	butalbital/ aspirin/caffeine
Lotusate	talbutal
Mebaral	mephobarbital
Nembutal	pentobarbital
Seconal	secobarbital
Solfoton	phenobarbital
Tuinal	amobarbital/ secobarbital

INSTRUCTIONS
Any of these medications can cause drowsiness and should not be used if you must drive or operate machinery. Never drink alcohol if you are taking a barbiturate.

INTERACTION
Studies have shown that phenobarbital and other barbiturates speed the body's elimination of both nifedipine and verapamil. If both a calcium channel blocker and a barbiturate are needed, the clinical response to the calcium channel blocker should be monitored; a higher dose could be required. *This interaction could be troublesome.*

Never take or stop medication without your doctor's advice.

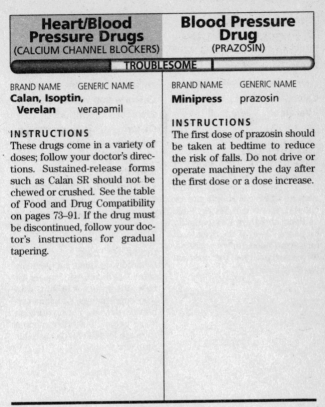

Heart/Blood Pressure Drugs
(CALCIUM CHANNEL BLOCKERS)

Blood Pressure Drug
(PRAZOSIN)

TROUBLESOME

BRAND NAME   GENERIC NAME
**Calan, Isoptin,
  Verelan**   verapamil

INSTRUCTIONS
These drugs come in a variety of doses; follow your doctor's directions. Sustained-release forms such as Calan SR should not be chewed or crushed. See the table of Food and Drug Compatibility on pages 73–91. If the drug must be discontinued, follow your doctor's instructions for gradual tapering.

BRAND NAME   GENERIC NAME
Minipress   prazosin

INSTRUCTIONS
The first dose of prazosin should be taken at bedtime to reduce the risk of falls. Do not drive or operate machinery the day after the first dose or a dose increase.

INTERACTION
When a person taking Minipress starts taking verapamil as well, blood levels of prazosin may increase by over 100 percent. Increased blood levels of Minipress could result in excessively low blood pressure.

A person starting on this combination should have blood pressure carefully monitored, so that the doctor can adjust the dose if necessary. The precautions for avoiding severe dizziness with the first dose of Minipress are appropriate when verapamil is added to the regimen. Lightheadedness can lead to falls, which may be very serious. *This interaction could be troublesome.*

Symptoms of Prazosin Overdose
Drowsiness, extremely low blood pressure, which may cause dizziness. Notify your physician of any symptoms.

Never take or stop medication without your doctor's advice.

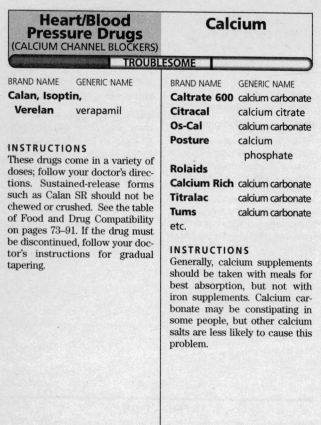

Heart/Blood Pressure Drugs (CALCIUM CHANNEL BLOCKERS)	**Calcium**

TROUBLESOME

BRAND NAME	GENERIC NAME
Calan, Isoptin,	
Verelan	verapamil

INSTRUCTIONS

These drugs come in a variety of doses; follow your doctor's directions. Sustained-release forms such as Calan SR should not be chewed or crushed. See the table of Food and Drug Compatibility on pages 73–91. If the drug must be discontinued, follow your doctor's instructions for gradual tapering.

BRAND NAME	GENERIC NAME
Caltrate 600	calcium carbonate
Citracal	calcium citrate
Os-Cal	calcium carbonate
Posture	calcium phosphate
Rolaids	
Calcium Rich	calcium carbonate
Titralac	calcium carbonate
Tums	calcium carbonate
etc.	

INSTRUCTIONS

Generally, calcium supplements should be taken with meals for best absorption, but not with iron supplements. Calcium carbonate may be constipating in some people, but other calcium salts are less likely to cause this problem.

INTERACTION

Calcium salts have been used in some cases of verapamil overdose or toxicity to reduce the effects of this calcium channel blocker. It is not clear if daily doses of calcium will modify the effectiveness of verapamil.

Tell your doctor if you plan to start or stop calcium supplements so that your clinical response can be monitored. The dose of verapamil may need to be adjusted.

Never take or stop medication without your doctor's advice.

Heart/Blood Pressure Drugs
(CALCIUM CHANNEL BLOCKERS)

Grapefruit Juice

TROUBLESOME

BRAND NAME	GENERIC NAME
Adalat,	
Procardia	nifedipine
Plendil	felodipine
Calan, Isoptin,	
Verelan	verapamil

INSTRUCTIONS
These drugs come in a variety of doses; follow your doctor's directions. Taking Adalat, Procardia, or Plendil with grapefruit juice could boost blood levels of the drug unexpectedly. See the table of Food and Drug Compatibility on pages 73–91. If the drug must be discontinued, follow your doctor's instructions for gradual tapering.

INSTRUCTIONS
Research on the effects of grapefruit juice on drug metabolism is still evolving. No one knows how many medications may be affected. To be on the safe side, do not take your medicines with grapefruit or grapefruit juice unless advised to do so by your physician.

INTERACTION
The first warning that grapefruit juice could interact with drugs came during a study of the blood pressure medicine Plendil (felodipine). Investigators were shocked to discover that blood levels of the drug jumped an astonishing 284 percent beyond predicted levels when the medicine was swallowed with grapefruit juice. Side effects were also far more prominent when grapefruit juice was used. Other studies have confirmed that grapefruit juice magnifies the drug's effects and side effects.

The same investigators found that blood levels of Procardia (nifedipine) were also 134 percent higher when the drug was taken with grapefruit juice than when it was taken with water. Apparently the flavonoids in the grapefruit juice slow the metabolism of these calcium channel blockers. *This interaction could be troublesome.*

Symptoms of Plendil or Procardia Toxicity
Headaches, facial flushing, low blood pressure, nausea, dizziness, confusion, fluid retention, nervousness, weakness, sleep problems, changes in heart rate or irregular heartbeat, and palpitations. Notify your physician of any symptoms.

Never take or stop medication without your doctor's advice.

Heart/Blood Pressure Drugs
(CALCIUM CHANNEL BLOCKERS)

Ulcer Drug
(H$_2$ ANTAGONIST)

TROUBLESOME

BRAND NAME   GENERIC NAME

Adalat,

Procardia   nifedipine

INSTRUCTIONS
These drugs come in a variety of doses; follow your doctor's directions. Taking Adalat or Procardia with grapefruit juice could boost blood levels of the drug unexpectedly. See the table of Food and Drug Compatibility on pages 73–91. If the drug must be discontinued, follow your doctor's instructions for gradual tapering.

BRAND NAME   GENERIC NAME

Tagamet   cimetidine

INSTRUCTIONS
Tagamet is usually taken with meals and/or at bedtime. Antacids may reduce absorption of Tagamet; do not take one for at least two hours after taking Tagamet.

INTERACTION
Cimetidine affects the liver's ability to metabolize many drugs. Nifedipine is vulnerable to this interaction. This combination of medications can lead to blood levels of nifedipine that are substantially higher than normal. This could lead to an exaggerated response to the blood pressure medicine. *This interaction could be troublesome.*

Studies on other calcium channel blockers are contradictory. It is possible that Tagamet increases levels of other calcium channel blockers such as verapamil or diltiazem slightly, but it does not appear that the effectiveness of these medications is likely to be affected.

Symptoms of Nifedipine Toxicity
Headaches, facial flushing, low blood pressure, nausea, dizziness, confusion, fluid retention, nervousness, weakness, sleep problems, changes in heart rate or irregular heartbeat, and palpitations. Notify your physician of any symptoms.

Never take or stop medication without your doctor's advice.

Ulcer Drug
(CIMETIDINE)

Tagamet

LIFE-THREATENING

Anticoagulant Coumadin
Asthma Drugs (theophylline) Bronkodyl Elixophyllin
Quibron-T Slo-Phyllin Theobid Theo-Dur Theolair
Theo-24 Uniphyl
Cancer Treatment BiCNU

DANGEROUS

Anticonvulsants Dilantin Mesantoin Peganone
Tegretol
Antifungal Agent Nizoral
Heart Medications Cardioquin Cordarone Ethmozine
procainamide Procan SR Pronestyl Quinaglute
Quinidex quinidine Quinora Tambocor

TROUBLESOME

Alcohol
Anti-Anxiety Drugs (benzodiazepines) Ativan
Dalmane Halcion Klonopin Librium Paxipam ProSom
Serax Tranxene Valium Xanax
Antidepressants (tricyclic) Adapin Anafranil
Asendin Elavil Norpramin Pamelor Sinequan Tofranil
Heart/Blood Pressure Drugs (beta-blockers) Inderal
Lopressor Normodyne
**Heart/Blood Pressure Drugs (calcium channel
blockers)** Adalat Procardia

Drugs on this list have the most serious known reactions with
Tagamet. Not every interaction is listed. Be sure to check with a health
professional before you take any other medication together with this
ulcer drug.

Ulcer Drug
(H₂ ANTAGONIST)

Anticoagulant
(WARFARIN)

LIFE-THREATENING

BRAND NAME	GENERIC NAME
Tagamet	cimetidine

INSTRUCTIONS
Tagamet is usually taken with meals and/or at bedtime. Antacids may reduce absorption of Tagamet; do not take one for at least two hours after taking Tagamet.

BRAND NAME	GENERIC NAME
Coumadin	warfarin

INSTRUCTIONS
Warfarin tablets can be swallowed with food or on an empty stomach. Try to avoid large variations in the quantity of vitamin-K–containing vegetables—such as broccoli, cabbage, or spinach—that you eat each day. Consuming much more or less than usual could change the action of the drug.

INTERACTION
Although warfarin may cause nausea, loss of appetite, stomach cramping, or diarrhea, taking Tagamet to treat these symptoms might trigger serious problems. Tagamet affects metabolism and increases Coumadin's blood-thinning potential. This prolongs prothrombin time (a measure of clotting) and could lead to serious hemorrhaging. *The interaction is potentially lethal.* Experts warn against this combination of drugs. If an ulcer medicine is needed with warfarin, Axid, Pepcid, or Zantac may be a safer alternative than Tagamet. Prothrombin time should be monitored when taking warfarin with an ulcer drug.
Symptoms of Warfarin Overdose
There may be no early warning signs of danger. Blood tests are essential. Symptoms include any unusual bleeding, including rectal or urinary tract bleeding, excessive menstrual bleeding, nosebleeds, bleeding around gums, bruising, red or tar-black stools, vomiting blood, and red or dark-brown urine. Notify your doctor immediately if you suspect a problem.

Never take or stop medication without your doctor's advice.

Ulcer Drug
(H₂ ANTAGONIST)

Asthma Drug
(THEOPHYLLINE)

LIFE-THREATENING

BRAND NAME   GENERIC NAME
Tagamet   cimetidine

INSTRUCTIONS
Tagamet is usually taken with meals and/or at bedtime. Antacids may reduce absorption of Tagamet; do not take one for at least two hours after taking Tagamet.

BRAND NAME

Aerolate	**Aquaphyllin**
Asmalix	**Bronkodyl**
Elixomin	**Elixophyllin**
Quibron-T	**Respbid**
Slo-bid	**Slo-Phyllin**
Theobid	**Theochron**
Theoclear	**Theo-Dur**
Theolair	**Theo-24**
Theovent	**Theo-X**
T-Phyl	**Uniphyl**

INSTRUCTIONS
Theophylline interacts with food in complex ways, so discuss this issue thoroughly with your doctor and pharmacist. Theophylline may upset the stomach. In some cases this problem can be alleviated by taking the drug with food. See the table of Food and Drug Compatibility on pages 73–91 for more information.

INTERACTION
One common side effect of theophylline is stomach upset, which may in some cases mimic the symptoms of an ulcer or chronic heartburn. If a patient taking theophylline is prescribed Tagamet for symptoms of stomach upset, blood levels of theophylline could reach toxic levels. *This interaction could be life threatening.*

Tagamet boosts blood levels of theophylline by a third to a half. Patients whose theophylline levels are already a bit high (over 15 mcg/ml) are at highest risk for trouble. Anyone who needs both of these medications should have blood levels of theophylline monitored closely. Notify your physician immediately of any symptoms of theophylline toxicity.

Symptoms of Theophylline Toxicity
Nausea, diarrhea, stomach pain, headache, insomnia, restlessness, and irritability. Severe toxicity (convulsions, heart rhythm changes, or death) may occur with no warning symptoms. Notify your doctor immediately if you suspect a problem.

Never take or stop medication without your doctor's advice.

Ulcer Drug (H$_2$ ANTAGONIST)	**Cancer Treatment**
LIFE-THREATENING	

BRAND NAME	GENERIC NAME	BRAND NAME	GENERIC NAME
Tagamet	cimetidine	**BiCNU**	carmustine

INSTRUCTIONS

Tagamet is usually taken with meals and/or at bedtime. Antacids may reduce absorption of Tagamet; do not take one for at least two hours after taking Tagamet.

INSTRUCTIONS

Like many chemotherapeutic drugs, BiCNU is given intravenously. Antinausea medicine can help reduce nausea and vomiting.

INTERACTION

BiCNU is a heavy-duty drug. Toxicity is a tradeoff in the fight against cancer. The one thing cancer patients don't need is extra problems. Because of the digestive upset BiCNU can cause, it is understandable that physicians might consider an acid controller such as Tagamet. But there are reports that such a combination could cause increased BiCNU bone marrow toxicity. *This side effect could be life threatening.*

It is not clear how Tagamet increases bone marrow suppression. It may be that this ulcer drug blocks normal metabolism of BiCNU or it may have a direct effect on bone marrow itself. No matter what the mechanism, Tagamet should probably not be used with BiCNU unless there are compelling reasons to take such a risk.

Symptoms of BiCNU Toxicity

Bone marrow toxicity creates blood diseases. Anemia, bleeding, and increased susceptibility to infections are signs of serious danger.

Never take or stop medication without your doctor's advice.

Ulcer Drug (H$_2$ ANTAGONIST)	**Anticonvulsants**

DANGEROUS

BRAND NAME	GENERIC NAME
Tagamet	cimetidine

INSTRUCTIONS

Tagamet is usually taken with meals and/or at bedtime. Antacids may reduce absorption of Tagamet; do not take one for at least two hours after taking Tagamet.

BRAND NAME	GENERIC NAME
Dilantin	phenytoin
Mesantoin	mephenytoin
Peganone	ethotoin
Tegretol	carbamazepine

INSTRUCTIONS

These drugs are best taken with food to reduce the likelihood of stomach upset.

INTERACTION

Tagamet appears to modify the metabolism of Dilantin and Tegretol. The same reaction seems likely also to affect Mesantoin and Peganone, although it has not yet been documented in the medical literature. The problem is that Tagamet affects liver enzymes so that they may be less capable of processing these anticonvulsants. As a result, blood levels can rise. This could lead to toxicity.

While Tagamet and Tegretol seem less likely to interact if Tegretol has been taken for longer than four weeks, physicians should be cautious when considering such a combination. Dilantin blood levels have climbed significantly when Tagamet was added to the regimen. Symptoms of overdose have been noted.

Symptoms of Dilantin or Tegretol Toxicity

Uncontrollable eye movements, unsteadiness on the feet, slurred speech, dizziness, muscle twitching, and confusion may be signs of toxicity. Notify your physician promptly of any symptoms.

Never take or stop medication without your doctor's advice.

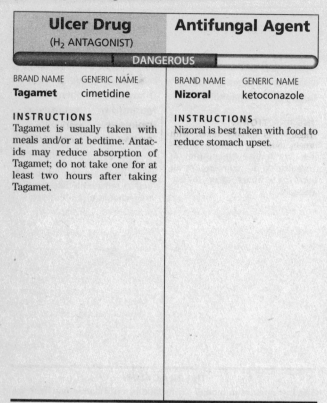

Ulcer Drug (H₂ ANTAGONIST)	Antifungal Agent

H_2 ANTAGONIST

DANGEROUS

BRAND NAME | GENERIC NAME
Tagamet | cimetidine

BRAND NAME | GENERIC NAME
Nizoral | ketoconazole

INSTRUCTIONS

Tagamet is usually taken with meals and/or at bedtime. Antacids may reduce absorption of Tagamet; do not take one for at least two hours after taking Tagamet.

INSTRUCTIONS

Nizoral is best taken with food to reduce stomach upset.

INTERACTION

Nizoral is often reserved for serious fungal infections because of its potential for liver toxicity. Some of these infections can be devastating or possibly even life threatening if not treated successfully.

Nizoral requires an acid environment to be absorbed effectively from the stomach. Drugs that make the stomach less acidic (Axid, Pepcid, Tagamet, and Zantac) appear to dramatically reduce absorption of Nizoral. This could lead to diminished effectiveness. Antacids and another acid-suppressing drug, Prilosec, could also hamper normal Nizoral absorption.

One reference recommends that doctors who must treat people who require Nizoral and a medication for ulcers consider the drug Carafate (sucralfate), which does not affect acidity.

Never take or stop medication without your doctor's advice.

Ulcer Drug
(H$_2$ ANTAGONIST)

Heart Medications

DANGEROUS

BRAND NAME	GENERIC NAME
Tagamet	cimetidine

INSTRUCTIONS
Tagamet is usually taken with meals and/or at bedtime. Antacids may reduce absorption of Tagamet; do not take one for at least two hours after taking Tagamet.

BRAND NAME	GENERIC NAME
Cardioquin	quinidine
Cordarone	amiodarone
Ethmozine	moricizine
Procan SR	procainamide
Pronestyl	procainamide
Quinaglute	quinidine
Quinidex	quinidine
Quinora	quinidine
Tambocor	flecainide

INSTRUCTIONS
Quinidine is best taken with food to reduce stomach upset. Procainamide is absorbed better on an empty stomach but it causes GI problems and may be taken at mealtime. Check with your physician and pharmacist on proper dosing for all these drugs; the dose must be individualized and timed carefully. Ethmozine should be started only in a hospital.

INTERACTION
Tagamet appears to have the potential to boost blood levels of these anti-arrhythmic medicines. When the ulcer drug is taken together with any of these heart medications, the potential for increased toxicity may rise. Because the dose is so critical to successful treatment with these powerful heart medications, anything that modifies the usual pattern could present a serious problem. *Arrhythmias might result, which could be life threatening.*

Experts recommend avoiding this combination unless it is essential. If Tagamet must be added to one of these heart medicines, blood levels must be monitored carefully, electrocardiographic tests considered, and dosage adjustments made if necessary.

Symptoms of Heart Medicine Toxicity
Except for subtle changes on an electrocardiogram, there may be no warning signs of serious danger. Heart palpitations, dizziness, fainting, chest discomfort, or shortness of breath require emergency treatment.

Never take or stop medication without your doctor's advice.

Ulcer Drug (H₂ ANTAGONIST)	**Alcohol**

TROUBLESOME

BRAND NAME GENERIC NAME	NAME
Tagamet cimetidine	beer

INSTRUCTIONS

Tagamet is usually taken with meals and/or at bedtime. Antacids may reduce absorption of Tagamet; do not take one for at least two hours after taking Tagamet.

NAME
beer
liquor
wine
medicines that contain alcohol

INSTRUCTIONS

The absorption and effects of alcohol are magnified if you drink on an empty stomach. Fatty food can delay alcohol absorption. If you drink, do so in moderation, and never drive.

INTERACTION

This interesting interaction is extremely controversial. Some researchers have demonstrated that people taking Tagamet have higher blood alcohol levels after several drinks than subjects not taking Tagamet. This reaction seems to affect only men because they have an enzyme in the stomach called alcohol dehydrogenase that breaks down some of the alcohol from a drink even before it is absorbed into the bloodstream. The data suggest that Tagamet deactivates this enzyme and enhances alcohol absorption. If this were true, people might have higher blood alcohol levels than they expect. But other research has contradicted this conclusion. An expert panel for the FDA decided that, although more work would be helpful, there is no reason to issue a warning at this time. Where does this leave patients? At this time there are no firm answers. If you take Tagamet and drink, be cautious . . . your blood alcohol levels might be higher than you think.

Symptoms of Alcohol Overdose

This interaction, if it occurs at all, probably has a modest effect on alcohol levels. Disorientation, unsteadiness, or loss of motor coordination would be symptoms to watch for.

Never take or stop medication without your doctor's advice.

Ulcer Drug
(H$_2$ ANTAGONIST)

Anti-Anxiety Drugs
(BENZODIAZEPINES)

TROUBLESOME

BRAND NAME	GENERIC NAME
Tagamet	cimetidine

INSTRUCTIONS
Tagamet is usually taken with meals and/or at bedtime. Antacids may reduce absorption of Tagamet; do not take one for at least two hours after taking Tagamet.

BRAND NAME	GENERIC NAME
Ativan	lorazepam
Dalmane	flurazepam
Doral	quazepam
Halcion	triazolam
Klonopin	clonazepam
Librium	chlordiazepoxide
Paxipam	halazepam
ProSom	estazolam
Restoril	temazepam
Serax	oxazepam
Tranxene	clorazepate
Valium	diazepam
Versed	midazolam
Xanax	alprazolam

INSTRUCTIONS
These drugs may be taken with food, especially if they upset the digestive tract.

INTERACTION
Tagamet can increase blood levels of benzodiazepines and prolong their stay in the body. Sedation and impairment could result, especially for older people. This interaction remains controversial since the data are contradictory. Be vigilant for any drowsiness or incoordination. Unsteadiness is a possible complication.

Symptoms of Benzodiazepine Overdose
This interaction could lead to symptoms of overdose such as disorientation, unsteadiness, confusion, slurred speech, drowsiness, dizziness, amnesia, and loss of motor coordination. Some other benzodiazepines may also be affected by cimetidine. Contact your physician if such symptoms occur.

Never take or stop medication without your doctor's advice.

Ulcer Drug (H₂ ANTAGONIST)	**Antidepressants** (TRICYCLIC)

TROUBLESOME

BRAND NAME	GENERIC NAME
Tagamet	cimetidine

INSTRUCTIONS
Tagamet is usually taken with meals and/or at bedtime. Antacids may reduce absorption of Tagamet; do not take one for at least two hours after taking Tagamet.

BRAND NAME	GENERIC NAME
Adapin, Sinequan	doxepin
Anafranil	clomipramine
Asendin	amoxapine
Aventyl, Pamelor	nortriptyline
Elavil, Endep	amitriptyline
Norpramin, Pertofrane	desipramine
Tofranil	imipramine
etc.	

INSTRUCTIONS
Usually these medications are better taken with food. A high-fiber diet may interfere with absorption, however. See page 22 for details.

INTERACTION

There is convincing evidence that Tagamet can increase blood levels of tricyclic antidepressants. This probably happens because the ulcer drug interferes with normal metabolism. Patients have reported increased side effects after such a combination. Symptoms included dizziness, drowsiness, and even psychosis.

Other ulcer medications (such as Zantac) have not been shown to have this effect. If Tagamet must be prescribed in combination with a tricyclic antidepressant, it is important to have blood levels of the antidepressant checked periodically.

Symptoms of Antidepressant Toxicity

People vary in their response to higher doses of tricyclics. Side effects may include confusion, dilated pupils, flushing, dry mouth, hallucinations, heart palpitations, and agitation. Older people may be especially vulnerable. Notify your physician of any symptoms.

Never take or stop medication without your doctor's advice.

Ulcer Drug (H$_2$ ANTAGONIST)	**Heart/Blood Pressure Drugs** (BETA-BLOCKERS)

TROUBLESOME

BRAND NAME	GENERIC NAME
Tagamet	cimetidine

INSTRUCTIONS

Tagamet is usually taken with meals and/or at bedtime. Antacids may reduce absorption of Tagamet; do not take one for at least two hours after taking Tagamet.

BRAND NAME	GENERIC NAME
Inderal	propranolol
Lopressor, Toprol	metoprolol
Normodyne, Trandate	labetalol

INSTRUCTIONS

Inderal and Lopressor are best taken with meals, but consistency is the most important factor. They should be taken at roughly the same time every day. Do not stop these medicines suddenly except on doctor's orders. Serious side effects could result.

INTERACTION

Tagamet appears to affect the liver's ability to metabolize certain beta-blockers such as Inderal and Lopressor. These drugs may not be eliminated as efficiently as expected, leading to increased blood levels. One study noted a doubling or even tripling impact on propranolol. The effect on metoprolol is more complicated. Some research has shown increased blood levels while other data show there is no problem. With such contradictory information, all we can suggest is prudent caution.

When blood levels of beta-blockers are substantially increased, there could be unwanted side effects. There have been reports of very slow heart rate and low blood pressure. If there is a compelling reason to take both Tagamet and Inderal or Lopressor simultaneously, blood pressure and pulse should be closely monitored. A physician may wish to reevaluate the standard dose of beta-blocker as well.

Symptoms of Beta-Blocker Toxicity

If beta-blocker blood levels get too high, people may experience side effects such as low blood pressure, dizziness, very slow heart rate, breathing difficulties, or heart failure. Notify your physician promptly of any symptoms.

Never take or stop medication without your doctor's advice.

Ulcer Drug (H₂ ANTAGONIST)	**Heart/Blood Pressure Drugs** (CALCIUM CHANNEL BLOCKERS)

TROUBLESOME

BRAND NAME	GENERIC NAME	BRAND NAME	GENERIC NAME
Tagamet	cimetidine	**Adalat, Procardia**	nifedipine

INSTRUCTIONS
Tagamet is usually taken with meals and/or at bedtime. Antacids may reduce absorption of Tagamet; do not take one for at least two hours after taking Tagamet.

INSTRUCTIONS
These drugs come in a variety of doses; follow the doctor's directions. Taking Adalat or Procardia with grapefruit juice could boost blood levels of the drug unexpectedly. See the table of Food and Drug Compatibility on pages 73–91. If the drug must be discontinued, follow your doctor's instructions for gradual tapering.

INTERACTION

Cimetidine affects the liver's ability to metabolize many drugs. Nifedipine is vulnerable to this interaction. This combination of medications can lead to blood levels of nifedipine that are substantially higher than normal. This could lead to an exaggerated response to the blood pressure medicine. *This interaction could be troublesome.*

Studies on other calcium channel blockers are contradictory. It is possible that Tagamet increases levels of other calcium channel blockers such as verapamil or diltiazem slightly, but it does not appear that the effectiveness of these medications is likely to be affected.

Symptoms of Nifedipine Toxicity
Headaches, facial flushing, low blood pressure, nausea, dizziness, confusion, fluid retention, nervousness, weakness, sleep problems, changes in heart rate or irregular heartbeat, and palpitations. Notify the physician of any symptoms.

Never take or stop medication without your doctor's advice.

Afterword

There have been many interactions reported since the hardcover edition of this book was published in 1995, so there is not enough room to list them all. Clearly this is a work in progress and will continue to expand over the years, but here are some of the more important new interactions you should know about. Because discoveries are reported continually, the list can never be considered complete. Please check all combinations with your physician and pharmacist and insist they take the time to do the necessary research to protect your health.

Food and Drug Debacle

Few issues have captured people's attention like food and drug interactions. Patients want to know how to take their medications correctly and are concerned that physicians and pharmacists rarely mention anything about meals or special prohibitions, such as grapefruit.

Perhaps the most tragic report we have is that of a young man who died as a consequence of combining **Seldane** (terfenadine) and grapefruit juice. He was in good health except for allergies that prompted his physician to prescribe the nonsedating antihistimine. He liked grapefruit juice and drank it several times a week. Neither his wife or young daughter liked it or drank it.

The day he died, he consumed two glasses of grapefruit juice as well as his medicine. The cause of death was determined to be terfenadine intoxication, even though he had taken his usual dose. His blood levels of **Seldane** were as high as those seen in other people who experienced fatal irregular heart rhythms due to **Seldane** overdose.

This case demonstrates that grapefruit interactions are no laughing matter. Although Seldane is no longer on the market because it interacts with so many things, there are other drugs that are also susceptible. We have heard of another lethal case that involved the antihistamine **Hismanal** (astemizole) combined with grapefruit juice. Grapefruit can also interact with other medications, including **Sular** (nisoldipine). One gentleman taking **Procardia XL** (nifedipine) and **Calan SR** (verapamil) landed in the hospital for a week after washing them down with a quart of grapefruit juice. According to Dr. J. David Spence, Director of the Stroke Prevention and Atherosclerosis Research Centre at the University of Western Ontario, Canada, any medication that interacts with erythromycin, ketoconazole, or itraconazole should also be suspected of a potential grapefruit interaction. This category includes the blood thinner **Coumadin** (warfarin), the heart drug **Rythmol** (propafenone), and the heartburn medicine **Propulsid** (cisapride).

Dr. Spence suspected that cholesterol-lowering medicines such as **Mevacor** (lovastatin) might be more toxic if taken with grapefruit juice. Subsequent research has confirmed that grapefruit juice has a profound impact on **Mevacor** (*Clin. Pharmacol. Ther.*, April 1998, pp. 397-402). This could lead to muscle breakdown which may become life threatening. In addition, **Zocor** (simvastatin) and **Lipitor** (atorvastatin) interact in a dangerous manner with itraconazole (*Clin. Pharmacol. Ther.*, March 1998, pp. 332-341; July 1998, pp. 58-65). Grapefruit could be expected to interact in a similar way with both of these cholesterol-lowering medications. In the future, all drugs metabolized through the enzyme CYP 3A4 should be tested for such an interaction. Grapefruit has already been shown to increase levels of the psychiatric medicine **Anafranil** (clomipramine), the anticonvulsant **Tegretol** (carbamazepine), and the estrogens 17-ß estradiol and ethinyl estradiol.

Grapefruit interactions have not been taken very seriously by the U.S. Food and Drug Administration. Canadian regulators have been no more responsive. Yet such interactions appear extremely important to us. New research suggests that there may be a cumulative impact. That is, if grapefruit is consumed on a regular basis the effect increases. Until grapefruit juice interactions are included in prescribing information, consumers are going to have to take personal responsibility for protecting themselves.

Are there other foods that, like grapefruit, have a significant effect on drug metabolism? This field of research is still very new, and we expect further discoveries. One that we find fascinating involves watercress and acetaminophen (**APAP**, **Panadol**, **Tylenol**, etc.). A single serving of watercress changed the metabolism of acetaminophen taken 10 hours later (*Clin. Pharmacol. Ther.*, Dec 1996, pp. 651-660). Blood levels were reduced; whether people would experience less pain relief from their **Tylenol** was not determined.

AIDS Drugs

The protease inhibitors **Crixivan** (indinavir) and **Norvir** (ritonavir) have made a big difference for many AIDS patients as part of a promising multidrug regimen. Doctors must be aware, however, that if the patient also has tuberculosis, the TB drugs **Mycobutin** (rifabutin) or **Rifadin** (rifampin) can reduce the effectiveness of the protease inhibitors, which boost blood levels and possible toxicity of the rifamycins. **Crixivan** and **Norvir** are also reported to raise blood levels of **Hismanal** (astemizole), increasing the risk of serious heart rhythm abnormalities. The protease inhibitors may also increase blood levels of benzodiazepines processed by CYP 3A4, leading to the possibility of marked sedation from **Dalmane** (flurazepam), **Halcion** (triazolam), **ProSom** (estazolam), **Tranxene** (clorazepate), **Valium** (diazepam), and **Xanax** (alsprazolam). **Norvir** has also been reported to raise blood levels of the pain relievers **Darvon** (propoxyphene) and **Demerol** (meperidine) to dangerous levels. These combinations are extremely hazardous. Other dangerous interactions with **Norvir** include **Ambien** (zolpidem), **Clozaril** (clozapine), **Enkaid** (encainide), **Feldene** (piroxicam), **Propulsid** (cisapride), quinidine, **Rythmol** (propafenone), **Tambocor** (flecainide), and **Vascor** (bepridil).

Another AIDS drug, **Videx** (ddI or didanosine), can reduce the effectiveness of certain antibiotics such as **Cipro** (ciprofloxacin) and antifungals such as **Nizoral** (ketoconazole) and **Sporanox** (itraconazole). These interactions are of concern because people with AIDS often need to be treated for opportunistic infections. Anyone taking medication for AIDS must be especially vigilant as dangerous drug interactions are quite common.

Cardizem

Many of the important interactions of **Cardizem** (dilti-azem), also prescribed under the names **Cardizem CD**, **Cardizem SR**, **Dilacor XR**, and **Tiamate**, are found in the charts on pages 403–418. **Cardizem** has also been found to quadruple blood levels of the cholesterol-low-ering drug **Mevacor** (lovastatin) (*Clin. Pharmacol. Ther.*, 1997, p. 201). Other cholesterol-lowering drugs that might conceivably be affected include **Zocor** (sim-vastatin) and **Lipitor** (atorvastatin). There has been rel-atively little research, but patients on **Cardizem** might wish to be cautious about other drugs affected by this enzyme (CYP 3A4), including cyclosporine and **Couma-din** (warfarin). **Propulsid** (cisapride) is also in this group of medications. One 45-year-old woman given **Propulsid** and **Cardizem CD** experienced a very dan-gerous change in heart rhythm (*Pharmacotherapy*, Mar/April 1998, pp. 381-385). **Cardizem** also raises blood levels of the heart rhythm regulator **Ethmozine** (moricizine).

Cognex

Cognex (tacrine) is prescribed for Alzheimer's disease. It requires careful adjustment of the dose. See page 322 for information about its interaction with the asthma drug theophylline. **Tagamet** (cimetidine) also interacts with **Cognex** and could increase the risk of side effects. The medication **Luvox** (fluvoxamine) prescribed for obsessive-compulsive disorder dramatically increases blood levels of **Cognex**. This is a potentially serious interaction that could lead to liver damage.

Cordarone

Cordarone (amiodarone) is a potent heart medicine

used to treat rhythm irregularities. It can interact with many other medications including **Coumadin** (warfarin), **Inderal** (propranolol), **Lopressor** (metoprolol), **Lanoxin** (digoxin), **Dilantin** (phenytoin), **Procan SR** (procainamide), **Cardioquin** (quinidine), **Norvir** (ritonavir), **Raxar** (grepafloxacin), **Zagam** (sparfloxacin), and **Theo-Dur** (theophylline). Anyone taking **Cordarone** needs to check with a physician and pharmacist if any other drug is prescribed.

Coumadin

Be sure to check the charts on **Coumadin** (warfarin) interactions earlier in this book (pages 224–245) since this anticoagulant interacts dangerously with a wide variety of other medications.

Most physicians and pharmacists were surprised to learn in 1998 that acetaminophen (APAP, **Panadol**, **Tylenol**, etc.) puts patients on **Coumadin** at significant risk of bleeding (*JAMA*, March 4, 1998, pp. 657–662). Although this interaction has been known for years (and was listed in the original hardcover edition of this book in 1995), the significance was not fully appreciated. The researchers discovered that as little as four regular-strength acetaminophen tablets daily for a week could elevate INR values (a test of blood clotting potential). They concluded, "Our data suggest that acetaminophen is an underrecognized cause of anticoagulant instability...Those patients taking warfarin who also require sustained high doses of acetaminophen need close monitoring of their INR levels."

Coumadin (warfarin) may also be affected by antifungal drugs such as **Diflucan** (fluconazole), **Nizoral** (ketoconazole), or **Sporanox** (itraconazole). Cholesterol-lowering medications such as **Mevacor** (lovastatin), **Lescol** (fluvastatin), and **Zocor** (simvastatin) can also interact with **Coumadin**. A possible interaction has also been reported with the heartburn drug **Propulsid** (cisapride). The anticoagulant effect of **Coumadin** is increased and this could lead to uncontrolled bleeding. We consider these drug interactions hazardous.

Dilantin

Dilantin (phenytoin) is an anticonvulsant with a number of potentially serious interaction (See pages 266–284). Four possible problems have come to our attention recently. The anti-herpes medication **Zovirax** (acyclovir) reduced the blood level and effectiveness of **Dilantin** in one seven-year-old patient, resulting in seizures. This combination has not, however been studied systematically. Such research was done on healthy adult volunteers to determine that **Sporanox** (itraconazole) can increase the concentration of **Dilantin**, and presumably its effects, while at the same time blood levels and effectiveness of the antifungal drug are diminished.

Two other drugs appear to raise blood levels of **Dilantin**: the antidepressant **Zoloft** (sertraline) and the antiplatelet drug **Ticlid** (ticlopidine). Symptoms such as dizziness, drowsiness, and trouble walking were reported in some cases. Any patient on **Dilantin** should have blood levels of the drug monitored closely if these medications must be started, stopped, or adjusted in dose.

Estrogens

Birth control pills and even postmenopausal replacement therapy can interact with a number of other medications (see Chapter Seven). There are now a few cases of women who have become pregnant while on oral contraceptives and the newer antifungal medicines **Sporanox** (itraconazole), **Nizoral** (ketoconazole) and **Diflucan** (fluconazole), which may be prescribed for vaginal yeast infection. One study has demonstrated a drop in blood levels of estrogen in women given the antibiotic **Dynabac** (dirithromycin). Although no pregnancies occurred in the women in the study, this is theoretically a possibility. Women who must take an antibiotic while taking birth control pills should add a barrier method to ensure additional contraceptive protection. **Norvir** (ritonavir) can also decrease blood levels of estrogens. Backup contraception is recommended. Grapefruit juice, on the other hand, can increase circulating levels of oral estrogens by about one-third.

Alcohol also appears to exert a powerful impact on circulating estrogen. A study published in the *Journal of the American Medical Association* (Dec. 4, 1996, pp. 1747-1751) found that women on postmenopausal estrogen replacement (specifically estradiol) had elevated levels of this hormone when they drank alcohol. The equivalent of one glass of wine doubled their blood estrogen. When the investigators administered the equivalent of three glasses of wine, estradiol jumped more than 300 percent.

Although this work is preliminary and does not reveal whether all forms of estrogen replacement therapy would be affected by alcohol, it does raise cautionary flags. Elevated estrogen may increase the risk of blood clots, which can lead to thrombophlebitis, stroke, pulmonary embolism, or heart attack.

The most controversial complication associated with estrogen is breast cancer. There is no consensus about the degree of risk, but the authors of the *JAMA* study suggest that, "The combination of ERT (estrogen replacement therapy) and alcohol ingestion may be additive and increase the risk of breast cancer more than either alone."

Fosamax

Fosamax (alendronate) has gained great popularity as a treatment for osteoporosis. Food, even coffee or orange juice, drastically reduces its absorption, however, so it must be taken with plain water at least half an hour before breakfast. Tea may also pose a significant problem, though its interaction potential has not yet been tested. Because **Fosamax** can also irritate the esophagus, it is important to take it with a full eight ounce glass of water and remain upright for 30 minutes after swallowing it.

Glucophage

Glucophage (metformin) has become a popular oral diabetes drug. It can interact with other medicines prescribed to lower blood sugar such as **DiaBeta** (glyburide) and **Precose** (acarbose). If combined therapy becomes necessary a very careful dosage regimen will have to be designed. **Tagamet** (cimetidine), **Lasix** (furuosemide), and **Procardia** (nifedipine) also interact with **Glucophage**.

A thickener in prepared low-fat foods such as sauces, salad dressings, and frozen yogurt, guar gum can interfere with absorption of **Glucophage**. One reader of our syndicated newspaper column reported that this interaction had a noticeable impact on his blood sugar control: "Since reading about guar gum, I have been avoiding it in prepared food formulations (salad dressings and fat-free ice cream). I think this has helped reduce my blood sugar

levels dramatically. Before that, **Glucophage** was dis-
appointingly ineffective."

A potentially deadly interaction may occur when a
person on **Glucophage** must undergo x-ray studies
with iodinated contrast media (used to study kidney,
heart, and brain, among other organs). **Glucophage**
must be discontinued two days before the procedure
and not restarted until two days afterwards, and then
only after kidney function has been tested and found
normal. Please discuss this regimen with your physician
whenever x-rays are ordered.

Halcion

Halcion (triazolam) and the injectable sedative **Versed**
(midazolam) are affected by antifungal agents such as
Nizoral (ketoconazole) and **Sporanox** (itraconazole).
They slow down metabolism of **Halcion** or **Versed** so
that side effects may be more common and last longer.
Increased sedation could be the consequence. Although
unreported at the time of this writing, **Diflucan** (fluconazole) may also interact in a similar manner.
Halcion is also affected by grapefruit.

Imitrex

Imitrex (sumatriptan) has become a very popular
migraine medicine. It generally works very well, but it
must not be combined with other migraine medicines
containing ergotamine or methysergide within the same
day. Brand names to watch for include **D.H.E. 45** (dihy-
droergotamine), **Ercaf**, **Ergomar**, or **Wigraine** (ergotamine), and **Sansert** (methysergide). MAO inhibitors
such as **Eldepryl** (selegiline), **Nardil** (phenelzine) or
Parnate (tranylcypromine) must have been discontin-

ued at least two weeks before a person can use **Imitrex** safely.

Inderal

Inderal (propranolol) can interact with many other medications (see pages 385–402). We were surprised to discover that it may also be affected by vitamin C. A small study has shown that 2,000 mg of vitamin C can reduce blood levels of **Inderal** by roughly one third. This may not seem significant, but a heart patient who must maintain a precise dosing schedule might discover that the enthusiastic use of vitamin C for a cold could diminish the benefits of propranolol.

Lanoxin

Lanoxin (digoxin) concentrations on the blood can be raised nearly 30 percent if it is taken together with the antidepressant **Serzone** (nefazodone). If there is no viable alternative to **Serzone**, the physician should monitor digoxin blood levels for possible toxicity. (See pages 363–374 for other digoxin interactions).

It has been known for some time that erythromycin can raise blood levels of **Lanoxin** in some people. Symptoms of **Lanoxin** overdose can result. A related antibiotic, **Biaxin** (clarithromycin), has now been shown to interact in a similar way (*Clin. Pharmacol. Ther.*, July 1998, pp. 123-128). **Prozac** (fluoxetine) may also elevate **Lanoxin** levels (*Arch. Int. Med.*, May 25, 1998, pp. 1152-1153).

The effect of the diabetes drug **Precose** (acarbose) on digoxin levels is confusing. The manufacturer of **Precose** tested this combination in healthy volunteers and found no interaction. One case reported in the medical literature, however, suggests that **Precose** may reduce absorption of **Lanoxin** in some individuals. Digoxin levels should be monitored carefully when **Precose** is started or stopped or the dose is changed.

Parlodel

Parlodel (bromocriptine) may become more toxic if it is taken together with phenylpropanolamine (PPA). This popular diet pill and decongestant is found in a great many prescription and over-the-counter products. Consequences of this interaction could include seizures, severe heart palpitations, and other heart problems. The migraine medicine **Midrin** (isometheptene) may also increase the toxicity of **Parlodel**.

Plendil

Plendil (felodipine) is a calcium channel blocker in the same family as **Procardia** (see pages 403–418). Grapefruit dramatically boosts blood levels of **Plendil**. Side effects can result, including flushing, headache, swelling of the legs, dizziness, and low blood pressure. Cyclosporine, used to prevent transplant rejection, also increases **Plendil** concentrations. The antifungal drug **Sporanox** (itraconazole) may have a similar impact on this blood pressure drug. There is a theoretical reason to believe that other antifungal agents such as **Nizoral** (ketoconazole) and **Diflucan** (fluconazole) might also impact **Plendil**. Certain antibiotics including erythromycin and **Biaxin** (clarithromycin) may also raise blood levels of **Plendil**, as can the acid-suppressor **Tagamet** (cimetidine).

Prilosec

Prilosec (omeprazole) has been given the green light by

the FDA to treat infectious ulcers (caused by *Helico-
bactor pylori*). This powerful acid-suppressing drug is
usually prescribed in conjunction with the antibiotic
Biaxin (clarythromycin). What may not be appreciated
by some prescribers is that these two drugs can interact,
potentiating each other. **Biaxin** boosts blood levels of
Prilosec while **Prilosec** increases blood and tissue concentrations of **Biaxin**. Because **Prilosec** is so effective
at reducing stomach acidity, it may alter the absorption
of certain other medicines. **Nizoral** (ketoconazole)
requires an acid environment for adequate absorption
and may not work as expected if taken while someone
is on **Prilosec**. Researchers came up with a clever con-
cept to counteract this problem. They had subjects take
Nizoral with Coca-Cola Classic to provide the missing
acid. For most people this helped measurably, but it cannot be counted upon for everyone.

Propulsid

Propulsid (cisapride) is a unique medicine for treating
night-time heartburn. Although not as popular as acid
suppressors such as **Pepcid** (famotidine), **Prilosec**
(omeprazole), **Tagamet** (cimetidine), or **Zantac** (ranitidine), the drug is making inroads, especially after an
intense direct-to-consumer advertising campaign. Since
Propulsid was introduced in 1993, millions of people
have taken it. But in June 1998, the FDA issued a star-
tling warning that **Propulsid** should be used only as a
last resort, after other treatments had failed. The problem is its propensity to interact with other medications.
In overdose or in some interactions, **Propulsid** can alter
heart rhythm in a potentially fatal way. Thirty-eight
deaths have been linked to **Propulsid**, although regulators are uncertain how many are directly due to the drug.

Some of the more troublesome interactions with **Propulsid** include antifungal compounds such as **Diflucan** (fluconazole), **Nizoral** (ketoconazole), and **Sporanox** (itraconazole). Some antibiotics are also very risky with **Propulsid**, including **Biaxin** (clarithromycin), erythromycin, and **TAO** (troleandomycin). **Luvox** (fluvoxamine) and the antidepressant **Serzone** (nefazodone) also interact. In one report, **Cardizem CD** (diltiazem) in combination with **Propulsid** caused a potentially fatal heart rhythm abnormality. **Propulsid** can boost blood levels and effects of the blood pressure medicine nifedipine (**Adalat** and **Procardia**). Protease inhibitors such as **Crixivan** (indinavir), **Norvir** (ritonavir), and **Viracept** (nelfinavir) should not be combined with **Propulsid**.

Although there is no mention in the medical literature, we worry about the possibility that **Propulsid** could interact with grapefruit. Until there is research to reassure us, we encourage grapefruit abstinence while on **Propulsid**. **Tagamet** (cimetidine) may also increase **Propulsid** concentrations, so one should resist any temptation to add OTC **Tagamet HB** if **Propulsid** doesn't give adequate symptom relief.

Prozac

Prozac (fluoxetine) nearly doubled the blood level of **Sandimmune** (cyclosporine) in one heart transplant patient and the dose of cyclosporine had to be reduced. When **Prozac** was discontinued, the level of cyclosporine dropped dramatically and the dose had to be readjusted. Other individual case reports suggest that **Prozac** may reduce the effectiveness of the anti-anxiety drug **BuSpar** (buspirone) in some people, and that it may combine with the cough suppressant dextromethorphan to trigger hallucinations. Because dextromethorphan is found in so many over-the-counter cough, cold, and flu remedies, this interaction bears watching. It has not been determined whether these cases are idiosyncratic or represent true drug incompatibilities, however. (Other **Prozac** interactions are on pages 285–296.)

Sandimmune

Sandimmune (cyclosporine) is prescribed primarily to prevent rejection of organ transplants. It is a tricky drug to administer and requires very careful monitoring to get the dose right. Grapefruit has a profound influence on cyclosporine levels (see page 53). Other drugs may reduce **Sandimmune** concentrations, including barbiturates (**Alurate**, **Amytal**, **Florinal**, **Mebaral**, **Nembutal**, phenobarbital, and **Seconal**), the anticonvulsants **Tegretol** (carbamazepine) and **Dilantin** (phenytoin), the antifungal drug **Lamisil** (terbinafine), the TB medicine rifampin (**Rifadin** and **Rimactane**), and the co-trimoxazale antibiotics (**Bactrim** and **Septra**). Medications that may increase blood levels of **Sandimmune** include **Biaxin** (clarithromycin), **Cardizem** (diltiazem), **Cardene** (ni-cardipine), erythromycin, **Diflucan** (fluconazole), **Nizoral** (ketoconazole), **Sporanox** (itraconazole), **Reglan** (metoclopramide), **Delta-Cortef** (prednisolone), prednisone, **Prozac** (fluoxetine), **Rocephin** (ceftriaxone), **Serzone** (nefazodone), and oral contraceptives. Anyone taking **Sandimmune** should check carefully with the transplant team when taking any other medications.

Serzone

Serzone (nefazodone) is a new-generation serotonin-based antidepressant in the **Prozac** (fluoxetine) family (see pages 285–296). **Serzone** appears to interact with many other medications including **Hismanal** (astemizole). This combination is potentially life-threatening. Another dangerous interaction involves the cholesterol-lowering drugs **Mevacor** (lovastatin), **Zocor** (simvastatin), and possibly **Lipitor** (atorvastatin). When taken in conjunction with **Serzone**, these medications may be more likely to cause muscle breakdown (rhabdomyolysis), which in severe cases could lead to kidney damage.

The sleeping pill **Halcion** (triazolam) and the anti-anxiety drug **Xanax** (alprazolam) are definitely affected by **Serzone** (blood levels go higher and increased sedation may occur). Similar medications that interact with **Serzone** include **Dalmane** (flurazepam), **Klonopin** (clonazepam), **Lanoxin** (digoxin), **Librium** (chlordiazepoxide), and **Valium** (diazepam). **Tegretol** (carbamazepine) is also affected by **Serzone** with concentrations of the anticonvulsant becoming elevated and side effects becoming more pronounced.

Synthroid

Synthroid (levothyroxine) is the most commonly prescribed thyroid supplement. Absorption can be diminished by iron, calcium carbonate, and the ulcer medicine **Carafate** (sucralfate). If the two must be taken together at least eight hours must separate **Synthroid** and **Carafate** to guarantee adequate blood levels of the hormone.

Tegretol

The anticonvulsant **Tegretol** (carbamazepine) interacts

with a large number of other medications. Please check the charts on pages 246–265. **Tegretol** also appears to be affected by the antidepressant **Serzone** (nefazodone). Concentrations of **Tegretol** rise and side effects are possible. One patient experienced slurred speech, drowsiness, excessive sleeping, loss of appetite, and diminished depth perception. The antifungal agent **Nizoral** (ketoconazole) may also increase blood levels of **Tegretol**, as can quinine. **Risperdal** (risperidone), which is used to treat schizophrenia, may be less effective when taken in combination with **Tegretol**. Grapefruit can boost blood levels of **Tegretol**.

Viagra

Viagra (sildenafil) was approved in 1998 for the treatment of impotence. The manufacturer warns that **Viagra** should never be taken by someone who is already on a nitrate-type heart medication. In addition to nitroglycerin (**Minitran**, **Nitro-Bid**, **Nitrodisc**, **Nitro-Dur**, **Nitrogard**, **Nitroglyn**, **Nitrol**, **Nitrolingual**, **Nitrong**, **Nitrostat**, **Transderm-Nitro**), nitrates include isosorbide mononitrate (**Imdur**, **ISMO**, and **Monoket**) and isosorbide dinitrate (**Dilatrate-SR**, **Isordil**, **Sorbitrate**). The combination of **Viagra** with a nitrate can lower blood pressure profoundly and precipitously, and may result in death. If someone who has taken **Viagra** suffers a cardiac event, it is important to tell the emergency medical personnel not to administer nitroglycerin. Although this is a standard treatment for a suspected heart attack, it could be lethal in the presence of **Viagra**.

Other interactions with **Viagra** have been less well-publicized. The antibiotic erythromycin (**E.E.S.**, **E-Mycin**, **ERYC**, **Ery-Tab**, **Erythrocin**, **Ilosone**, **PCE**) can raise blood levels of **Viagra** by 182 percent, which may increase the risk of side effects. Antifungal drugs such as **Nizoral** (ketoconazole) and **Sporanox** (itraconazole) also increase circulating levels of the impotence drug, as does **Tagamet** (cimetidine). Several other medications, including the antibiotic **Biaxin** (clarithromycin), blood pressure pills like **Cardizem** (diltiazem) and **Calan** (verapamil), and the antidepressant **Serzone** (nefazodone), might be expected to interact with **Viagra** and should be used with caution. We also counsel caution with respect to grapefruit, since this food may affect metabolism of the drug.

About the Authors

Joe Graedon

Pharmacologist Joe Graedon is a best-selling author, nationally syndicated newspaper columnist, host of an award-winning internationally syndicated radio talk show, and lecturer at the University of North Carolina School of Pharmacy. He is president of Graedon Enterprises, Inc., a corporation providing pharmaceutical and health care information services.

Joe Graedon received his B.S. from Pennsylvania State University in 1967 and went on to do research on mental illness, sleep, and basic brain physiology at the New Jersey Neuropsychiatric Institute in Princeton. In 1971 he received his M.S. in pharmacology from the University of Michigan. Following his medical anthropologist wife Teresa to Mexico, he taught clinical pharmacology to second-year medical students at the Benito Juárez Unversity of Oaxaca. While in Mexico, he started work on *The People's Pharmacy* (St. Martin's Press, 1976; revised 1985, 1996, 1998), a popular book on medicines that would eventually go on to become a *New York Times* number one best-seller.

Joe's other books, coauthored with Dr. Terry Graedon, include *The People's Pharmacy-2* (Avon, 1980), *The New People's Pharmacy #3: Drug Breakthroughs of the '80s* (Bantam, 1985), *50+:*

The Graedons' People's Pharmacy for Older Adults (Bantam, 1988), and *Graedons' Best Medicine: From Herbal Remedies to High-Tech R_x Breakthroughs* (Bantam, 1991), *The People's Guide to Deadly Drug Interactions* (St. Martin's Press, 1995, 1997). *No Deadly Drug* (Pocket Books, 1992), coauthored with Dr. Tom Ferguson, is Graedon's first novel. Joe also coauthored with Dr. Ferguson *The Aspirin Handbook: A User's Guide to the Breakthrough Drug of the '90s* (Bantam, 1993). The total number of the Graedons' books in print well exceeds two million. Joe and Teresa were contributors to the 1997 edition of *The Merck Manual of Medical Information Home Edition*.

Joe has lectured at Duke University School of Nursing, the University of California School of Pharmacy (UCSF), and the University of North Carolina School of Pharmacy. He served as a consultant to the **Federal Trade Commission** from 1978 to 1983, and was on the Advisory Board for the **Drug Studies Unit** at UCSF from 1983 to 1989. He is a member of the **Board of Visitors** of the School of Pharmacy at the University of North Carolina, Chapel Hill. He is a member of the **American Association for the Advancement of Science**, the **Society for Neuroscience**, and the **New York Academy of Science**. For more than a decade Joe and Terry contributed a regular column on self-medication for the journal *Medical Self Care*. Joe is an editorial adviser to *Men's Health Newsletter.* Joe and Terry's newspaper column, **The People's Pharmacy**, is syndicated nationally by King Features. *The People's Pharmacy* radio show won a Silver Award from the Corporation for Public Broadcasting in 1992. It is syndicated to more than 500 radio stations in the United States and abroad on public radio, the InTouch Radio Reading Service, and the American Services Network.

Joe's features on health and pharmaceuticals have been syndicated nationally to public television stations via Intraregional Program Service member exchange. He is considered the country's leading drug expert for consumers. He has been a guest expert on *Donahue, 20/20, Geraldo, The Oprah Winfrey Show, Sally Jessy Raphael, Live with Regis and Kathie Lee, Today, Good Morning America, CBS Morning News, Sonia Live, The Home Show, Everyday with Joan Lunden, The Larry King Show,* and *The Tonight Show with Johnny Carson.* He lives in Durham, North Carolina, with his wife and coauthor, Teresa. Joe speaks frequently on issues of pharmaceuticals, nutrition, and self-care.

Teresa Graedon

Medical anthropologist Teresa Graedon is a best-selling author, syndicated newspaper columnist, and host of an award-winning internationally syndicated radio talk show. Teresa Graedon received her A.B. from Bryn Mawr College in 1969, graduating magna cum laude with a major in anthropology. She attended graduate school at the University of Michigan, receiving her A.M. in 1971. She received a fellowship from the Institute for Environmental Quality (1972–1975), which enabled her to pursue doctoral research on health and nutritional status in a migrant community in Oaxaca, Mexico. Her doctorate was awarded in 1976.

Teresa taught at Duke University School of Nursing with an adjunct appointment in the Department of Anthropology from 1975 to 1979. Since that time she has taught courses periodically in medical anthropology and international health at Duke University. From 1982 to 1983 she pursued postdoctoral training in medical anthropology at the University of California, San Francisco.

Dr. Graedon has coauthored with Joe Graedon the following books: *The People's Pharmacy-2* (Avon, 1980), *The New People's Pharmacy #3: Drug Breakthroughs of the '80s* (Bantam, 1985), *Totally New and Revised The People's Pharmacy* (St. Martin's Press, 1985), *50+: The Graedons' People's Pharmacy for Older Adults* (Bantam, 1988), *Graedons' Best Medicine: From Herbal Remedies to High-Tech R_x Breakthroughs* (Bantam, 1991), and *The Aspirin Handbook: A User's Guide to the Breakthrough Drug of the '90s* (Bantam Books, 1993). The total number of her books in print exceeds two million.

Teresa is a member of the **Society for Applied Anthropology**, the **American Anthropological Association**, the **Society for Medical Anthropology**, and the **American Public Health Association**. The newspaper column she writes with Joe, **The People's Pharmacy**, is syndicated nationally by King Features. In 1992 *The People's Pharmacy* radio show won a Silver Award from the Corporation for Public Broadcasting. It is syndicated nationally and is heard on more than 500 radio stations in the United States and abroad on public radio, the InTouch Radio Reading Service, and the American Services Network.

Index

For greater ease in locating the interactions of interest to you, please note that entries in the Guides to Dangerous Drug Interactions are indicated in bold. Entries in tables are indicated in italicized numerals.